P9-AEX-844

WITHDRAWN

CONSUMER HEALTH

Making Informed Decisions

J. Thomas Butler, EdD, CHES (ret.)
Delaware State University

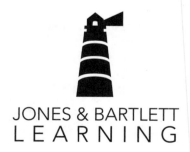

JONES & BARTLETT
LEARNING

World Headquarters
Jones & Bartlett Learning
5 Wall Street
Burlington, MA 01803
978-443-5000
info@jblearning.com
www.jblearning.com

Jones & Bartlett Learning Canada
6339 Ormindale Way
Mississauga, Ontario L5V 1J2
Canada

Jones & Bartlett Learning International
Barb House, Barb Mews
London W6 7PA
United Kingdom

Jones & Bartlett Learning books and products are available through most bookstores and online booksellers. To contact Jones & Bartlett Learning directly, call 800-832-0034, fax 978-443-8000, or visit our website, www.jblearning.com.

Substantial discounts on bulk quantities of Jones & Bartlett Learning publications are available to corporations, professional associations, and other qualified organizations. For details and specific discount information, contact the special sales department at Jones & Bartlett Learning via the above contact information or send an email to specialsales@jblearning.com.

Production Credits
Publisher, Higher Education: Cathleen Sether
Senior Acquisitions Editor: Shoshanna Goldberg
Senior Associate Editor: Amy L. Bloom
Editorial Assistant: Prima Bartlett
Associate Marketing Manager: Jody Sullivan
Production Manager: Julie Champagne Bolduc
Production Assistant: Sean Coombs
V.P., Manufacturing and Inventory Control: Therese Connell
Rights and Photo Research Manager: Katherine Crighton
Permissions and Photo Researcher: Anna Genoese
Cover Design: Kristin E. Parker
Cover Image: Pills © Lepas/Dreamstime.com
Composition: Laserwords Private Limited, Chennai, India
Printing and Binding: Malloy, Inc.
Cover Printing: Malloy, Inc.

To order this product, use ISBN: 978-1-4496-4645-5

Library of Congress Cataloging-in-Publication Data
Butler, J. Thomas.
 Consumer health : making informed decisions / J. Thomas Butler.
   p. cm.
 Includes bibliographical references and index.
 ISBN 978-0-7637-9339-5 (pbk.)
 1. Medical care. 2. Health promotion. 3. Consumer education. 4. Medical care--United States. I. Title.
 RA410.5.B87 2012
 362.1--dc22
                          2011006265

6048
Printed in the United States of America
15 14 13 12 11   10 9 8 7 6 5 4 3 2 1

Dedicated to the memory of my dad, Kenneth J. Butler. What a guy!

Brief Contents

Chapter 1. Being a Good Consumer 1

Chapter 2. The American Health Care System 19

Chapter 3. Health Fraud 47

Chapter 4. Health Insurance 67

Chapter 5. Medications 87

Chapter 6. Complementary and Alternative Medicine 105

Chapter 7. Dietary Supplements 135

Chapter 8. Weight Management 159

Chapter 9. Advertising 183

Chapter 10. Consumer Protection 215

Contents

PREFACE   XIII

ACKNOWLEDGMENTS   XV

Chapter 1   *Being a Good Consumer* *1*

Chapter Objectives   1
Shopping   1
Grocery Shopping   2
Characteristics of Good Consumers   5
Evaluating Information   7
The World Wide Web as an Information Source   10
Choosing a Primary Care Physician   11
Using Health Care Responsibly   12
Making Intelligent Decisions   16
Summary   16
Key Terms   17
Study Questions   17
References   17

Chapter 2   *The American Health Care System* *19*

Chapter Objectives   19
Medical Care in the United States   19
Quality of Care in America   22
Disparities in the Health Care Delivery System   23
A Costly System   24
Key Indicators for Measuring Performance of the Health System   29
  Healthy Lives   29
  Quality of Care   30
  Access   30
  Efficiency   31
  Equity   31

Improving America's Health Care System   32
Quality Assurance   36
Universal Health Care   38
   National Health Service   39
   Single-Payer Model   39
   Insurance Exchanges   39
Selecting a Health Care Facility   40
   Selecting a Hospital   40
   Selecting a Senior Living Facility   41
Summary   43
Key Terms   43
Study Questions   44
References   44

Chapter 3   *Health Fraud* 47
   Chapter Objectives   47
   Identifying Health Fraud   47
   Health Quackery   50
   Insurance or Health Care Fraud   54
   Weight Loss Fraud   56
   Fitness Fraud   56
   HIV/AIDS Fraud   57
   Diabetes Fraud   58
   Arthritis Remedy Fraud   58
   Victimizing Cancer Victims   58
   Sexual Enhancement Products   59
   Influenza Scams   60
   Aging Scams   60
   Home Genetic Tests   60
   Combating Health Fraud   62
   Summary   63
   Key Terms   63
   Study Questions   64
   References   64

Chapter 4   *Health Insurance* 67
   Chapter Objectives   67
   Health Reform—2010   68
      Exchanges   72
      Fairness in Coverage: Toward Universality   72
      Cutting Costs   73
   Selecting a Health Insurance Plan   75
   Traditional Health Insurance   76
   Managed Care   77
      Health Maintenance Organizations   77
      Preferred Provider Organizations   78

    Point of Service   78

    COBRA   79

   Government-Sponsored Health Insurance   80

    Medicare   80

    Medicaid   81

    State Children's Health Insurance Program   82

   Supplemental Plans   82

   Tax-Advantaged Options   83

    Health Savings Accounts   83

    Health Reimbursement Arrangements   83

    Flexible Spending Accounts   84

   Getting the Most from Your Health Insurance   84

   Summary   85

   Key Terms   85

   Study Questions   86

   References   86

Chapter 5   Medications **87**

   Chapter Objectives   87

   Prescription Drugs   88

   Generic Prescription Drugs   91

   Internet Prescriptions   93

   Drugs from Canada   95

   Counterfeit Drugs   95

   Orphan Drugs   97

   Nonprescription Medications   97

   A Word About Pain Relievers   100

   Behind-the-Counter Medications   100

   Disposing of Unused Medicines   101

   Summary   102

   Key Terms   102

   Study Questions   103

   References   104

Chapter 6   Complementary and Alternative Medicine **105**

   Chapter Objectives   105

   Why the Two Sides of "Medicine"?   106

   Categories of CAM   108

   How Popular Is CAM?   110

   Examples of Alternative Therapies   112

    Homeopathy   112

    Naturopathy   114

    Ayurveda   116

    Reiki   118

    Yoga   118

    Chiropractic   120

Acupuncture   122

Reflexology or Zone Therapy   125

Religious-Based Practices   126

Herbs and Dietary Supplements   127

Why Are Alternative and Complementary Treatments So Popular?   129

Should You Consider an Alternative or Complementary Therapy?   129

Summary   131

Key Terms   131

Study Questions   132

References   132

Chapter 7   Dietary Supplements *135*

Chapter Objectives   135

What Are Dietary Supplements?   135

Reducing Risk When Using Supplements   136

Research on Dietary Supplements   140

Vitamins and Minerals   141

Amino Acids   147

What About Herbs?   148

Regulation of Dietary Supplements   149

Summary   156

Key Terms   157

Study Questions   157

References   157

Chapter 8   Weight Management *159*

Chapter Objectives   159

America's Weight Problem   159

Standard Recommendations for Weight Control   162

The Role of Physical Activity in Controlling Weight   163

The Mediterranean Diet   164

Very-Low-Calorie and Low-Calorie Diets   164

Commercial Weight Loss Programs   165

Weight Watchers   166

Jenny Craig   167

OPTIFAST   168

Medifast   168

Nutrisystem   169

Volumetrics Diet   169

Online Commercial Weight Loss Programs   170

Organized Self-Help Programs   170

Carbohydrate-Restricted Diets   170

The Atkins Diet   171

The South Beach Diet   173

Possible Negative Effects of Restricted Carbohydrate Diets   173

Diet Pills and Drinks   174
  Available Without a Prescription   175
  Prescription Weight Loss Products   177
Fad Diets   177
Do Diet Programs Work?   178
Bariatric Surgery   178
  Restrictive Procedures   178
  Malabsorptive Procedures   179
Summary   179
Key Terms   179
Study Questions   180
References   180

Chapter 9   Advertising *183*
Chapter Objectives   183
Types of Advertising   184
Advertising Techniques and Tricks   185
  Word-of-Mouth Marketing   185
  Testimonials and Endorsements   186
  Weasel Words   187
  Attention Grabbers   187
  Appeal to Basic Human Weaknesses and Fears   188
  Visual Imagery   188
  Statistics   188
  Comedy   188
  Sex   189
  Product Placement   189
The Scope of Advertising   190
Advertising of Prescription Drugs   191
Advertising of Nonprescription Drugs   195
Targeting Special Groups   196
Marketing to Children   197
Unmeasured Media   205
Infomercials   205
Internet Advertising and Marketing   208
Summary   209
Key Terms   210
Study Questions   211
References   211

Chapter 10   Consumer Protection *215*
Chapter Objectives   215
Federal Consumer Protection   216
  U.S. Federal Trade Commission   216
  Consumer Product Safety Commission   217

U.S. Food and Drug Administration   218
Patient Safety Organizations   220
Environmental Protection Agency   221
U.S. Department of Agriculture   222
United States Postal Inspection Service   223
State and Local Governmental Protection   224
Nongovernmental Protection Agencies   225
Better Business Bureau   225
Consumer Federation of America   227
Consumers Union   228
AARP   228
National Consumers League   228
The National Consumer Protection Technical Resource Center   229
Health Research Group and Public Citizen   229
Accrediting and Certification Agencies   229
The Joint Commission   230
National Committee for Quality Assurance   230
URAC   230
Community Health Accreditation Program   231
Other Accrediting or Certification Organizations   231
Summary   231
Key Terms   232
Study Questions   232
References   232

GLOSSARY   235

INDEX   241

PHOTO CREDITS   251

Preface

What is it that instructors and students want and need from a textbook? As a person who has taught in higher education for almost four decades and who has taught consumer health for many years, I have observed that college teaching and learning have changed over time. What we want now is not what we once wanted. "Teaching from the book" was acceptable in the past. Today's instructors and students need more flexibility and more creativity. Today's textbook is the centerpiece of a course, an important tool, but not the course itself.

With that in mind, this text is written so that the content is current and well documented. It is written so that the instructor can build the course around the text. Instead of devoting entire chapters to consumer issues related to specific diseases or conditions, such as cancer, cardiovascular disease, or HIV/AIDS, the text weaves diseases and health conditions into discussions about fraud, alternative and complementary treatments, advertising, and the economics of health care. It allows the instructor and student to apply the concepts and examples to specific diseases. The goal is to provide students with the information and the decision-making skills to utilize health resources in the most beneficial ways.

While there is no need to utilize chapters in the exact sequence that they are presented, there is logic to the order of the presentation. The first chapter, "Being A Good Consumer," discusses skills necessary to being an effective consumer, including the abilities to evaluate information, make decisions, and protect oneself. The next three chapters discuss health care and related topics, including quality of the health care system, comparison of the American system with the systems of other developed nations, fraud perpetrated against the system and the individual, health insurance, and insurance reform. Chapter 5 discusses issues related to medications—over-the-counter and prescription. Chapter 6 addresses complementary, alternative, and integrative therapies. Some instructors may choose to assign this chapter, which will satisfy neither strong advocates nor strong detractors of alternative therapies, at the same time they assign Chapter 2, Chapter 3, or Chapter 5. Chapter 7 addresses dietary supplements. Instructors may assign it concurrently with Chapter 5, Chapter 6, or Chapter 8 ("Weight Management"). The instructor may choose to teach Chapter 9 on advertising before or concurrent with other topics. The same is true with the final chapter on consumer protection.

Tables, figures, and boxes provide condensations of large amounts of information. The intent is to present topics in a thought-provoking manner without dwelling on minute details that may be obsolete in a short time. Key terms are defined in each chapter and in the glossary. Creative instructors will adapt the text, PowerPoint presentations, and sample student activities, which are available as free instructor downloads, to their teaching styles and to the many learning styles of their students.

This book is also accompanied by extensive student and instructor resources. To learn more, visit: http://go.jblearning.com/butler.

Acknowledgments

The author wishes to thank the reviewers for their careful work and comments. Their contributions have increased the value and quality of this book.

Tania B. Basta, PhD, MPH, CHES, Ohio University

Cindy Connelley, Assistant Professor, Husson University

Martha A. Dallmeyer, PhD, Bradley University

Miriam J. Evans, MEd, CHES, South Carolina State University

Ari Fisher, Instructor, Louisiana State University

Debra C. Harris, PhD, MST, University of Wisconsin, Oshkosh

Joseph Hudak, PhD, MPH, Ohio University Eastern

Kimberly A. Parker, PhD, MPH, MA, CHES, Texas Woman's University

Sister Marguerite Polcyn, OSF, PhD, Lourdes College

Dhitinut Ratnapradipa, PhD, Southern Illinois University

Kerry Whipple, PhD, CHES, University of North Carolina at Wilmington

Chapter 1

Being a Good Consumer

Chapter Objectives

The student will:

- List and discuss the characteristics of good consumers.
- Discuss strategies to get the best value for your money when shopping for food.
- Discuss consumers' responsibility to report fraudulent or irresponsible practices on the part of merchants and health care providers.
- Discuss the characteristics of products certified to be "fair trade."
- Discuss the characteristics of sound scientific studies.
- Evaluate the quality of informational resources on the World Wide Web by following guidelines listed in this chapter.
- Discuss the process of selecting a primary care physician.
- Explain how to use health care responsibly.
- List some guidelines for safe shopping on the World Wide Web.
- List some ways to avoid problems when purchasing exercise equipment.
- Discuss the process of making intelligent decisions.

There are many pitfalls that can affect individuals who shop or use goods and services related to health. As we shall see in Chapter 10, there are a number of consumer protection agencies, both public and private. However, the good consumer is a responsible consumer. He or she never takes information on faith. The good consumer asks questions and seeks expert advice.

Being a responsible consumer means that you have a certain amount of skepticism. There are many sources of information available, some good, some not so good. A smart consumer searches out valid sources of information and then attempts to verify what he or she learns from the source.

The wise consumer takes responsibility for his or her own health. This does not mean that you should self-treat every illness, although there are many conditions that can be treated by the informed consumer. It means that, when going for health care, the consumer is prepared and curious, inquiring of the health care provider for information necessary to make decisions. The effective patient participates fully in his or her health care and the decisions related to it.

Shopping

Many people shop as entertainment, for the sheer joy of the experience. These people may or may not be searching to fill a specific need and may not even be seriously considering a purchase. They may be vulnerable to **impulse buying**, a purchase that the shopper does not really need and may later regret buying. These shoppers may find it useful to leave their money or credit card at home and simply enjoy the experience.

In contrast, the serious shopper is one who is attempting to fill a need. The shopper usually has a limited amount of money to spend and a limited amount of time to shop. For these people, it is important to realize that shopping is really a quest for information. You may obtain information from an advertisement, a friend, a salesperson, a label, a magazine article, the Internet, or several other sources. You may gain information from actual use of the product, such as trying on a dress, test driving a car, or taking advantage of a promotion at a fitness center. Shoppers should understand that accessing any of these sources of information has costs. These costs may include transportation costs and time. Only the consumer can place a value on his or her time.

Another cost is called **opportunity cost**. This is something you give up when you decide to do something else. For example, you may give up valuable time with your family in order to gain information about a product. A wise consumer takes into consideration what he or she is trading for the information obtained.

The key to successful shopping is to weigh the cost versus the benefit. Would you drive to five different stores to price vitamins if you knew that you would save only a dollar? On the other hand, spending an hour or two on the Internet gaining information about the hospitals in your area is shopping time well spent. The key to effective shopping is to be able to determine when you have gained enough

information to make a wise purchase without incurring more costs than you gain in savings.

It is to your advantage to expend more shopping costs, including time, when purchasing something that costs a lot of money, when you believe the difference between prices and quality of items is large, or when you do not have much money to spend. It is also wise to spend more in shopping costs if what is gained improves chances of health or safety.

Grocery Shopping

Shopping for food is one of the most important functions in a family. There are many choices of where to obtain food and what food to purchase. Many people in developed countries like the United States and Canada purchase food in supermarkets. Large supermarkets often avoid low-income or inner city areas, leaving residents to purchase food at convenience stores or small "mom-and-pop" stores. These stores usually offer limited choices and high prices.

Where available, farmers' markets offer fresh fruit and vegetables at reasonable cost. Produce at these markets sometimes may cost a few cents more than supermarket produce, but it is worth it for the freshness and added shelf life. Consumers can often find produce at a farmers' market that is not available at supermarkets. Federal law requires farmers' markets to be operated by the farmers themselves, by municipalities, or by nonprofit organizations. Despite the law, some commercial entities imitate farmers' markets. Some merchants at these markets sell organic food, although much produce may not meet the federal guidelines for that distinction. Farmers' markets offer a good option for obtaining nutritious foods while patronizing area farmers.

Supermarkets provide many choices for shoppers. Many of those choices are convenient, but expensive and less nutritious. For example, packaged or frozen vegetables may lose much of their nutritional value in processing, and, with added packaging, they are more expensive by volume than fresh vegetables. Processed meat products are usually high in sodium and fat.

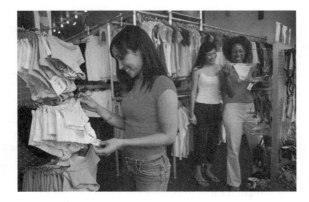

While shopping can be a social and enjoyable experience, it is really a search for information.

Supermarkets are laid out with a plan in mind—to lead the customer to spend more money. Today's supermarkets may include floral departments, delis, bookstores, banks, pharmacies, video stores, and more. Such stores have the goal of exposing shoppers to more products through their layouts. One way they do this is by influencing traffic flow. A good example is the placement of the bakery. The bakery is usually located far from the front door. This accomplishes two purposes. First, if you are going to the bakery to pick up a specific item, you are forced to pass several other items that you may not have otherwise considered buying. Second, the aroma of the bakery wafting through the store may influence customers who had no intention of visiting the bakery to do so. Some stores pump out canned odors of baking long after the actual baking is finished.

Markets targeting upscale customers often include a combination of free-flowing departments. Free-flowing areas allow more customer interaction. In order to lengthen the time spent in the store, the upscale grocery store pattern may include more entertainment and design elements. Some contain cafés and dining areas. These elements contribute to an enjoyable shopping experience, and an enjoyable shopping experience produces more sales.

Keeping the shopper in the store for as long as possible and promoting impulse buying are the primary goals of the construction and layout of supermarkets. Items are placed on the ends of each aisle with a colorful sign, leading the consumer to believe that they are on sale; they probably are not. Some products are placed in more than one section; for example, salad dressing may be placed in the heart of the store but also in the produce section, where the most expensive brands are displayed. Produce is displayed in bright light, often having been recently sprayed with water or with wax applied to the peels so that the light is reflected and the produce is more appealing. Both sides of the checkouts are lined with candies, magazines and tabloids, and useless gadgets; these are called **point-of-sale displays** and are designed to entice impulse purchases. Items at the checkout are often more expensive than the same

items in other places in the store, candy being a good example.

The inside perimeter of supermarkets are very similar to one another. Usually, the produce section, with its bright colors, greets the customer at the front door. As you move around the store you come to the meat counter, deli, bakery, if there is one, and dairy section. Dairy products are usually farthest away from the front door because most families purchase cheese, milk, or butter most frequently. Forcing the customer to pass many other products increases the likelihood of impulse buying.

Supermarkets are often laid out in order of price so that the customer encounters the most expensive items at the beginning of the visit and the cheapest at the end. We are much more likely to spend money on accessories and other related items if we have just decided to buy an expensive item. In comparison, these items seem cheaper than had we encountered them first. Similar items are grouped—for example, picnic supplies with charcoal or spaghetti sauce with spaghetti.

The middle of the store usually contains the frozen food section and shelves of canned and packaged food as well as paper goods, cleaning supplies, and personal health and grooming products. The placement of products is not accidental. The most expensive brand name products are usually at eye level where they are easiest to see with their colorful labels. As your eye goes to the floor, you find cheaper brands, store brands, and generics. Store brands are sometimes placed higher if they actually bring more profit to the store. The most frequently purchased items are often placed in the middle of the aisle. This requires the shopper, even if he or she intends to purchase only one item, to pass numerous other items.

One final trick in supermarket geography is the shuffle. Stores like to reorganize the placement of products. Just when a customer learns the location of the items he or she buys regularly, they are moved. This requires the customer to be exposed to a whole new set of items.

Pricing information at supermarkets is usually on the shelf instead of the product. Wise consumers read the shelf label to make sure the product has not been placed in the wrong location. Labels that give unit pricing (e.g., per ounce) are useful to the consumer. Markets sometimes like to confuse the consumer with inconsistent unit pricing, pricing one item per ounce and another by pound or kilogram.

Good consumers read labels when shopping. The nutrition box provides useful information and allows for comparison of the nutritional value of similar food products. Many consumers try to buy whole wheat bread for the fiber and nutrients. However, bread products labeled "multigrain," "wheat," or "sprouted" are not whole wheat and do not provide the nutritional benefits of whole wheat. A look at the ingredients will reveal the words "100 percent whole wheat" as opposed to "enriched wheat flour," which is white flour. Similarly, if a package is labeled "juice," then it must be 100 percent juice. Words like "juice cocktail" and "juice drink" indicate a very small percentage of real juice and usually a lot of sugar. There are a number of ingredients that are really sugar but are camouflaged by names like high fructose corn syrup, rice syrup, organic dehydrated cane juice, molasses, sorghum syrup, lactose, and dextrose.

TIPS FOR SUPERMARKET SHOPPING

1. Walk the periphery of the store, picking up items that you need—bread, milk, produce. Then stand at the end of each aisle and read the aisle names and group item tags. If you don't need anything from that aisle, avoid it. If you do, walk straight to the item, grab it, and return to the end of the aisle.
2. Avoid the center aisles where the canned, boxed, and frozen foods are located. Processing and packaging add much to the price and the nutritional value is much less than for fresh food.
3. Leave the kids at home. Children use their "pester power" to nag parents into buying things they don't need or want. However, when children are old enough, take them along to use the shopping experience as a teachable moment.
4. Check out fliers and internet offers before you go shopping. If an item is on sale, say frozen chicken breasts, plan to buy two if you can store them.
5. Use a list and stick to it. This will reduce impulse buying. However, if a real bargain appears, take advantage if you can use the item before it spoils or expires.
6. Avoid the free samples. Of course, they taste good. You'll end up buying something you didn't plan to buy. These samples are never fresh fruit.
7. Use coupons wisely. They can cut your overall expenses, but don't buy something you don't need just to save a few cents.
8. Don't shop when you are hungry. Those free samples and other enticements are more effective when you have an empty stomach.
9. Remember, fresh is better than canned or processed. This includes fruits, vegetables, and meats.
10. Items at the end of aisles are usually not on sale. Banners and tags protruding from shelves may or may not indicate a real sale price. Keeping track of what you paid for an item in the past will help you determine if it is really on sale.
11. Look for expiration or sell-by dates.
12. Keep an eye on the scanner to make sure you are charged correctly. When you get home, look at your receipt to double-check pricing and coupon redemption.
13. Practice good decision-making skills.

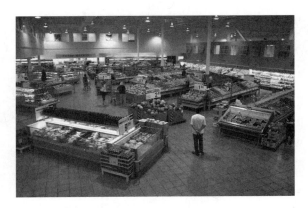

The layouts of supermarkets are consistent and designed to keep the shopper in the store longer so that he or she spends more money. In most supermarkets, a colorful, well-lighted produce department is near the entrance.

Characteristics of Good Consumers

Good consumers are intelligent consumers. They exhibit the following characteristics:

1. ***They are skeptical and demand evidence of claims.*** Smart consumers understand that companies frequently use biased or incomplete data to substantiate their claims. Companies may use surveys laden with loaded questions to elicit a desired response. Marketers also overgeneralize the effects of their products. Friends sometimes inadvertently lead consumers to wrong conclusions by asserting that a product caused an event simply because the use of the product and the occurrence of the event happened near the same time. Skeptical consumers take friends' advice with a measure of caution.

2. ***They are socially aware.*** How you spend your money influences the products and services available to you. Wise consumers take time to learn about origins of the food they eat or the business practices of a store they frequent. They prefer products that promote sustainable livelihoods for producers, environmental conservation, and economic viability. They avoid products produced by child labor. Intelligent consumers make a conscious effort to buy food, clothing, and other products made by ethical manufacturers and produced in humane factories. By employing these socially conscious practices, consumers can contribute to social change.

3. ***They are environmentally aware.*** They use paper instead of plastic and they recycle, conserve, and reuse.

4. ***They shop for economy.*** When going out to shop, they try to plan ahead by making a list of what they need. They purchase all nonperishables, slow-perishables, and fast-ingestibles in bulk. Buying in bulk helps reduce the environmental damage and costs of packaging. Buying directly from the producer, such as a farmer, helps cuts costs and helps to inspire the production of better-quality goods and services by local farmers, factories, and merchants.

5. ***They seek reliable sources of information.*** They understand that advertising has the goal of selling products and services, and they are skeptical of information provided in ads. They evaluate information carefully. Wise consumers seek out sources of information that are unbiased.

6. ***They are patient.*** It sometimes takes time to find quality products and services at reasonable cost. Whenever possible, consumers take the time to investigate the benefits and risks of the product or service. They do not fall for high-pressure sales tactics. If the deal "has to be made today," or is a "limited time offer," it probably is not a deal at all.

7. ***They communicate effectively.*** They follow the advice in the box on page 13, always prepare for medical visits, and ask appropriate questions. They are assertive in making sure they get their questions answered.

8. ***They select health care practitioners carefully and use those practitioners wisely.*** They seek out physicians, dentists, and other practitioners who are properly trained

and possess the appropriate degrees. Asking friends and relatives for recommendations may not inform us about the professional competence of health care practitioners, but it may inform us about how professionals interact with patients, how long you have to wait for an appointment or in a waiting room, and the general "feel" of the experience. Wise consumers investigate whether or not the doctor participates in their health insurance plan. They use alternative health care sparingly and in consultation with their physician. Wise consumers keep track of their health issues by keeping a health journal, recording their medical history, doctor visits, immunizations, test dates and results, allergies, and medications. They write down any questions about their health and take the questions to their next health care appointment. Smart consumers consider themselves partners in their own health.

9. *They practice good health habits, taking a proactive role in their health.* They make daily decisions to improve their health. Wise consumers of health care have a healthy lifestyle; this helps to lower the costs of health care. Regular exercise, balanced diet, avoidance of tobacco products, moderate drinking, safe and responsible sexual behavior, and observing safety precautions promote health and reduce costs. Intelligent consumers keep track of recommended medical tests and screenings and the recommended intervals to have them.

10. *They take an active role in the management of their health problems.* They learn about their health problems by seeking out the best sources of information. They follow their physicians' advice but become informed about their health problems. If information from a physician contradicts that from another valid source, wise consumers attempt to resolve the differences even if it means seeking a second medical opinion. They understand their health insurance plan. Health insurance plans vary in their coverage; consumers should fully understand limitations. Wise consumers read all of the literature sent out by their insurer and ask questions about vague or unclear language; such literature may contain substantial changes in policies and practices. If indicated, the consumer will consider changing plans.

11. *They read and understand contracts.* Contracts, some of which contain warranties or guarantees, can be complicated and are always written to favor the person who wrote them. Good consumers read them carefully and ask questions, even if it means seeking the advice of an attorney, when committed to a long-term and/or high-cost item. This would include, for example, memberships in fitness programs or weight reduction clubs. Oral contracts, as the old saying goes, "are worth the paper they are written on." Health insurance plans are usually quite complicated and full of industry and legal terms with which most consumers are unfamiliar. The least a good consumer would do is read the information carefully. Health insurance contracts are usually quite complicated and full of industry and legal terms with which most consumers are unfamiliar. The least a good consumer would do is read the information carefully.

12. *They report unethical or fraudulent practices.* Whether it is a physician who practices in an unethical manner or questionable practices by a merchant, the wise consumer reports practices that can harm others. Failing to do so can put other patients at risk. The medical board of the state will accept complaints on physician practices. The Federation of State Medical Boards provides a complete list of medical boards at http://www.fsmb. org/directory_smb.html. If the consumer suspects Medicare or Medicaid fraud, it can be reported confidentially by calling 1-800-HHS-TIPS (1-800-447-8477) or by sending email to HHSTips@oig.hhs.gov.

The local Better Business Bureau also takes complaints about interactions between customers and private businesses. The Joint Commission, an accreditation organization, accepts consumer complaints about health care facilities on its Web site or by calling 1-800-994-6610.

Evaluating Information

There is a huge amount of health information available to consumers. Some of it is valuable, while much of it is merely opinion or is presented in a way to sell a product or a book. Celebrities frequently set themselves up as experts, and many consumers believe that because the media grant these stars an interview they have credibility. Usually, they have no more credibility than the average person. Intelligent consumers search out information generated by legitimate medical and scientific studies, rather than well-known people who are given a podium because of their fame or a publishing contract because their celebrity attracts sales. See the box for some examples of celebrity forays into giving advice about health and medicine.

Conscientious consumers carefully search for information about health-related services and products. However, the quality of available information varies a great deal. Consumers should look

CELEBRITY ADVICE ABOUT HEALTH

Celebrities frequently offer advice about health practices and products. This advice may go beyond simply serving as a paid spokesperson for a product to offering medical advice and criticizing medical practice. It should be understood that few celebrities have the medical credentials to provide useful, reliable information about health. A few examples include:

- Actor Tom Cruise made headlines by claiming that "psychiatry is pseudoscience" and "there is no such thing as a chemical imbalance in a body." He also criticized the use of antidepressants in the treatment of postpartum depression. **The truth** is that psychiatry is an accepted medical specialty, medications are frequently used to overcome chemical imbalances in the nervous system, and postpartum depression responds well to antidepressants such as Paxil, Zoloft, and Prozac.
- Actress Suzanne Somers has written over a dozen books, mostly about health and aging. Some of her books advocate for unproven alternative cancer "cures" and she rails against chemotherapy. She also encourages readers to use "bioidentical" hormones instead of synthetic ones and hints that they can help women recapture the sexuality, beauty, and health of youth. **The truth** is that chemotherapy has cured many forms of cancer for many people for many years. Alternative therapies are those that have not been shown under clinical trials to be effective. Ms. Somers offers her personal experience as proof of these therapies' effectiveness, but one example does not substitute for science. Several doctors, including three quoted in one of her books, sent a letter to Somers and her publisher charging that the claims in her book about hormones are misleading, inaccurate, and downright dangerous for women to follow.
- Jenny McCarthy, an actress and former *Playboy* magazine model, has written books linking childhood vaccinations with autism. **The truth** is that medical authorities, supported by research, reject the assertion.
- Television personality Bill Maher expressed opposition to the flu vaccine on his cable program, questioning why someone would let a doctor "stick a disease into your arm."

(continues)

The truth is that flu vaccines, except for the inhaled flu mist, contain killed viruses that cannot cause the flu. While it is true that a small number of people have reactions to the vaccines, vaccines are very safe and provide protection, though not total, against a disease that kills tens of thousands of people yearly.

- Actress Demi Moore used a beauty treatment that involved what she described as "highly trained medical leeches" to detoxify her blood. **The truth** is that leech therapy has proven to assist in the reattachment of body parts, but their use in beauty treatment is unproven. They carry some forms of bacteria that can cause infections when they puncture the skin.
- Talk show host Oprah Winfrey and model Kate Moss have advocated cleansing the body with a "detox diet." Moss promoted a 21-day diet of soy, poultry, fish, brown rice, steamed vegetables, lentils, beans, and green tea. **The truth** is that there is a paucity of clinical studies looking at the validity of detox diets. Until there is evidence that they provide some benefit, the safe assumption is that they do not. If a person is concerned about chemicals in food, he or she can avoid junk food and choose organic produce.
- Singer and actress Beyonce Knowles, appearing on the *Oprah Winfrey Show,* said that she used the Master Cleanse diet to lose weight for a movie. The "Master Cleanse" is a liquid diet that purports to cleanse and detoxify the body while stimulating healthy tissue growth. **The truth** is that diets that border on fasting may rob the body of necessary nutrients. Reducing calories and increasing physical activity are the keys to healthy weight loss. Knowles said that she regained the weight, a typical conclusion to using extreme diets.
- Heather Mills, former wife of singer Paul McCartney, was quoted as saying, "Every day there's a new report warning that obesity levels in children are out of control ... the fact that those kids who drink the most milk gain the most weight should cause alarm bells...." **The truth** is that there is no scientific link between childhood weight increases and increases in milk consumption. Moreover, dietary patterns characterized by increased dairy consumption may protect against developing obesity, including in people who are already overweight.
- Carole Caplin, style adviser to Cherie Blair, the wife of former British Prime Minister Tony Blair, said that women should be informed about how to avoid breast cancer by "keeping the lymph system clear and unclogged." **The truth** is that the statement has no meaning. It is not based on knowledge of the anatomy of the human body or of breast cancer.

for scientific studies, knowing characteristics of those that provide meaningful, useful information. Studies testing the safety and effectiveness of drugs, the usefulness of a device, or the safety of a product should be conducted using the scientific method. See the box on page 9. Key factors for consumer consideration include:

- *Clinical studies.* These studies involve human beings as subjects. While it is true that the early stages of testing of drugs may involve animals, the results have little

value unless studies have been done using humans. Studies done solely in test tubes and petri dishes or exclusively using non-human species do not prove benefits to humans.

- *Sample size.* In the early stages of drug trials, small numbers of people are administered the drug. This is to determine side effects and other safety concerns while putting few people at risk. However, studies done using large groups of human subjects yield information that is more likely to stand up to scrutiny.

- *Randomized, controlled trials.* Human subjects in these trials are usually divided into groups. One or more groups receive the treatment being investigated. Another group receives no treatment or an inactive substance called a **placebo**. This group is referred to as the control group. Participants are assigned to groups randomly. Having control and treatment groups allows for comparison of the treatment with no treatment, so that conclusions can be drawn about its real effect.
- *Double-blind studies.* In these studies, neither the researchers nor the human subjects know who is receiving the

treatment under investigation and who is receiving the placebo. This reduces the effects of bias or expectations.

Good scientific studies appear in peer-reviewed journals. This means that they are not published until they are reviewed by an independent group of experts. They also identify the original source of information contained in the article. While the results of scientific studies may appear in newspapers and other general news sources, so do studies that may generate readership while not adhering to these characteristics. It is good practice to look for replicated studies, ones that have been repeated by different investigators with similar results. One or two small studies usually are not enough to make a definite decision about the efficacy of a product.

THE SCIENTIFIC METHOD

The scientific method is a way to solve a problem, answer a question, and/or determine if events are related, causal, or unrelated.

The first step in the scientific method is determining the problem or research question. The question should be clear and one that can be solved by experimentation. It identifies and clarifies the problem. A good research question allows us to identify the dependent variable(s) and the independent variable(s). An independent variable is a factor that is intentionally manipulated by the researcher. Manipulation may include giving or withholding a treatment. The dependent variable is one that may change as a result of the manipulation of the independent variable. Often, research questions ask if the manipulation of the independent variable affects the dependent variable.

The second step involves observation and information gathering about the issues related to the question. This usually means reading what is known about the variables.

The third step is formulating a hypothesis, a prediction of the answer to the research question.

The fourth step is conducting an experiment. It is often a measurement of the dependent variable as the independent variable is manipulated. The experiment should be designed so that variables are controlled and bias is minimized. This is usually done by ensuring adequate size and random selection of sample, or appropriateness of the individuals from which data are collected; using a controlled group; and employing accurate and objective measurement instruments.

The fifth step is to analyze data collected in the experiment to determine if the hypothesis is confirmed. Data are often organized in charts or graphs.

The sixth step is drawing a conclusion about the question, frequently accompanied by recommendations.

The seventh step is communicating the results, usually in the form of a written report.

The World Wide Web as an Information Source

The content of information on the World Wide Web is virtually unregulated. Anyone can set up a Web site and, barring slander, load it with any information he or she chooses. While commercial sites face some regulation, it is entirely possible to place erroneous information on the Web, and no regulatory agency would be the wiser. Opinion can be passed off as fact. Claims can be made without substantiation. The competent consumer should use the following as guidelines when evaluating Web information:

- *Be skeptical.* Take little at face value. Verify with trusted sources of information if your health is at stake. **Quackery** abounds on the Internet, so be wary of claims of a quick, easy cure. Another good sign that the information is questionable is the writing style. Use caution if there are lots of exclamation points, talk of break-throughs or miracles, or guarantees.
- *Check out the sponsor of the site.* Sites created by national nonprofit organizations, universities, major medical centers, and governmental organizations are usually reputable, although governmental sites may be polluted by political motives. Commercial sites exist to sell product; be cautious of their information. The advertisements on the site may indicate a bias. Any reputable health Web site will make it easy to learn who is responsible for the site.
- *Determine the site's objectives.* Is education the primary motive, or is making a sale the objective? Avoid sites that do not clearly distinguish scientific evidence from opinion or advertisement. Many sites may seem health-oriented but actually push a political agenda.
- *Find out if the information is current.* Look for a date of posting or last update. Web sites should be reviewed and updated regularly. Older material may not include recent findings, such as newly discovered side effects of treatments or advances in the field. Dates of updates are usually on the bottom of the page.
- *Check out the domain suffix.* Sites whose Uniform Resource Locators (URL) end in .edu are usually run by universities or schools; those ending in .org are maintained by not-for-profit groups, usually those whose focus is research, service, or teaching the public; those ending in .gov are maintained by state or federal agencies; those ending in .mil are part of the U.S. military; and those ending in .com or .biz are usually commercial sites and are often selling products. However, site endings can sometimes be misleading.
- *Look for the original source of material presented on the site.* Medical facts and figures should have references and citations. Opinions should be clearly set apart from information that is based on research.
- *Look for the Web site's linking policy.* Some Web sites link to no other sites, some only to verifiable sites that meet certain criteria, and some to any site that asks or pays for a link. This policy is often found in a home page section titled "About This Web Site."
- *Familiarize yourself with the site's policy on personal information.* This is usually contained in a privacy statement. Web sites have the ability to determine the path—i.e., other Web sites—being used to get to the site. They also collect personal information if a visitor subscribes or becomes a member. Any Web site asking for personal information should explain exactly what the site will and will not do with the information.

There are a number of excellent sources of information on the Internet. Many of these are run by government agencies and recognized organizations such as the Mayo Clinic or the American Medical Association. The Federal Citizen Information Center (2009) indicated that the following are generally recognized as reliable Web-based information sources:

- HealthFinder.gov and MedlinePlus.gov provide information on health issues, health care programs, and organizations.
- InteliHealth.com offers information and advice from Harvard Medical School.
- MedicareNewsWatch.com offers a quick reference to Medicare Advantage programs available in your local area.
- MayoClinic.com offers an index of diseases and more.
- MLAnet.org, the Web site of the Medical Library Association, offers links to Web sites suggested by librarians.
- Mentalhelp.net links to a broad range of mental health topics.

Choosing a Primary Care Physician

Your **primary care physician** (PCP) is your partner in health. It is important to choose a doctor who fits your needs, bearing in mind that your insurance coverage may limit your choices. Some **managed care** plans limit your choice of physicians, but generally there is a lengthy list. In recent years, a specialty called family medicine has been developed; these specialists are usually PCPs. In addition, doctors who specialize in internal medicine generally take care of the general health of adults. General practitioners are considered not to focus on any one medical specialty. Any of these may be considered a PCP, depending on the insurance plan.

Begin your search by talking to people you trust. If you are moving to another area or if you know physicians in your area, ask for recommendations from them—good doctors usually recommend good doctors. Family, friends, and coworkers may be good sources of information. Bear in mind that these people are usually not capable of evaluating the medical education or effectiveness of a physician, but they can provide valuable information about charges, length of time it takes to get an appointment, promptness of a doctor, and general doctor-patient interactions.

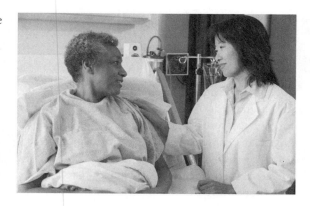

Doctor-patient interaction is an important variable in selecting a physician.

There are other good sources of information about primary care physicians. Try the following:

- Your state medical licensing board can provide information about complaints or disciplinary action against the doctor.
- The American Board of Medical Specialties can provide information about certification. All doctors must be licensed to practice medicine, but not all are board certified.
- Your state insurance department carries a registry of complaints that have been filed relative to insurance and medical practice.
- The *Directory of Medical Specialists,* available at most libraries, carries current professional and biographic information about more than 400,000 practicing physicians. Remember that many primary care physicians do have certification in specialties.

Once you obtain the names of some physicians who interest you, it is a good idea to call their offices to get more information. It is likely that you will not necessarily be satisfied with all of the information you receive from any one doctor's office, but weighing pros and cons is part of the process. A few questions you may ask include:

- Is the doctor taking new patients?
- Will the doctor treat my children?
- Is the doctor in my insurance plan? (If you are a Medicaid or Medicare patient,

be sure to ask if the doctor will accept the payments offered by these plans.)

- When the doctor is away, who takes care of his or her patients?

After narrowing your search to a few physicians, it is a good idea to set up an appointment for an interview, a sort of "get acquainted" session. Some physicians charge for this appointment, but it is usually worth it to understand office policies and to determine if the doctor is a good match for you and your family.

Using Health Care Responsibly

There was a time when many patients went passively to their doctor, received treatment (or did not), and went home. Patients may not have understood their diagnoses or the treatment. They usually asked few questions. Doctors were viewed as all-knowing experts, sometimes as magicians or even godlike. Those days are behind us. Physicians want and expect patients to be active participants in their own care and to make informed decisions about the treatments they receive.

Patients should always be prepared for appointments with physicians. You should write down all the medications you take, including over-the-counter medicines and dietary supplements. Write down your symptoms and any questions you have for the doctor. Family members should accompany patients whose memory or thought processes are impaired. Doctor-patient appointments are shrinking in length, and the patient should be ready to make the most of the time with the doctor.

Physicians and other deliverers of health care sometimes make errors. These errors generally fall into the following categories:

- Medication errors—preventable mistakes in prescribing and delivering medication to patients
- Surgical errors
- Diagnostic inaccuracies—incorrect diagnoses that may lead to incorrect or ineffective treatment or unnecessary testing

- System failures—inconsistencies in the organization of health care delivery and the way resources are provided to the delivery system

The degree of damage is illustrated by examining the damage done by only one category of error—medication errors. Medication errors encompass all mistakes involving prescription drugs, over-the-counter products, vitamins, minerals, or herbal supplements. The Committee on Identifying and Preventing Medication Errors of the Institute of Medicine of the National Academies (Aspden, Wolcott, Bootman, & Cronenwett, 2006) estimated that medication errors alone cause injury to 1.5 million people each year. The extra medical costs of treating drug-related injuries occurring in hospitals alone amount to at least $3.5 billion a year. In addition, there are costs associated with lost productivity and other health costs. The Committee estimated that a conservative 400,000 preventable drug-related injuries occur each year in hospitals, 800,000 occur in long-term care settings, and roughly 530,000 occur just among Medicare recipients in outpatient clinics.

HealthGrades (2008) analyzed patient data for Medicare patients from 2004 to 2006. The analysis revealed that during that two-year period, over 238,000 potentially preventable deaths occurred during patient safety incidents. The estimated cost to the Medicare program was about $8.8 billion.

While it is unreasonable to believe that all errors will be prevented, there are many actions that patients can take to reduce the likelihood of occurrence. The box on page 13 contains information from the Agency for Healthcare Research and Quality that will help the consumer assist in the reduction of medical errors.

Consumers can purchase virtually anything via the World Wide Web. While this provides much convenience, it also presents risk. The following are some guidelines for Internet shopping:

- Purchase from known, trusted Web sites. Merchants that are established and well known are more likely to deal fairly with consumers. Read reviews left by other shoppers. Observe ratings, but do not take them at face value since there may be many reasons for lower ratings.

What Can You Do? Be Involved in Your Health Care

1. **The single most important way you can help to prevent errors is to be an active member of your health care team.**

   That means taking part in every decision about your health care. Research shows that patients who are more involved with their care tend to get better results. Some specific tips, based on the latest scientific evidence about what works best, follow.

Medicines

2. **Make sure that all of your doctors know about everything you are taking, including prescription and over-the-counter medicines, and dietary supplements such as vitamins and herbs.**

   At least once a year, bring all of your medicines and supplements with you to your doctor. "Brown bagging" your medicines can help you and your doctor talk about them and find out if there are any problems. It can also help your doctor keep your records up to date, which can help you get better quality care.

3. **Make sure your doctor knows about any allergies and adverse reactions you have had to medicines.**

   This can help you avoid getting a medicine that can harm you.

4. **When your doctor writes a prescription, make sure you can read it.**

   If you can't read your doctor's handwriting, your pharmacist might not be able to either.

5. **Ask for information about your medicines in terms you can understand—both when your medicines are prescribed and when you receive them.**

   - What is the medicine for?
   - How am I supposed to take it, and for how long?
   - What side effects are likely? What do I do if they occur?
   - Is this medicine safe to take with other medicines or dietary supplements I am taking?
   - What food, drink, or activities should I avoid while taking this medicine?

6. **When you pick up your medicine from the pharmacy, ask: Is this the medicine that my doctor prescribed?**

   A study by the Massachusetts College of Pharmacy and Allied Health Sciences found that 88 percent of medicine errors involved the wrong drug or the wrong dose.

7. **If you have any questions about the directions on your medicine labels, ask.**

   Medicine labels can be hard to understand. For example, ask if "four doses daily" means taking a dose every six hours around the clock or just during regular waking hours.

8. **Ask your pharmacist for the best device to measure your liquid medicine. Also, ask questions if you're not sure how to use it.**

   Many people do not understand the right way to measure liquid medicines. For example, many use household teaspoons, which often do not hold a true teaspoon of liquid. Special devices, like marked syringes, help people to measure the right dose. Being shown how to use the devices helps even more.

(continues)

9. **Ask for written information about the side effects your medicine could cause.**

   If you know what might happen, you will be better prepared if it does—or, if something unexpected happens instead. That way, you can report the problem right away and get help before it gets worse. A study found that written information about medicines can help patients recognize problem side effects and then give that information to their doctor or pharmacist.

Hospital Stays

10. **If you have a choice, choose a hospital at which many patients have the procedure or surgery you need.**

    Research shows that patients tend to have better results when they are treated in hospitals that have a great deal of experience with their condition.

11. **If you are in a hospital, consider asking all health care workers who have direct contact with you whether they have washed their hands.**

    Handwashing is an important way to prevent the spread of infections in hospitals, yet it is not done regularly or thoroughly enough. A recent study found that when patients checked whether health care workers washed their hands, the workers washed their hands more often and used more soap.

12. **When you are being discharged from the hospital, ask your doctor to explain the treatment plan you will use at home.**

    This includes learning about your medicines and finding out when you can get back to your regular activities. Research shows that at discharge time, doctors think their patients understand more than they really do about what they should or should not do when they return home.

Surgery

13. **If you are having surgery, make sure that you, your doctor, and your surgeon all agree and are clear on exactly what will be done.**

    Doing surgery at the wrong site (for example, operating on the left knee instead of the right) is rare, but even once is too often. The good news is that wrong-site surgery is 100 percent preventable. The American Academy of Orthopaedic Surgeons urges its members to sign their initials directly on the site to be operated on before the surgery.

Other Steps You Can Take

14. **Speak up if you have questions or concerns.**

    You have a right to question anyone who is involved with your care.

15. **Make sure that someone, such as your personal doctor, is in charge of your care.**

    This is especially important if you have many health problems or are in a hospital.

16. **Make sure that all health professionals involved in your care have important health information about you.**

    Do not assume that everyone knows everything they need to.

17. **Ask a family member or friend to be there with you and to be your advocate (someone who can help get things done and speak up for you if you can't).**

    Even if you think you don't need help now, you might need it later.

18. **Know that "more" is not always better.**

    It is a good idea to find out why a test or treatment is needed and how it can help you. You could be better off without it.

19. **If you have a test, don't assume that no news is good news.**

    Ask about the results.

20. **Learn about your condition and treatments by asking your doctor and nurse and by using other reliable sources.**

Source: 20 tips to help prevent medical errors. (2000, February). Patient Fact Sheet. AHRQ Publication No. 00-PO38. Agency for Healthcare Research and Quality, Rockville, MD. Retrieved from http://www.ahrq.gov/consumer/20tips.htm

- Use independent evaluations, such as those by *Consumer Reports*.

- Do not use a debit card. Credit cards generally offer better protections for the consumer. Both credit and debit cards allow you to dispute charges to your account, but your money is tied up while you dispute the charges made with your debit card. Web sites are sometimes "hacked" and customers' credit or debit card information stolen. Major credit cards usually offer a zero liability policy, meaning if you notify the issuing bank of unauthorized transactions, you pay nothing. Most debit cards do not offer the same policy. Do not send your credit card number to anyone by e-mail.

- Use sites that do price comparisons. Many shopping Web sites allow consumers to purchase from a number of vendors at the same time. This allows for sorting the results by the lowest price. It also can provide vendor or store ratings. Examples are PriceGrabber.com, Shopping.com, and PriceSCAN.com.

- Set up a secondary e-mail address for registering or buying at online stores. When purchasing online, customers are prompted to enter an e-mail address. This allows the store to contact you with order confirmations and tracking information. However, they also allow the vendor to continue to send you more e-mail. Using a secondary, free e-mail address eliminates this problem for your main address.

- Never purchase from an unsolicited e-mail and do not reveal personal information or credit card information to anyone who contacts you by e-mail.

- Understand the company's privacy statement. Internet companies often sell or trade personal and commercial information about clients, leading to junk e-mail, solicitations, and, occasionally, identity theft. (Brick-and-mortar companies and some nonprofit agencies also trade in client information.)

- Read and understand the return policy. If it is unclear, ask questions by e-mail or phone.

- Shop only at sites that display the secure symbol. When you are directed to the "Check Out" section, make sure that the URL begins with "https:". Https provides much better protection by encrypting and decrypting user page requests as well as the pages that are returned by the Web server. The use of https protects against eavesdropping and third-party attacks.

Making Intelligent Decisions

Intelligent consumers make intelligent decisions. Unfortunately, many consumers act on impulse, often making decisions that they soon regret. Making decisions is a process that follows a logical progression of steps. The steps are:

1. *Identify the decision to be made.* This includes identifying the goals and objectives it should achieve. It also includes identifying your needs. For instance: Do I really need this service? How often will I use this product? Do I need the best or will a slightly lower quality product meet my needs?

2. *Identify your own values.* Your values may help you limit your choices. The decision you eventually make should fit your own values.

3. *Obtain information.* Get the facts, but remember that you cannot get all the facts. Get as many facts as possible about a decision *within the limits of time imposed on you and your ability to process them,* but remember that virtually every decision must be made in partial ignorance. Lack of complete information must not be allowed to paralyze your decision (Harris, 2008). Use the best sources of information available.

4. *Develop a list of alternatives.* List all the possible choices you have, including the choice of doing nothing.

5. *Consider the pros and cons of each alternative.* List the good things and not-so-good things about each alternative. This step requires you to consider the benefits of each alternative as well as the risks. You should carefully examine each alternative in light of its relative benefit. It often helps to rate the various alternatives against one another. This helps to determine if something might be nice but not really necessary.

6. *Make a decision.* After carefully considering all of the alternatives and their relative worth, you must decide on one course of action. Once you have made the choice, implement it.

   In some cases, decisions affect future events, or sometimes similar situations arise and you must make a similar choice. In these cases, it helps to observe a seventh step.

7. *Evaluate the decision.* Take an objective look at the decision you have made in light of the goals and objectives you identified in Step 1. This evaluation can be a useful information source for future decision.

SUMMARY

People shop for several reasons, but the good consumer uses shopping as a method of gaining information. Balancing costs, including time and transportation costs, with what is gained from shopping is the key. Good consumers are intelligent consumers who exhibit several characteristics not seen consistently in average or poor consumers.

Wise consumers are skeptical and seriously evaluate health information before accepting or acting upon it. They understand the importance of clinical, randomized, controlled, double-blind studies that employ large samples of subjects. Good consumers also evaluate information on the World Wide Web carefully, realizing that it is easy to place inaccurate information on the Web. They are just as careful when purchasing products and services on the World Wide Web, selecting merchants prudently and using practices that enhance security.

Choosing and using medical care is a responsibility that good consumers take seriously. They select and use a primary care physician wisely, using reliable sources of information.

Making decisions is a process. Following a planned set of steps increases the likelihood that decisions about health and consumerism will be seen as positive over time.

Key Terms

Impulse buying: a spur-of-the-moment, unplanned purchase

Managed care: a system of delivering and financing health care that is designed to reduce cost and control the use of health care

Opportunity cost: something you give up when you decide to do something else

Placebo: substance used in medical treatment that has no pharmaceutical effect on the problem it is being used to treat

Point-of-sale displays: displays set up at places where payment is made

Primary care physician: the physician who handles most of your care and who makes referrals to specialists

Quackery: promotion of health practices or remedies that have no compelling scientific basis

Study Questions

1. What are some important characteristics of a good consumer?
2. How would you apply the characteristics of a good consumer when food shopping?
3. How do you shop for economy?
4. How can you take an active role in your own health care?
5. Where can you report fraudulent business practices?
6. What are the characteristics of good studies that evaluate products and services?
7. How can you evaluate information on the Internet?
8. How do you select a primary care physician?
9. What are the impacts of medication and medical errors?
10. What are some guidelines for purchasing on the World Wide Web?
11. What are the steps in sound decision making?
12. How would you apply the steps in sound decision making when shopping for food?

References

Aspden, P., Wolcott, J. A., Bootman, J. L., & Cronenwett, L. R. (Eds.). (2006). *Preventing medical errors.* Washington, DC: National Academies Press.

Federal Citizen Information Center, U.S. General Services Administration. (2009). *2009 consumer action handbook.* Washington, DC: U.S. General Services Administration.

Harris, R. (2008). *Introduction to decision making.* Retrieved from http://www.virtualsalt.com/crebook5.htm

HealthGrades. (2008). *The fifth annual HealthGrades patient safety in American hospitals study.* Retrieved from http://www.healthgrades.com/media/dms/pdf/patientsafetyinamericanhospitalsstudy2008.pdf

Chapter 2

The American Health Care System

Chapter Objectives

The student will:

- Discuss the structure of the medical care system in the United States.
- Describe the quality of the U.S. health care system.
- Describe health disparities in the U.S. health care system.
- Describe how lack of access to health insurance affects overall health and health care.
- Compare the U.S. health care system to those of other industrialized countries.
- List some measures of quality in a health care system.
- Describe ways to improve the system.
- Describe quality assurance methods in today's health care system.
- Compare arguments for and against a universal health care system.
- List some measures contained in the health care reform legislation of 2010 that may improve the health care system.
- Discuss the processes of selecting a hospital and senior living facility.

Medical Care in the United States

The health care delivery system in the United States is composed of many types of provider groups and institutions. There are 213 federal hospitals and 5,010 **community hospitals** in the United States (American Hospital Association, 2010b). The majority of America's community hospitals, about 59 percent, are nongovernmental and not-for-profit. About 18 percent are private, for-profit institutions. The rest are operated by state or local governments (American Hospital Association, 2007). In addition, there are specialty hospitals that concentrate on special populations like children or specific diseases like cancer.

Most hospitals have emergency departments that will quickly provide urgent medical care to persons who are very ill or injured people. Emergency medical care is quite expensive and should be reserved for true emergencies. Paramedics, emergency medical technicians (EMTs), and some nurses are highly trained in emergency medical care. They often accompany the patient to the emergency room in the ambulance and begin to administer crisis care during the transport. Some hospitals provide care that is so sophisticated that they are referred to as trauma centers.

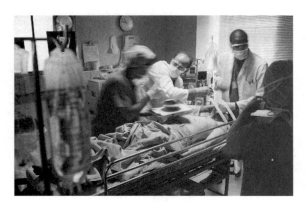

The emergency room serves as a bridge, stabilizing a patient before full hospital admission. They also provide outpatient care when primary care is not available.

Most hospitals offer services beyond traditional inpatient treatment. According to the American Hospital Association (2010b), 61 percent of hospitals offer home health service, 62 percent offer **hospice care**, and 22 percent offer Meals on Wheels.

Some of the larger teaching hospitals and county hospitals have clinics that provide health care at a reduced rate. These clinics provide some forms of medical care such as immunizations and contraceptives for families who cannot afford private care and who do not have insurance. Some clinics are general care and some are specialty clinics, such as prenatal care or cardiology clinics.

Clinics often afford experience for interns or residents as they serve a rotation there. Departments of public health also run community health clinics. These clinics are usually open to all, but they are used primarily by people who have no health insurance and people whose income is low. They are often located in rural or low-income areas where there are few medical services available.

Acute care clinics, or minor emergency care clinics, are usually located in the community and often close to a hospital. In general, they provide care for people who are ill or injured but not serious enough to need an emergency room. They are sometimes called walk-in clinics because patients can be seen without an appointment. Many people who do not have primary care physicians receive acute care at these facilities.

Aspiring physicians complete four years of college and then pass tests to demonstrate their qualifications before being admitted into medical school. Medical school is usually four more years of study. Medical students do clinical studies in a hospital, including a year of internship, then several years as a resident, learning under the supervision of experienced physicians. They may choose to specialize in a branch of medicine, or they may choose to become a primary care or internal medicine doctor. The box defines several medical specialties. Physicians may go into private practice or they may practice at hospitals or clinics.

DEFINITIONS OF MEDICAL SPECIALTIES

Allergy and immunology: evaluation, physical and laboratory diagnosis, and management of disorders involving the immune system, including asthma, eczema, adverse reactions to food, drugs, and insect stings and bites

Anesthesia: application of pharmacology and physiology to dull sensation or awareness and manage the airway of patients receiving treatment

Cardiology: diagnosis and treatment of conditions related to the heart and blood vessels

Dermatology: care and treatment of the skin, hair, and nails

Emergency medicine: urgent medical care for acute medical or surgical conditions or injuries

Endocrinology: diagnosis and treatment of conditions relating to the endocrine system (i.e., hormones and glands), including diabetes and thyroid conditions

Family medicine: continuing, comprehensive health care for the individual and family; often serves as the primary care physician

Gastroenterology: diagnosis and care of diseases of the digestive system, including the stomach, intestines, liver, and pancreas

Geriatrics: care and treatment of the elderly

Gynecology: care for women, particularly the health of women's reproductive organs

Hematology: diagnosis and treatment of disorders of the blood and blood-forming organs

Hepatology: a branch of gastroenterology involving the liver and biliary tract

Infectious diseases: diagnosis and treatment of conditions caused by biological agents

Intensive care: continuous monitoring and treatment of seriously ill patients using special medical equipment and services

Internal medicine: general medical care of adults, usually 18 years of age and older

Neonatology: care and development of newborn babies and the treatment of their diseases

Nephrology: care and treatment of diseases of the kidneys

Neurology: diagnosis and treatment of diseases, disorders, and injuries to the brain, spinal cord, nervous system, and related structures

Obstetrics: medical care during pregnancy and delivery and for a short period thereafter

Oncology: diagnosis and treatment of cancer and other malignant diseases

Ophthalmology: diagnosis and treatment of eye diseases and conditions

Orthopedics: diagnosis and treatment of diseases and conditions affecting the bones, joints, muscles, and tendons

Otorhinolaryngology: care and treatment of diseases of the ears, sinuses, nose, throat, and upper airway

Palliative care: deals with pain and symptom relief and emotional support in patients with terminal illnesses

Pathology: interpretation of laboratory tests on blood, urine, and other body fluids

Pediatrics: medical care of infants, children, and adolescents

Physical medicine and rehabilitation: care designed to provide functional improvement and restoration after injury, illness, or congenital disorders

Plastic surgery: elective cosmetic surgery and reconstructive surgery after traumatic mutilation or disfigurement

Podiatry: treatment of diseases of the foot and ankle

Preventive medicine: health care to delay or avert disease or illness

Proctology: care of the rectum, anus, and colon

Psychiatry: diagnosis, treatment, and prevention of cognitive, perceptual, emotional, and behavioral disorders; may include treatment of substance abuse and addictive disorders

Pulmonology: treatment of diseases and disorders of the lung

Radiology: use of x-ray, ultrasound, computerized tomography, and magnetic resonance imaging for diagnostic purposes

Radiology, nuclear: use of radioactive isotopes in diagnosis and/or treatment

Rheumatology: diagnosis and treatment of diseases of the joints, including arthritis and autoimmune diseases

Sports medicine: care and prevention of injuries and diseases acquired in sports

Surgery, general: surgery involving the skin, endocrine glands, abdomen, and breasts; usually, a precursor to more specialized surgery

Urology: deals with urinary tracts of males and females and the male reproductive system

Most private practice physicians have privileges to practice at one or more hospitals. A large majority of physicians work in physician-owned private practices. Less than one-fourth of all physicians work in practices of ten or more physicians, and nearly 60 percent work in groups of fewer than five (Kane, 2004).

Nurses and medical assistants help physicians provide health care in hospitals, clinics, and private offices. Often, nurses are the first person to see a patient, recording the medical history and checking vital signs. They may also draw blood for laboratory tests and conduct minor procedures. If the patient is admitted to a hospital, nurses and medical assistants administer many treatments that have been ordered by a physician. They must be licensed by graduating from a nursing training program, usually at a college or university, and passing a licensing exam. Nursing school is from two to four years depending on the type of license or degree.

Quality of Care in America

Many Americans believe that they live in a nation that delivers the best, most comprehensive health care in the entire world. They would be mistaken. While it may be true that the United States has some of the best-equipped hospitals and the best-trained physicians in the world, the system falls far short of what is attainable (The Commonwealth Fund, 2008).

Infant mortality rate (IMF) and life expectancy at birth (LEB) are two measures of the health of a nation that reflect the quality of the health care delivery system. According to the U.S. Central Intelligence Agency (2010), the United States ranks forty-fifth among the nations of the world in IMF and forty-nineth in LEB.

In 2000, the World Health Organization evaluated the health care delivered in 191 nations. In the analysis, WHO developed three primary goals for what a good health system should do:

- Good health: "making the health status of the entire population as good as possible" across the whole life cycle

- Responsiveness: responding to people's expectations of respectful treatment and client orientation by health care providers
- Fairness in financing: ensuring financial protection for everyone, with costs distributed according to one's ability to pay

WHO (2000) also distinguished between the overall "goodness" of health systems, described as "the best attainable average level" and fairness, described as "the smallest feasible differences among individuals and groups." The United States ranked number 37, behind such countries as Italy, Andorra, Oman, Colombia, United Arab Emirates, and Costa Rica. On the positive side, WHO ranked the United States first among the 191 nations in the category of responsiveness, the extent to which caregivers are responsive to the client/patient expectations with regard to non-health areas such as being treated with dignity and respect.

In a study involving 1,536 children in 12 metropolitan areas, Mangione-Smith et al. (2007) produced some startling data about the medical care received by children. Children were found to receive appropriate outpatient medical care only 47 percent of the time. They received indicated care for acute medical problems 67.6 percent of the time, appropriate care for chronic conditions 53.4 percent of the time, and appropriate preventive care only 40.7 percent of the time. McGlynn et al. (2003) found that adults received appropriate care only 54.9 percent of the time. The Institute of Medicine (IOM; 1999) stated that at least 44,000 people, and perhaps as many as 98,000 people, die in hospitals each year as a result of medical errors that could have been prevented. In addition, there are about 99,000 deaths per year from hospital-acquired infections (Klevins et al., 2007), most of which could have been prevented. The IOM concluded, "Even using the lower estimate, preventable medical errors in hospitals exceed attributable deaths to such feared threats as motor-vehicle wrecks, breast cancer, and AIDS." These findings raise questions about the quality and safety of health care in the United States.

Emergency room care in America may be sliding in quality. In 2010, about half of all urban and teaching hospitals reported that their emergency departments were "at" or "over" capacity (American Hospital Association, 2010a). In a study by Johns Hopkins University (Vanlandingham, Powe, Marone, Diener-West, & Rubin, 2005), two-thirds of hospital emergency department directors who responded reported that on-call coverage is inadequate to meet the needs of their patients. On-call coverage problems were reported more often in urban (73 percent) than rural (60 percent) hospitals and were similar in geographic regions of the country. The greatest shortage of specialists was in hand surgery. Among hospitals where hand surgery coverage is perceived to be very or extremely important for overall patient outcomes, 69 percent of hospitals had less than full-time coverage. Hospitals also had less than full-time coverage for plastic surgery (52 percent), neurosurgery (49 percent), ear, nose, and throat (44 percent), and psychiatry (42 percent). On-call coverage shortages were related to the proportion of uninsured patients in the hospital emergency department, but not to the supply of specialists. The researchers concluded that the shortage of on-call coverage is an emerging trend that threatens the integrity of the health care safety net, placing patients at potential risk for injury.

In a study of the health care systems in seven industrialized nations, Schoen, Osborn, Doty, Bishop, Peugh, and Murukutla (2007) found that, among adults in seven countries, U.S. adults reported the highest overall error rates, including lab and medication errors. One-third of U.S. patients with chronic conditions reported a medical, medication, or lab test error in the past two years, compared with 28 percent of patients in Canada and 26 percent in Australia. Patient-reported errors were highest for patients seeing multiple doctors or with multiple chronic illnesses.

In response to the problem of medical errors, the state of Massachusetts announced a new policy in 2009. Under the policy, five state agencies, including Medicaid, have adopted uniform nonpayment policies for costs associated with 28 serious reportable health care events, with the goal of advancing quality care. Under the new guidelines, state agencies and their contractors will not pay for certain serious reportable health care events. These largely preventable events include surgery on the wrong body part; surgery on the wrong patient; care ordered by or provided by someone impersonating a physician, nurse, pharmacist, or other licensed provider; and patient death or serious disability associated with a medication error. It remains to be seen if this policy will affect overall health care or if other states will adopt similar policies.

Disparities in the Health Care Delivery System

Healthy People 2020 (U.S. Department of Health and Human Services, 2009) contains the health objectives for the United States to be reached by 2020. It sets the course for federal and state efforts to improve the health status of Americans. The document continued the themes established in *Healthy People 2010* (U.S. Department of Health and Human Services, 2000). One of the four overarching goals of the recent document is to achieve health equity, eliminate disparities, and improve the health of all groups. Despite enormous resources that were committed to eliminating disparities in the past, they continue.

Access to health care, defined as the availability and timely use of health services to produce the optimum outcomes, is vital to overall health and wellness. Attaining full access to health care involves three discrete steps:

- Gaining entry into the health care system
- Gaining access to sites of care where patients can receive needed services
- Finding providers who will meet the needs of individual patients and with whom patients can develop a relationship based on mutual communication and trust (Bierman, Magari, Jette, Splaine, & Wasson, 1998)

All three of these steps are largely dependent on whether or not an individual has health insurance. Among 30 industrialized nations, only the United States, Mexico, and Turkey have not achieved near universal health care coverage (Organisation for Economic Co-operation and Development, 2009).

In the United States, racial and ethnic minorities and low-income populations experience serious disparities in rates of insurance and access to health care (Agency for Healthcare Research and Quality, 2009). Four in ten low-income Americans do not have health insurance, and nearly half of all uninsured people in the United States are poor. About one-third of the uninsured have a chronic disease, and they are six times less likely to receive health care for a health problem than the insured (Kaiser Family Foundation, 2009). In contrast, 94 percent of upper-income Americans have health insurance (Agency for Healthcare Research and Quality, 2009). More than one in three Hispanics and American Indians and just under one in five African Americans are uninsured (Kaiser Family Foundation, 2009). In comparison, only about one in eight whites lacks health insurance (Agency for Healthcare Research and Quality, 2009). Health care reform legislation, the Health Care and Education Reconciliation Act of 2010 (HCERA) that revised the previously passed Patient Protection and Affordable Care Act (PPACA), has the potential to shrink the disparities.

Uninsured patients are about twice as likely to leave a hospital emergency department without being seen as patients with private insurance. In addition, African Americans were about 50 percent more likely to leave without being seen as whites (Agency for Healthcare Research and Quality, 2009).

A primary care provider and a facility where a person receives regular care substantially improve health outcomes. However, Hispanics are only half as likely as whites to have a usual source of care. Half of Hispanics and more than a quarter of African Americans do not have a regular doctor, as compared with only one-fifth of whites. Low-income Americans are three times less likely to have a usual source of care compared with those with higher incomes (HealthReform.gov, 2009).

A Costly System

The United States has by far the most expensive health care system in the world, based on health expenditures per capita and on total expenditures as a percentage of gross domestic product (University of Maine, 2001). We spend more on health care than any other country. Moreover, resources are allocated unequally, inefficiently, and wastefully. The money spent does not yield the value we expect.

The United States spends a disproportionate amount of its gross domestic product (GDP) on health care, and a greater percentage of GDP on health care than any other country. Table 2.1 illustrates large and consistent increases in expenditures. In 1940, after the Great Depression had ended and as the world was plunging into war, we spent about 4 percent of the U.S. GDP on health care. By 1985, we were spending over 10 percent of GDP on health care. Without major adjustments, we are projected to spend almost 20 percent of GDP on health care in the year 2019. This means that one-fifth of every dollar produced in goods and services in the United States will be spent on health care. The Organisation for Economic Co-operation and Development (2009) reported that in 2007, other industrialized countries spent 6 to 11 percent of GDP on health care, with an average of 9 percent, far lower than the percentage of GDP spent in the United States.

Table 2.1 demonstrates growth in terms of real dollars. In 1985, health care expenditures in the United States were just over $439 billion. By the year 2000, expenditures had grown to over $1.3 trillion. In 2008, we spent over $2.3 trillion on health care, a figure that is projected to expand to over $4.7 trillion in 2019. The data in Table 2.1 for the years 2010, 2014, and 2019 are based on estimates of the cost after passage of the health reform legislation of 2010. Many of the provisions of the law go into effect in 2014. We will discuss this legislation later in this chapter.

The amount of money spent on health care per person is illustrated in the right-hand column of Table 2.1. A steady and rapid increase is occurring

TABLE 2.1 HEALTH CARE EXPENDITURES

Year	GDP in Billions	Health Care Expenditures in Billions	%GDP	Amt. Per Capita
1929	$ 103.4	$ 3.6	3.5	$ 29.49
1935	72.2	2.9	4.0	22.65
1940	100.0	4.0	4.0	29.62
1950	286.2	12.7	4.4	81.86
1960	526	27.5	5.2	148
1970	1,039	74.9	7.2	356
1975	1,638	133.1	8.1	605
1980	2,790	253.4	9.1	1,100
1985	4,220	439.3	10.4	1,818
1990	5,803	714.0	12.3	2,813
1993	6,657	912.6	13.7	3,469
1998	8,747	1,190.0	13.6	4,297
2000	9,817	1,353.6	13.8	4,790
2002	10,470	1,603.4	15.3	5,560
2005	12,434	1,973.3	15.9	6,649
2007	13,841	2,300.3	16.0	7,600
2008	14,441	2,338.7	16.2	7,681
2009*	14,283	2,472.2	17.3	8,047
2010**(est.)	14,789	2,632.4	17.8	
2014**(est.)	17,966	3,358.8	18.8	
2019**(est.)	22,460	4,716.5	21.0	

Sources: Centers for Medicare & Medicaid Services, Office of the Actuary: Data from the National Health Statistics Group. *NHE summary including share of GDP*. Retrieved from http://www.cms.hhs.gov/NationalHealthExpendData/02.National HealthAccountsHisorical.asp#TopofPage

*Centers for Medicare & Medicaid Services. (2010). *National health expenditure projections, 2009–2019*. Retrieved from http://www.cms.hhs.gov/NationalHealthExpendData/proj2009.pdf

**Centers for Medicare & Medicaid Services. (2010). *Estimated financial effects of the "Patient Protection and Affordable Care Act," as amended* (Memorandum April 22, 2010). Retrieved from http://www.cms.gov/ActuarialStudies/Downloads/ PPACA_2010-04-22.pdf

and can be emphasized by the fact that the per-person expenditure will double between 2005 and 2019. Figure 2.1 demonstrates the rate of annual growth in health care spending in the United States, a rate that is much greater than inflation, the economy as a whole, and workers' earnings. Figure 2.2 depicts how the health care dollar is spent in America.

Utilization of health care and the accompanying costs are not spread evenly among the population. In 2002, 5 percent of the civilian noninstitutionalized population accounted for 49 percent of overall U.S. health care spending. Among this group, annual medical expenses, not including health insurance premiums, equaled or exceeded $11,487 per person. The average expenditure was

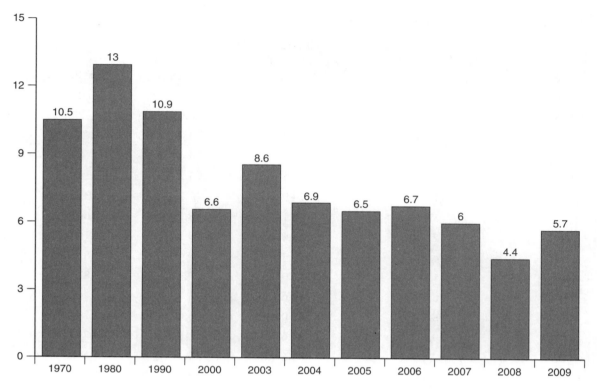

FIGURE 2.1 ANNUAL PERCENTAGE GROWTH RATES IN HEALTH SPENDING, UNITED STATES
Source: Centers for Medicare and Medicaid Services, Office of the Actuary.

about $35,543 for the top 1 percent. In contrast, the 50 percent of the population with the lowest expenses accounted for only 3 percent of overall U.S. medical spending. For this group, annual medical spending was below $644 per person (Conwell & Cohen, 2005).

In 2002, persons over the age of 65 made up about 13 percent of the U.S. population, but they consumed 36 percent of the total U.S. personal health care expenses. The average health care expense in 2002 was $11,089 for those older than age 65 and $3,352 for those between the ages of 19 and 64 (Keehan, Lazenby, Zezza, & Catlin, 2004). In studying insurance company data on 3.75 million enrollees and data from the Medicare Current Beneficiary Survey, Alemayehu and Warner (2004) found that 8 percent of health care expenses occurred before age 20, 13 percent during young adulthood (20–39 years), 31 percent during middle age (40–64 years), and 49 percent after age 65. Both of these reports

clearly indicate that health care expenses go up dramatically with advancing age.

Other reasons for the exceptionally high cost of health care in the United States can be attributed to a number of factors, ranging from costs of medical technology and prescription drugs to the high administrative costs of the complex multiple-payer system in the United States (Woolhandler & Himmelstein, 1997; University of Maine, 2001). There appears to be a shift from nonprofit to for-profit health care providers, including for-profit hospital chains, that has also contributed to the rise in costs.

In 2007, an estimated 45.3 million Americans, over 15 percent of the population, had no health insurance, as reported by the U.S. Bureau of the Census (2008). Another 16 million people are considered underinsured (Schoen, Doty, Collins, & Holmgren, 2005). People without health insurance are much less likely than those with insurance to receive recommended preventive services and

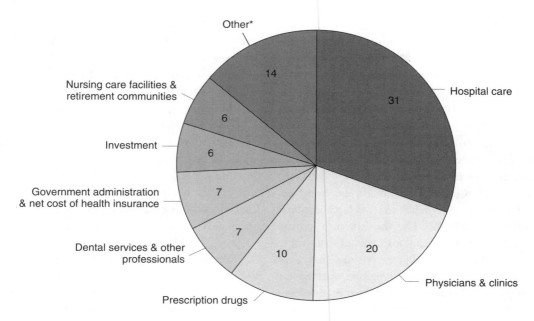

Other*

14

Hospital care

31

Nursing care facilities &
retirement communities

6

Investment

6

Government administration
& net cost of health insurance

7

Dental services & other
professionals

7

10

20

Prescription drugs

Physicians & clinics

*Includes medical goods, government and public health activities, home health care, and other health, residential, and personal care.

Figure 2.2 Percentages of US health care expenditures, 2009

Source: Centers for Medicare and Medicaid Services, Office of the Actuary, National Health Services Group. Retrieved from http://www.cms.gov/NationalHealthExpendData/downloads/PiechartSourcesExpenditures2009.pdf.

medications, are less likely to have access to regular care by a personal physician, and are less able to obtain needed health care services. Consequently, Americans receive appropriate preventive, short-term, and long-term health care as recommended by professional guidelines in only about 55 percent of the instances in which those recommendations would apply (McGlynn et al., 2003). The uninsured are more likely to suffer preventable illnesses, more likely to suffer complications of those illnesses, and more likely to die prematurely (Ayanian, Weissman, Schneider, Ginsburg, & Zaslavsky, 2000; McWilliams et al., 2007). Delayed treatment frequently results in more expenses as conditions worsen and services such as intensive care become necessary. Uninsured individuals are more likely to use emergency rooms for care, a practice that increases costs by large measure. As the American College of Physicians—American Society of Internal Medicine (2001) pointed out, "People without health insurance tend to live sicker and die younger than people with health insurance."

There is a reciprocal relationship between health care costs and drops in health insurance. Just as people without insurance use the system in ways that cost more in the long run, rising health care costs correlate to drops in health insurance coverage (Kaiser Family Foundation, 2004).

While most hospitals, especially government-owned institutions, write off a portion of their

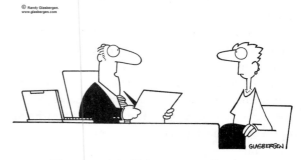

"We can contain health insurance costs if you're willing to let your coworkers diagnose you with information they find on the Internet."

Source: © Randy Glasbergen, used with permission from www.glasbergen.com.

costs for treating the uninsured, shifting the costs of treating the uninsured to those who are insured is common. This results in increased costs for taxpayers and higher premiums for those with private insurance.

In March 2010, President Barack Obama signed into law the Health Care and Education Reconciliation Act of 2010. This act was the result of the conference report of the two branches of Congress relating to the Patient Protection and Affordable Care Act that made some changes to the PPACA. We refer to the legislation as the HCERA/PPACA. The health care reform law seeks to reduce the number of uninsured Americans. Some of the key provisions that went into effect soon after passage include offering tax credits to small businesses to make employee coverage more affordable, prohibiting new health plans from denying coverage to children with **preexisting conditions** and providing access to affordable insurance for those who are uninsured because of preexisting conditions, banning insurance companies from dropping people from coverage when they get sick, and extending coverage for young people up to their twenty-sixth birthday through their parents' insurance.

Another issue facing the American health care system is the aging of the population. The "Baby Boomer" generation, the largest cohort of the population, is reaching retirement age. With age comes higher prevalence of chronic diseases and greater need for medical care. This means more health care providers will be necessary. Yet the United States does not have national policies to guide the training, supply, and distribution of health care providers to meet future needs for particular specialties of medicine, such as primary care (American College of Physicians, 2008).

Technological innovation is a major strength of American medicine. It has provided some of the most clinically effective diagnostic and treatment options in the history of medical practice. Yet that same strength has a downside. Technology is expensive and contributes to driving up the cost of medical care. The more technology is disseminated into practice, the higher the per capita utilization and the more the spending. The United States

has no effective public policies to control the spread of technology, which often occurs before adequate evaluation of its effectiveness (American College of Physicians, 2008). Technological progress accounts for a large share of the rise in the U.S. health care expenditures illustrated in Table 2.1 (Cutler & McClellan, 2001).

Before new technology hits the practice setting, it should be evaluated at least for clinical effectiveness and possibly for cost effectiveness. The United States has no centralized authority for conducting or coordinating these evaluations. Various public and private organizations, including the Agency for Healthcare Research and Quality, the Medicare Coverage Advisory Committee, the Veterans Administration, and the Blue Cross/Blue Shield Association, conduct technological assessments. Evaluations of clinical effectiveness and determinations of best practices are also offered by professional organizations, including the American College of Physicians and nongovernmental organizations such as the American Heart Association. A coordinated assessment system would reduce duplication of efforts, thus cutting costs.

Access to health technology and its use is mostly controlled by health insurers and **health maintenance organizations** (HMOs). These organizations are usually for-profit businesses. They are free to base their coverage decisions on any available evaluations, to make their own assessments or purchase them from private companies, or to ignore research findings. These decisions to purchase or use technology may be based to a large extent on profit rather than on best medical practices.

The source of all of this money is another issue of interest. Figure 2.3 depicts the sources of health care funding. About 46 percent of the costs of health care are currently paid in some form by the taxpayer, either through state, federal, or Social Security taxes. Noteworthy is the fact that even with a major percentage of costs borne by government programs, mostly Medicare and Medicaid, federal government underpayment to the 5,010 community hospitals totaled $32.4 billion (American Hospital Association, 2009a).

The HCERA/PPACA was passed with the promise to bring down health care costs. One

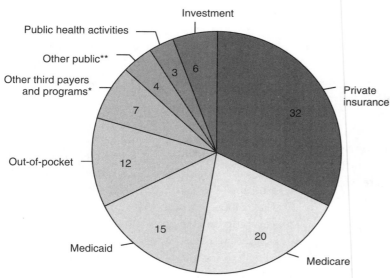

FIGURE 2.3 PERCENTAGE OF SOURCES OF THE U.S. HEALTH CARE DOLLAR, 2009

Note: Out-of-Pocket includes copays, deductibles, and treatments not covered by private health insurance.

Source: Centers for Medicare & Medicaid Services, Office of the Actuary, National Health Services Group. Retrieved from http://www.cms.gov/ NationalHealthExpendData/ downloads/PieChartSources Expenditures2009.pdf.

*Includes worksite health care, other private revenues, Indian Health Service, workers' compensation, general assistance, maternal and child health, vocational rehabilitation,Substance Abuse and Mental Health Services Administration, school health, and other federal and state local programs.

**Includes Veterans Administration, Department of Defense, and CHIP

of the measures included is a requirement that health plans annually report on the share of premium dollars spent on medical care. If those in the individual and small group market spend less than 80 percent of premiums on medical services, and plans in the large group market fail to spend at least 85 percent of premiums on medical services, they will be required to provide rebates to policy holders. There are also provisions that will crack down on fraud, waste, and abuse in the Medicare, Medicaid, State Children's Health Insurance Program, and private insurance.

Key Indicators for Measuring Performance of the Health System

International comparisons on most key indicators of the public's health have shown that the United States has poorer health outcomes in the aggregate than many other industrialized countries (American College of Physicians, 2008).

The Commonwealth Fund Commission on a High Performance Health System (2008; Schoen, Davis et al., 2006) identified 37 indicators of

"high performance" for measuring health care systems. The Commission then arranged the indicators into five main groups and rated the U.S. system according to the five groups with a composite score. When compared with international benchmarks on a scale of 1 to 100, the U.S. 2008 ratings were:

Healthy lives	72
Quality	71
Access	58
Efficiency	53
Equity	71
Total	65

The Commission concluded that the quality of care in the United States is highly variable, and opportunities are routinely missed to prevent disease, disability, hospitalization, and mortality. Let us examine the Commission's findings further.

Healthy Lives

The Commission developed several performance indicators to reflect the system's ability to achieve the goal of helping "everyone, to the extent possible, lead long, healthy, and productive lives," including preventable mortality, life expectancy, and certain health-related limitations faced by adults and children. The United States scored 72 out of 100 in this area overall in 2008, up slightly over 2006. Among 19 industrialized countries, the United States ranked fifteenth in 2006 on "mortality from conditions amenable to health care," or deaths before age 75 that are potentially preventable with timely, effective care (Schoen, Davis et al., 2006). The U.S. rate was more than 30 percent worse than the Commission's benchmark—the top three countries. The United States also ranked at the bottom for healthy life expectancy and last on infant mortality in 2006. The U.S. fell to last place in 2008 among 19 industrialized nations on deaths that might have been prevented with timely and effective care (The Commonwealth Fund, 2008).

Quality of Care

A high-performance health care system provides care that is necessary, appropriate, and of high quality. The standard of care would be practicing medicine consistent with evidence of clinical effectiveness. Errors would be kept to a minimum. Indicators of high quality include provision of patient-centered care, low nursing home admissions and readmission rates, low rates of medical errors, and low preventable death rates. The United States scored well in 2006 on providing the "right care" for a given condition and for provision of preventive care like Pap smears and mammograms, but low on long-term care management, safe care, and patient-centered care.

The Commission's conclusions were backed up by two published studies. According to data on medical records from 12 metropolitan areas of the United States, children received about 46.5 percent of the care they needed, including 67.6 percent of the indicated care for acute medical problems, 53.4 percent of the indicated care for chronic medical conditions, and 40.7 percent of the preventive care (Mangione-Smith et al., 2007). Examination of adults' medical records in 12 metropolitan areas revealed that the recommended care was offered and delivered only 54.9 percent of the time, with little difference in the proportion of recommended acute care, care for chronic conditions, screening, and follow-up (McGlynn et al., 2003).

Access

In a high-performance health care system, services would be available and accessible to all members of the population. The Commonwealth Fund Commission identified indicators of access to care that included affordability, health insurance coverage, ability to see a physician and obtain the needed medical attention, families spending less than 10 percent of income on out-of-pocket medical costs and premiums, minimal number of patients with problems with medical bills and debts, and health system participation. Between 2006 and 2008 the access score of the United States dropped from 67 to 58. The poor score was attributed to the rising rates of uninsured and underinsured Americans and the rise in health care costs in relation to the growth in income. As of 2007, 75 million adults ages 19 to 64—42 percent—were either uninsured or underinsured during the year (The Commonwealth Fund, 2008). By 2009, 50.7 million Americans were not insured at all, including 7.5 million children under 18 (DeNavas-Walt, Proctor, & Smith, 2010). The health reform legislation of 2010 may eventually influence the causes of uninsurance and underinsurance.

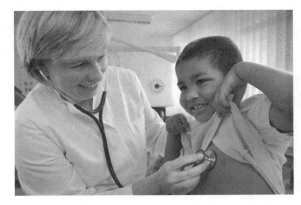

Primary care, such as well child care given children, is critical to quality, equity, and efficiency of a health care system.

Efficiency

The Commonwealth Fund Commission's indicators of efficiency included low rates of overuse, inappropriate use, or waste; minimal expenditures for administrative and regulatory cost; and use of information tools, such as electronic medical records, to support care. These indicators illustrate that quality, access, and costs are interconnected—i.e., poor quality contributes to higher costs, and poor access undermines quality, while simultaneously contributing to less efficient care. The Commission (2008) reported that U.S. patients were three to four times more likely than patients in other developed countries to have duplicate tests or that medical records or test results were not available at the time of their appointment. The United States lags far behind the leading nations in the use of electronic medical records. Less than 15 percent of U.S. hospitals have electronic capabilities to store and use physician notes, less than 17 percent use electronic systems for computerized physician order entry for medications, and about 60 percent have electronic alert systems for drug allergies and drug-drug interactions (American Hospital Association, 2009b). U.S. health insurance administrative costs are much higher than in other countries with mixed private/public insurance systems, when viewed as a share of total health spending. The Commonwealth Fund Commission (2006b) noted that the United States has poor performance in terms of measures of national health expenditures, administrative costs, the use of information technology, and the use of multidisciplinary teams.

Equity

The Commission used several measures of equity, including differences based on income, insurance status, and geography (urban or rural), as well as differences among demographic characteristics such as age, gender, race, and ethnicity. Minimal differences among groups in terms of access to and quality of health services would be expected in a well-operating health system. Among the nations studied, the United States ranked last in equity in 2006. A major inequity was demonstrated in

access and quality based on income. Differences were especially obvious between low-income or uninsured populations and high-income and insured populations. In the United States, access to health care is directly related to income and race (Battista & McCabe, 1999). Minorities, low-income, or uninsured adults and children are more likely to wait when sick, to encounter delays and poorly coordinated care, and to have untreated dental caries, uncontrolled chronic disease, avoidable hospitalizations, and worse outcomes than white, higher-income, or insured counterparts (The Commonwealth Fund, 2008).

The Commission found that compared with citizens in five other industrialized nations, Americans face higher out-of-pocket costs, are less apt to have a long-term physician, are less able to see a doctor on the same day when sick, and are less apt to get their questions answered or receive clear instructions from a doctor.

The Commonwealth Fund Commission found that the capacity to innovate and improve the system is a critical element in attaining high performance. Such a system would include a skilled and motivated workforce, emphasizing primary care. It would support a culture of quality improvement and continuous learning that rewards recognition of opportunities to reduce errors and improve outcomes. Investment in public health initiatives, research, information necessary to inform and drive health care decisions, and having an infrastructure that supports and encourages innovation and prepares sufficient numbers of well-trained health care professionals would surely pay off in quality over time. The Commission concluded that their evaluation results make a compelling case for change. Simply put, we fall far short of what is achievable on all major dimensions of health system performance. The overwhelming picture that emerges is one of missed opportunities—at every level of the system—to make U.S. health care truly the best that money can buy (The Commonwealth Fund, 2006b).

Billions of dollars in waste could be saved if our health care system were improved. The Commonwealth Fund Commission (2008) estimated that $100 billion a year could be saved by lowering insurance administrative costs. Hundreds of thousands of deaths could be prevented by improving system quality, accessibility, and efficiency.

Improving America's Health Care System

The HCERA/PPACA, while open to amendments, repeal, or legal challenges before full enactment, is directed at alleviating many of the problems in the U.S. health care system. This section will address some solutions to the problems in the system, including some of those embedded in the legislation.

Primary care is key to a quality health care system. Systems that have a high level of primary health care are associated with better overall mortality rates, including premature death from asthma and bronchitis, emphysema and pneumonia, and cardiovascular diseases (Macinko, Starfield, & Shi, 2003). The U.S. system has seen a reduction in the number of **primary care physicians** and fewer medical students committed to that career track. Currently, about one-third of physicians work in primary care (Docteur, Suppanz, & Woo, 2003).

Promoting patient-centered primary care is offered as a way of making the system more effective (Davis, Schoen, Guterman, & Shih, 2007). However, before this can be attained, there must be incentives for physicians to go into primary care, a field that has less earning potential than specialties such as cardiology, surgery, and neurology.

The United States has very limited control over the supply of physicians and the specialties they choose. The government has limited funding to support primary care training programs and scholarship programs with service obligations, such as the National Health Service Corps and the Indian Health Service. However, the federal government can influence physician supply somewhat through Medicare reimbursement of graduate medical education residency training positions. In Canada and the United Kingdom, the government has

much more leverage to manipulate the health care workforce supply, including controlling both training capacity and employment opportunities. This type of control over the supply of different types of physicians is a characteristic of health care systems that perform well. The HCERA/PPACA contains provisions to encourage aspiring medical students to practice primary care medicine. The laws support development of training programs that focus on primary care such as medical homes, team management of chronic disease, and models that integrate physical and mental health services.

Increasing the ratio of primary to specialty care physicians would make it easier and more efficient to implement preventive health care. It is obvious that preventing illness is preferable to treating that illness from both humanitarian and financial perspectives. Primary care physicians, because of their regular contact with patients, can be more effective at preventive medicine.

Controlling the type of physician being prepared is intertwined with controlling the supply of physicians. In recent years, many physicians have exited the profession for a variety of reasons that include high medical malpractice insurance premiums and reduced professional satisfaction because of increased influence of insurance companies on the practice of medicine. While the HCERA/PPACA may affect a portion of the problem, more incentives must be provided to make the arduous training period required to be a physician worthwhile in terms of both income and job satisfaction.

Related to control of supply of physicians is the need for a societal investment in the education of health professionals, including nurses, physician assistants, and physical therapists. This could ensure a robust workforce of health care providers that are well trained and present in sufficient numbers. The HCERA/PPACA increases the capacity for nursing education, supporting training programs, providing loan repayment and retention grants, and creating a career ladder to nursing. There are grants to employ and provide training to family nurse practitioners who provide primary care in federally qualified health centers and nurse-managed health clinics.

As we have seen, there are tremendous disparities in the health care received by different groups of people. The HCERA/PPACA attempts to maximize funding for health care professionals who commit to practice in underserved areas. The laws provide state grants to providers in medically underserved areas. There is increased flexibility in the use of funding to support training in outpatient settings and to ensure the availability of residency programs in underserved, including rural, areas. There is funding to recruit and train providers in rural areas.

Currently, much control over care is exerted by the insurance or **managed care** organizations (MCOs; see Chapter 4). Before performing a test or procedure, physicians often must verify that an insurer will cover the cost. This is essentially asking for permission to practice in a manner consistent with the physician's training and professional judgment. This situation is exacerbated by the fact that often the company representative who makes the determination is not a physician. Replacing physicians' judgment with that of a company who is committed to making profits is a recipe for failure. An important key to reforming the American health care system is removing health care decisions from those who have a financial interest in delivering fewer services.

Many consumers view managed care as "managed costs," under the assumption that managed care companies are more interested in controlling costs than ensuring the appropriate and high-quality care we expect. Yet, it does not appear that managed care companies manage costs very well. According to 1996 Medical Expenditure Panel Survey data, there were no statistically significant differences in the concentration of health care expenses between those enrolled in health maintenance organizations and other types of gatekeeper plans than those enrolled in **indemnity insurance** or **preferred provider organizations** (Berk & Monheit, 2001).

IMMEDIATE COST-SAVING MEASURES IN THE HEALTH CARE AND EDUCATION RECONCILIATION ACT OF 2010

Many of the provisions of the act will be delayed for several years. However, some went into effect within months of the signing of the bill. By encouraging preventive care, primary prevention, fairness, and other cost-effectiveness measures, these immediate effects can, in the long term, reduce costs.

- Free preventive care under Medicare by eliminating copayments for preventive services and exempting preventive services from deductibles under Medicare
- Incentives to Medicare and Medicaid beneficiaries to complete behavior modification programs
- Requirement of new plans to provide preventive services with no copayments and required exemption of preventive services from deductibles, including immunizations; preventive care for infants, children, and adolescents; and additional preventive care and screenings for women
- A Prevention and Public Health Fund to expand and sustain funding for prevention and public health programs
- Requirement of Medicaid coverage for tobacco cessation services for pregnant women
- Access to effective internal and external appeals processes regarding decisions by the health insurance plan for subscribers to new plans
- Requirement of plans in individual and small group markets to spend 80 percent of premium dollars on medical services, and of plans in large group markets to spend 85 percent

(continues)

- Increased funding for community health centers so that more patients can receive services at these low-cost facilities
- Grants to small employers that establish wellness programs
- New investment to increase the number of primary care practitioners
- New programs to support school-based health centers and nurse-managed health clinics
- Assistance to states in establishing offices of health insurance consumer assistance to help people with filing complaints and appeals

Sources: The White House. (2010). *Key provisions of health reform that take effect immediately.* Retrieved from http://www.whitehouse.gov/healthreform/immediate-benefits

Emergency Nurses Association. (2010). *Patient Protection and Affordable Care Act & Health Care and Education Reconciliation Act.* Retrieved from http://www.ena.org/government/healthcarereform/Documents/AnalysisFinalHRCBills.pdf

Health education is closely linked with preventive medicine. More physicians, clinics, and hospitals should employ and utilize the services of professionally trained health educators. It is not enough to assume that a health care practitioner has the skills to provide adequate health education. The HCERA/PPACA established a grant program to support the delivery of evidence-based and community-based prevention and wellness services. Health education should be an integral part of any such effort.

The Institute of Medicine's Committee on the Consequences of Uninsurance (2004), after extensive study of the health care system, concluded that lack of health insurance coverage is a major stumbling block to having the best possible system. The Committee offered the following principles for guiding the debate and evaluating various strategies:

1. Health care coverage should be universal.
2. Health care coverage should be continuous.
3. Health care coverage should be affordable to individuals and families.
4. The health insurance strategy should be affordable and sustainable for society.
5. Health insurance should enhance health and well-being by promoting access to high-quality care that is effective, efficient, safe, timely, patient-centered, and equitable.

Equity and continuous access are important components of a well-performing health care system. Health insurance coverage is a critical element in those components. Without health insurance, many people postpone treatment until a minor illness becomes worse, harming their health and producing greater costs. The health reform legislation was promoted on the promise of reducing the number of uninsured in the United States by two-thirds.

A **single-payer health care** system has the potential to reduce administrative costs. However, the HCERA/PPACA did not initiate such a system. Nevertheless, reducing the costs of insurance administration should be a priority. This would increase competition and lower costs. The HCERA/PPACA contains provisions for achieving these ends.

Improving access to information on the quality and costs of health care, and promoting better information on the cost effectiveness of health care technology and procedures, would increase the effectiveness of the market. Information allowing the application of market principles would bring down costs.

Highest level systems are based on models that emphasize and deliver care that stresses coordination and integration. In these systems, there are decision-support systems for clinicians, seamless care transitions, and integration at every level of care (The Commonwealth Fund, 2006a). These characteristics are gradually making their way into American medicine. The specialist known as a **hospitalist** completes medical school, usually specializing in internal medicine, family practice, or pediatrics. Hospitalists coordinate or assume much of the care of a hospitalized patient. There are many advantages of hospitalists in the care of hospitalized patients. One advantage is that hospitalists have more expertise in caring for complicated hospitalized patients on a daily basis. They are also more available most of the day in the hospital to meet with family members and are able to follow up on tests, answer nurses' questions, and deal with problems that may arise. In many instances, hospitalists may see a patient more than once a day to ensure that care is going according to plan and to explain test findings to patients and family members (Nabili, 2010). The use of hospitalists seems to improve patient safety, reduce financial strains on primary care physicians, and improve efficiency and cost effectiveness of hospitals.

The United States lags behind better performing health care systems in the implementation of electronic health records (EHR), or electronic medical records, and systems. EHR systems are an important element in an integrated health care system. They can be used to order tests, prescribe medications, and access patients' test results. They can provide electronic alerts to physicians and other care providers about potential problems concerning drug interactions and dosages. They can issue reminders to patients about preventive or follow-up care and can even be used to provide patients with test results. EHR systems can generate lists of patients who are due for tests or preventive care or sort patients by diagnosis or by health risk. Denmark has developed a comprehensive EHR system that connects nearly all physician practices and hospitals electronically, allowing physicians to electronically prescribe and share patient information. In 2006, between 79 percent and 98 percent of physicians in Australia, New Zealand, the United Kingdom, and the Netherlands, all nations with high-performing systems, had sophisticated EHR systems. Less than half of physicians in the United States had EHR systems (Schoen, Davis et al., 2006). Hand-scrawled prescriptions and misread test orders have resulted in countless negative patient episodes. EHR

systems have the potential for greatly reducing these errors. The HCERA/PPACA mandates the development of a plan to integrate reporting on quality of care with reporting of meaningful use of EHR.

Currently, the market power of insurers, providers, pharmaceutical companies, device manufacturers, and other suppliers allows them to set prices above competitive market levels. The ability of government to negotiate prices, especially for prescription medications, is an important key to controlling health care costs and for ensuring that patients get the medications they need. This is the case in Belgium, Canada, Japan, and with the U.S. Veterans Administration. However, when Congress passed legislation that authorized Medicare Part D, a program to provide prescription drug coverage, it specifically prohibited the government from negotiating prices with the pharmaceutical companies. With the huge volume that the Medicare program generates, the savings could be substantial. The Veterans Administration has negotiated drug prices for years, saving billions of taxpayer dollars.

Tort reform has been a conversation piece in the U.S. Congress for decades. Currently, the health care system and its malpractice insurers are operating in an environment that encourages avoidance of lawsuits, often leaving physicians to deliver elements of care out of fear of being sued as much as in the best interests of the patient. Americans have become very litigious. Health care providers are often the target of these lawsuits. In the real world, babies are born with problems and people die. We often react to these events by seeking legal counsel. While there is no doubt that health care providers sometimes make errors, often resulting in catastrophic outcomes, it is also true that the system that allows for a high number of questionable lawsuits and enormous financial awards is driving up costs of health care. Physicians may order tests just to make sure that "all the bases are covered" or perform a Caesarian section at the first sign of fetal stress in case they would ever have to mount a defense against a malpractice charge. Often, even if the insurer thinks the physician acted responsibly, the insurer will reach a negotiated settlement with the plaintiff rather than incur the legal expenses of defending the physician. This may lead to increases in the physician's premiums for medical malpractice insurance that may be passed on to patients or to patients' insurance companies. The HCERA/PPACA awards five-year demonstration grants to states to develop, implement, and evaluate alternatives to current tort litigations. There is no easy answer to this problem, but it is time that we have a national discussion about it and its implications. The demonstrations funded by HCERA/PPACA are a tentative first step toward that discussion.

Quality Assurance

Hospitals and health plans are accredited by private accreditation organizations. For example, The Joint Commission (TJC) develops standards of performance for a wide range of health care facilities and awards accreditation based on compliance with those standards. Accreditation is a coveted achievement for hospitals and other facilities.

Hospitals that are accredited by TJC must have professional review committees composed of active physicians who evaluate selected cases to ensure the quality of care at the hospital. A utilization committee determines the appropriateness of hospital admissions and lengths of hospital stays. Audit committees look for defective or unnecessary care. Tissue committees review the work done in surgery.

Hospitals may discipline physicians by reducing, suspending, or revoking hospital treatment privileges. These actions could substantially affect a doctor's ability to practice and earn, especially in communities with few hospitals.

Local, county, and state medical societies do not have the power to take away a physician's right to practice medicine. However, they may reprimand or expel members who violate accepted medical practice or in other ways defame the profession. This action is an embarrassment because it is brought about by peers in the full view of

colleagues. In the case of specialists, it may reduce their referrals.

Physicians are certified by specialty boards that are independent of the medical societies. To maintain board certification, the physician participates in an extensive process that involves completing accredited education and specialty training and periodic oral and written exams to demonstrate competency (American Board of Medical Specialties, 2008).

In order to practice medicine, a physician must be licensed in the state in which he or she wishes to practice. State licensing boards have the authority to revoke or suspend a license. Revocation by one state does not necessarily disqualify a physician from practicing in other states. In recent years, licensing laws have been tightened somewhat.

The National Practitioner Data Bank (NPDB) and the Healthcare Integrity and Protection Data Bank (HIPDB) are government data banks. NPDB was created by Congress. According to the NPDB-HIPDB Web site (2008): "The intent [of NPDB] is to improve the quality of health care by encouraging State licensing boards, hospitals and other health care entities, and professional societies to identify and discipline those who engage in unprofessional behavior; and to restrict the ability of incompetent physicians, dentists, and other health care practitioners to move from State to State without disclosure or discovery of previous medical malpractice payment and adverse action history. Adverse actions can involve licensure, clinical privileges, professional society membership, and exclusions from Medicare and Medicaid."

The NPDB is primarily an alert or flagging system intended to facilitate a comprehensive review of health care practitioners' professional credentials. The information contained in the NPDB is intended to direct discrete inquiry into, and scrutiny of, specific areas of a practitioner's licensure, professional society memberships, medical malpractice payment history, and record of clinical privileges. Licensing boards, professional societies, hospital administrators, and malpractice insurance carriers are required to report certain actions against physicians to the NPDB. New regulations went into effect on March 1, 2010, requiring the NPDB Public Use Data File to include selected variables from reports on adverse licensing actions against all health care practitioners and health care entities and certain actions taken by peer review organizations and private accreditation organizations in addition to selected variables from medical malpractice payment, clinical privileges, professional society membership, U.S. Drug Enforcement Administration (DEA) reports, and Medicare and Medicaid exclusion actions taken by the U.S. Department of Health and Human Services Office of Inspector General (NPDB-HIPDB, 2010).

The HIPDB was created by the secretary of the U.S. Department of Health and Human Services, acting through the Office of Inspector General (OIG), as directed by the Health Insurance Portability and Accountability Act of 1996 to combat fraud and abuse in health insurance and health care delivery. The HIPDB collects information about criminal convictions, license and certification actions, civil judgment related to health care but not malpractice, and exclusion from federal and state health care programs. State and federal agencies and health plans may access and review the information held by the HIPDB. The HIPDB is primarily a flagging system that may serve to alert users that a comprehensive review of a practitioner's, provider's, or supplier's past actions may be prudent. The HIPDB is intended to augment, not replace, traditional forms of review and investigation, serving as an important supplement to a careful review of a practitioner's, provider's, or supplier's past actions (NPDB-HIPDB, 2009).

States regulate insurance companies, but the federal government regulates self-insured employer benefit plans. According to Kofman and Pollitz (2006), "Because of the importance of health insurance to the general public welfare, states have been regulating private health insurance companies and products since the late 19th century. State insurance regulation has sought to promote several policy objectives, such as assuring

the financial solvency of insurance companies, promoting risk spreading, protecting consumers against fraud, and ensuring that consumers are paid the benefits that they are promised." The federal government has historically respected the state's role in regulating insurance. In 1944, the U.S. Congress explicitly recognized this role in the McCarran-Ferguson Act, which said "the business of insurance ... shall be subject to the laws of the several States...." Since the early 1970s, however, the federal government has taken a more active role in areas of insurance regulation that traditionally had been reserved by the states. In 1974, the federal government became the primary regulator of health benefits provided by employers. In the 1980s and 1990s, Congress established minimum national standards for group health insurance.

Every state has adopted certain basic standards for health insurance that apply to all types of health insurance products, including requiring insurers to be financially solvent and capable of paying claims. Standards require prompt payment of claims and other fair claims handling practices. Other aspects of health insurance regulation, however, vary by state and by the type of coverage purchased. These include external review and appeals, covered benefits, access to health insurance, and rating patients based on projections of future health care needs. As a result of a 1974 federal law called the Employee Retirement Income Security Act (ERISA), health benefits offered by private employers are not regulated by states. While ERISA allows states to regulate health insurance policies that employers may purchase, employers that self-insure are not subject to state regulation. The types of state consumer protections discussed above do not apply to self-insured job-based health coverage (Kofman & Pollitz, 2006).

The federal government has more recently gotten involved in the regulation of health insurance. Congress has adopted standards for employer-sponsored group health plans. Most of these have been incorporated into ERISA and the federal tax code. The most significant were added by the

Consolidated Omnibus Budget Reconciliation Act (COBRA) in 1986 and by the Health Insurance Portability and Accountability Act of 1996 (HIPAA). COBRA applies to employers with 20 or more employees and gives workers and their dependents a right to continue job-based health coverage under certain circumstances. HIPAA was written to improve access to health insurance and to prohibit discrimination against people with medical needs. Generally, HIPAA sets a minimum federal floor of consumer protections to apply to all private health insurance, with exceptions for state and local government employers. Enforcement is by both state and federal governments.

Medicare, private insurers, and employers are starting to use pay-for-performance programs to pay hospitals and physicians based on the quality of services provided. Some states, along with private and public insurers, have made performance ratings of hospitals available to the public, and a few health plans are beginning to rate physician groups and individual physicians (Citizens' Health Care Working Group, 2005). The agencies that administer Medicare and Medicaid may terminate a practitioner's participation in those programs. Typical grounds for exclusion are fraud and overutilization. The HCERA/PPACA established a hospital value-based purchasing program in Medicare to pay hospitals based on performance on quality measures.

Managed care organizations, being nongovernmental, have more leverage. They can terminate the participation of a provider or refuse to renew a contract if the provider does not meet the MCO's standards.

Universal Health Care

Reforming the American health care system has been discussed for decades. Rhetoric intensified as the costs of health care continued to grow and more and more Americans were without health insurance. During the 2008 presidential campaign, health reform took center stage. Universal coverage and a "public option" were proposed. Neither was included in the HCERA/PPACA.

Proponents argue that health care is a basic human right and that a country as wealthy as the United States should make sure that all of its citizens have access to health care. They point out that the United States is the only industrialized nation that does not have universal health care and offer examples of individuals whose lives have been shattered because of inability to obtain or keep health insurance. They frequently point out the accessibility and convenience of the universal health care systems in Canada and Great Britain. They claim that freedom to choose health care providers would be enhanced because people are now often forced to see only providers on their insurer's panel.

Supporters also point out that nations that have a national universal health care system spend less of their wealth on health care even as their citizens have higher levels of health as measured by several indicators. Recall that the United States spent over 17 percent of GDP on health care in 2009, a far higher percentage than other countries.

Those who oppose a universal health care system do so on ideological grounds, claiming that such a system is "socialized medicine." They also note that the only way to support it is through taxation and that everyone's tax burden would increase. Many in the opposition believe that costs would increase, especially during the implementation phase. Opponents also claim that people who live in nations with universal health care often have to wait for long periods of time for surgeries and other procedures. Another point of disagreement is the notion that individuals may lose the freedom to choose their own physicians.

There are two models that have been discussed for over 30 years in the United States. The two models are the "national health service" and the "single-payer model." The Patient Protection and Affordable Care Act of 2010 included neither of these models, but it contained a compromise known as "health insurance exchanges." Nevertheless, we will explore the two models because other industrialized countries have them and much of the HCERA/PPACA will not be implemented for years, leaving time for changes.

National Health Service

This is the approach taken by Great Britain. Under this model, the government is both the health care deliverer and the insurer. If a national health service were implemented in the United States, the government might own or lease facilities—e.g., hospitals, laboratories, and clinics. It could own office buildings or lease them to physician groups. Health care providers would be either employees of the government or independent contractors. The system would be funded by taxes. While other countries with this type of system do not usually do so, the government could also impose **deductibles** and **copayments**. Having a national health service does not necessarily mean the total elimination of health insurance companies. Some individuals in Great Britain opt for private insurance.

Some physicians have experience with this type of employment. In the 1970s, after passage of the Health Maintenance Organization Act, some HMOs contracted with physicians to work as employees of the company in the so-called closed panel model.

In this model, doctors receive a fixed salary and have fixed working hours, much like other employees. Physicians do not have to maintain their own offices with the attendant costs of leasing, utilities, and staff. However, the earning potential of physicians could be lessened in this approach. It is not clear how physicians' legal liability would be impacted by the change in employment status. The government would probably assume most of the responsibility for medical malpractice insurance premiums.

It is less likely that physicians would practice defensive medicine in a national health service. Questionable and unnecessary tests would probably be done less frequently. This would reduce costs. In addition, there would be much less administrative cost associated with this model.

Critics claim that choice of physicians and treatment locations would be reduced. They also worry that, given that there is no or little cost that the patient would experience directly at the time of the service, people would abuse and overuse the system.

Single-Payer Model

This is the model that is practiced in Canada. In this model, the role of insurance companies is eliminated. Physicians and other health care providers operate in a **fee-for-service** paradigm. If this model were adopted in the United States, facilities would remain as they are under the current system—i.e., some private, some state or locally owned. There would be a single conduit for paying for services, funded by taxes. This conduit could be a part of the federal government, similar to Medicare.

This model would virtually eliminate the lobbying power of the insurance industry. Instead of private insurance companies determining prices and fees, either the government or a diverse board representing consumers, providers, business, and government would assume that role.

Both the U.S. General Accounting Office and the Congressional Budget Office have issued reports stating that a single-payer system would pay for itself due to reduced administrative costs, as well as having universal access to health care, especially preventive care (Physicians for a National Health Program, 1999). Proponents also assert that it would reduce fraud and waste by concentrating the financial aspects in a single payer with authority to monitor costs, records, and performance. Finally, they contend that the model is not socialized medicine, because it is a payment system, not a health care delivery system.

Opponents to the single-payer system point out that the federal government has been unable to control fraud and waste in other programs, including Medicare and Medicaid. Therefore, it makes little sense to assume that the government will be any more effective with a much larger program and responsibility.

Insurance Exchanges

A third model for making health care more universal is contained in the HCERA/PPACA. Under provisions of the acts, the states will be eligible for federal financial support for developing statewide or multiple substate **exchanges** or forming multistate, regional exchanges. These exchanges would be a menu of insurance plans. A state may also contract with a private, nonprofit entity to operate its exchange. If a state fails to act or to meet minimum standards, the federal government may operate within the state. The HCERA/PPACA allows and encourages individuals who are not covered by employer-based health insurance to enroll in a health insurance plan through the exchange. At annual enrollment, each participating employee would choose among the various health plans offered in the exchange. The employee would pay more or less depending on the premium of the chosen plan.

Once the exchanges begin to operate, they will want to offer leading health plans to attract and serve subscribers. The health plans will want to meet the exchanges' requirements and specifications, in order to gain access to customers. This, if it goes as planned, will offer a marketplace of insurance coverage and choices for individuals and families. Choice intensifies competition among health plans by making comparison shopping easy and by lowering barriers for new competitors. Exchange choice also would serve to increase competition and lower cost.

Selecting a Health Care Facility

Most of us will have to use a hospital, nursing home, or other health care facility in our lifetimes. Perhaps we will have to make these decisions for ourselves, our family members, or others for whom we have assumed responsibility. As we have seen, medical errors plague the system; not all hospitals are equal in this regard. Since these facilities are integral parts of the health care system, we shall discuss some of the elements that can assist us in choosing a facility. Keep in mind that the steps in decision making discussed in Chapter 1 apply here.

Selecting a Hospital

If your doctor recommends hospital treatment, there are a number of questions that good physi-

cians welcome and that patients should ask. For example:

- How did the physician arrive at the diagnosis? Would it be appropriate to order additional tests to confirm the diagnosis?
- What are the treatment options and what are the risks and benefits of each?
- Are there outpatient options? What are the risks and benefits of them as compared with inpatient treatment?
- Why is this hospital the physician's choice?
- Does the treatment require highly technical or sophisticated treatment? Can this hospital deliver this treatment? Could another?
- What are the side effects and complications that could occur with the treatment? Do they require specialized treatment? Will the staff and facilities at this hospital be able to deliver this care?
- What is the hospital's experience with the type of health problem and required treatment? Does it require specialized skills on the part of the staff? Are there hospitals that have more experience and higher success rates with this diagnosis and treatment?

Patients have a role to play in selecting hospitals. However, much of the responsibility for choosing a hospital rests with the physician. This is a good reason to select a physician in whom you have confidence. Most physicians have admitting privileges at only one or a few hospitals; this limits choice. If your primary care physician refers you to a specialist, you have the opportunity to inquire about which hospitals the specialist uses. This is a good point for patient input in the selection of the specialist and the hospital. The PCP will usually favor specialists who practice in one of his or her hospitals and with whom the PCP is familiar. This works in the patient's favor if he or she wants the PCP to remain involved in the care.

It is important to choose a physician who practices at a highly rated hospital for two reasons. First, this will enhance your chances of being admitted to such a hospital if the need arises. Second, it enhances your chances that your doctor will be a top-quality professional. Superior hospitals attract superior physicians. Similarly, it is important to choose a health insurance plan that allows use of highly rated hospitals. Patients should check with both the physician and the insurer to make sure that the insurer will cover costs charged by the hospital. This is crucial if you are in a network with a limited choice of facilities.

Patients can obtain much information well before the actual need for hospitalization, such as the accreditation status of nearby hospitals. Patients can also find impartial rating information about hospitals. *U.S. News & World Report* publishes an annual report on the quality of care at hospitals that offer highly specialized and complex services as well as more routine ones. *Consumers' Checkbook* is a nonprofit consumer information and services resource. It provides ratings for nearly every short-term hospital for acute inpatient care in the United States except veterans and military hospitals. HealthGrades offers ratings of physicians, hospitals, and nursing homes. Ratings are presented by locality and health problem.

Selecting a Senior Living Facility

Most of us will have to deal with the stressful issues relating to entering or assisting a family member to enter a retirement community or nursing home. Eldercare Locater (http://www.eldercare.gov) provides information and referral services for those seeking local and state support resources for the elderly; it is a good place to start. The decision-making process described in Chapter 1 is applicable to this situation. For every family, there are specific factors that affect the choice. These factors include location, costs, payment method, medical needs, availability of special care units, mobility of the resident, and need for social interaction. Location is one of the most important factors. Residents and their families often prefer a facility that is close to the family's home. Another consideration is the special services or features of the facility. For those with disabilities, specialized care units may be a requirement.

There are several choices for the elderly if they are leaving their primary residence. Retirement communities or homes form one option. These are generally reserved for people who can take care of their basic needs but want to live around people of similar age and with similar interests. Residents live in private dwellings, often apartments. Food service is usually available but the resident is free to prepare meals in his or her residence. Some level of health care is available and there is usually an arrangement with a hospital or clinic to provide medical care if necessary. Assisted living communities provide more health care, although residents may have as much independence as they choose. These facilities can provide help with the activities of daily living, such as bathing, dressing, and grooming. They also coordinate services by outside health care providers, administer medications if necessary, and monitor resident activities to help to ensure their health, safety, and well-being. For those requiring the highest level of care, there are nursing homes or skilled nursing facilities. These facilities have registered nurses who help provide around-the-clock care to people who can no longer care for themselves due to physical, emotional, or mental conditions. A physician supervises each patient's care, and a nurse or other medical professional is almost always on the premises. Skilled care may also include physical, occupational, or speech therapy. Nursing homes also provide custodial care, such as bathing, toileting, eating, and getting in and out of bed.

Whenever possible, the person who is moving to the facility should be involved in the choice. The first step in making the decision is determining the needs of the senior. This usually requires the advice of the PCP. Second, obtaining referrals can be very helpful. They may come from the family physician, social workers, hospital discharge planners, clergy, and family friends who have firsthand knowledge about choosing a facility.

Once the level of care is decided, the type of facility can be determined. At that point, based on referrals and information searches, the family can reduce the choices to a relative few. The best way to determine an appropriate match of a facility with patient needs is through visits. The first visit and tour should be arranged with the administrator so that you can ask specific questions about costs, insurance, staffing, management of volunteers, and medical care. All questions should be answered to your satisfaction. Make unannounced visits at various times of the day and different days of the week. Introduce yourself to family members you see arriving and departing and ask them the pros and cons of the facility. Ask residents what they like and dislike about the facility. The following are some issues to be explored on your visits:

- Licensure and accreditation: Does the facility hold a current license from the state? Does the administrator hold a state license? (If not, cross the facility off the list.) Ask to see the last three inspection reports. What credentials do caregivers possess? The Commission on Accreditation of Rehabilitation Facilities gives approval to aging services.

- Location: Are the senior and the family happy with the location? Is it close to a hospital? Is the area safe and free from crime? Are there shopping centers and entertainment opportunities nearby?

- Patient services: Does the facility have a written description of patient and family rights and responsibilities that is readily available? Does the patient's physician make regular visits to the facility? Does the facility have an arrangement with a nearby hospital for emergency transportation and admission? Are the physical therapy staff all academically prepared for the job? Is a social worker available to assist patients and family? Is there a 24-hour emergency response system? Ask to see it. Is a registered nurse available at all times? If not, what are the qualifications of the staff in his or her absence? Are barbers and beauticians available? May patients worship as they choose on a regular basis? Are arrangements made to assist residents who celebrate religious holidays?

- Facility appearance: Is the entire facility clean? Are there unpleasant odors? Do you feel welcome when you enter the facility? Are the grounds neat and well kept? Are there outside areas that the residents can use comfortably? Is there a room for private visits with family and friends? Are exterior doors locked during daytime and evening hours?

- Staff attitudes: Is the environment warm and pleasant? Do staff members demonstrate interest, respect, and affection for residents? Do staff members respond quickly to calls for assistance? Are visiting hours convenient? Do administrators take the time to answer questions and discuss problems?

- Dining and food service: Is the dining room attractive? Are the tables and chairs comfortable and safe? Can wheelchairs easily navigate the room? Does a dietician help in meal planning? Is the food varied, tasty, fresh, and attractively served? Is there enough time to eat? Is the quantity sufficient? If residents need help eating, is it cheerfully provided? If needed, is food delivered to residents' rooms? Are beverages and healthy snacks available all day?

- Living quarters: Does each bedroom have a window? If there are more than one resident in a room, is there a privacy curtain? Is there a nurse call button? Are personal items encouraged in the rooms? Is the bed easily accessible? Are bathrooms easily accessible to the bedroom? Do bathrooms have hand rails and call buttons? Is there a walk-in shower? Do tubs have no-slip surfaces and bathing chairs if needed?

- Activities: Are activities planned? Are all residents encouraged to participate? Are patients' preferences included in activity planning? Are outside trips planned? Are there intergenerational events with local schools, scout troops, and youth organizations? Do volunteers work with patients? Make sure the volunteers are trained.

- Costs: Are meals covered in the basic fee? Are most services covered in the basic rate? If not, what services are not covered? Does the facility accept Medicare, Medicaid, and/or other insurance? What is the policy on returning advance payments?

Nursing Home Compare, operated by the U.S. Department of Health and Human Services, will help you compare facilities in many states. The URL is http://www.medicare.gov/nhcompare/home.asp.

Once you have gained all the information you need, it is time to compare the facilities' pros and cons. It may be necessary to have another conversation with the family member's physician. It is very important that the resident be involved in the gathering of information and the selection of the facility.

Admissions contracts are complicated legal documents. It is advisable to have an attorney review them before signing.

SUMMARY

The health care system of the United States is a multilayered entity. Spending on health care in the United States is higher on a per capita basis than in any other nation, and the cost is rapidly rising. The quality of the system, according to authoritative estimates using a variety of measures, is much less than other industrialized nations and much worse than it should be, given the costs.

Racial and ethnic minorities and low-income populations suffer serious disparities in access to health care. Too many Americans are denied access to health care because of lack of health insurance.

Quality assurance is attempted on several levels. Accreditation is a way to improve institutional quality. Individual practitioners are subject to licensing requirements and discipline by professional societies and hospitals where they practice.

A number of steps could be implemented to improve the system, including models that would provide universal health care. Among these steps are increasing the number of primary care practitioners, providing incentives for people

to purchase health insurance and for insurers to make it more widely available, implementing widespread use of electronic health records, and increasing preventive services and health education.

After extensive study, a panel at the University of Maine (2001) concluded:

> There is a growing recognition that the major problems of rising costs and lack of access constitute a real crisis. However, the search for solutions has not been easy or clear cut. Policymakers often attempt to address the symptoms of our health care crisis through short-term, patchwork solutions, under the pressure of time and the constraints of political decision-making, rather than analyzing the system itself as a whole.

Passed in 2010, the Patient Protection and Affordable Care Act, together with the Health Care and Education Reconciliation Act, form effort to reduce these inequities and increase the quality of health care while reducing overall costs.

KEY TERMS

Access to health care: the availability and timely use of health services to produce the optimum outcomes

Acute care clinics: facilities, open to patients with less serious injuries, that accept patients without appointments

Community hospitals: nonfederal, short-term general and special hospitals whose facilities and services are available to the public

Copayment: a flat fee that an insured person pays for each use of the health care system

Deductible: the amount of money a policy holder pays each year before the health insurance policy begins paying

Exchange: a marketplace of health insurance plans from which consumers may choose

Fee-for-service: a plan in which charges are made for each single service that is provided

Health maintenance organization: type of prepaid medical service in which subscribers pay a monthly or yearly fee for all health care and the organization controls costs and access to specific services

Hospice care: medical services, emotional support, and spiritual resources for family members and people who are in the last stages of a terminal illness

Hospitalist: a physician who coordinates or assumes much of the care of a hospitalized patient

Indemnity insurance: a type of health insurance that requires the subscriber to pay certain charges, such as copayments and deductibles, and which allows the insured to choose his or her health care provider

Managed care: a system of health care delivery with the goal of reducing costs and use

Preexisting condition: a health problem existing before your health insurance goes into effect

Preferred provider organization: a type of managed care organization of health care providers and hospitals that have contracted with an insurer or a third-party administrator to provide health care at reduced rates to the insurer's or administrator's clients

Primary care: the entry point for patients into the health care system; it includes diagnosis and treatment of acute and chronic illnesses and is performed and managed by a personal physician in collaboration with other health professionals

Primary care physician: the physician who handles most of your care and who makes referrals to specialists

Single-payer health care: a system in which there is one insurer of health care, the government

STUDY QUESTIONS

1. Describe the training and education of a physician.
2. What are some weaknesses of the U.S. health care system?
3. What are some problems related to lack of health insurance?
4. Why are health disparities a major focus of the health care system?
5. How are health insurance and health disparities related?
6. How does the United States compare with other industrialized nations in financial expenditures for health care?
7. What are some steps that we could take to improve the U.S. health care system?
8. How is quality assured in the health care system?
9. What are some arguments for and against a universal health care system in America? What is your opinion?
10. Do you think the Patient Protection and Affordable Care Act of 2010 will improve the U.S. health care system? Why or why not? What provisions do you think are positive? Are there any provisions that will have negative impact?
11. How do you select a hospital?
12. How do you select a living facility for an elderly person?

REFERENCES

Agency for Healthcare Research and Quality. (2009). *National healthcare disparities report, 2008*. Rockville, MD: U.S. Department of Health and Human Services.

Alemayehu, B., & Warner, K. E. (2004). The lifetime distribution of health care costs. *Health Services Research, 39*(3), 627–643.

American Board of Medical Specialties. (2008). *The importance of board certification*. Retrieved from http://www.abms.org/Who_We_Help/Consumers/importance.aspx

American College of Physicians. (2008). Achieving a high-performance health care system with universal access: What the United States can learn from other countries. *Annals of Internal Medicine, 148*(1), 55–75.

American College of Physicians—American Society of Internal Medicine. (2001). *Statement for the record of the Ways and Means Subcommittee hearing on the nation's uninsured*. Retrieved from http://acponline.org/hpp/ways_means.htm

American Hospital Association. (2007). *Fast facts on US hospitals*. Retrieved from http://aha.org/aha/resource-center/Statistics-and-Studies/fast-facts.html

American Hospital Association. (2009a). *American Hospital Association underpayment by Medicare and Medicaid fact sheet.* Retrieved from http://www.americanhealthsolution.org/assets/Uploads/Blog/09medicunderpayment1.pdf

American Hospital Association. (2009b). *Annual Survey with Information Technology Supplement.* Washington, DC: American Hospital Association.

American Hospital Association. (2010a). *AHA Rapid Response Survey, Telling the Hospital Story Survey.* Chicago: American Hospital Association.

American Hospital Association. (2010b). *Chartbook: Trends affecting hospitals and health systems.* Retrieved from http://www.aha.org/aha/research-and-trends/chartbook/index.html

Ayanian, J. Z., Weissman, J. S., Schneider, E. C., Ginsburg, J. A., & Zaslavsky, A. M. (2000). Unmet health needs of uninsured adults in the United States. *JAMA, 284*(16), 2061–2069.

Battista, J. R., & McCabe, J. (1999). *The case for universal health care in the United States.* Retrieved from http://cthealth.server101.com/the_case_for_universal_health_care_in_the_united_states.htm

Berk, M. L., & Monheit, A. C. (2001). The concentration of health expenditures, revisited. *Health Affairs, 20*(2), 9–18.

Bierman, A., Magari, E. S., Jette, A. M., Splaine, M., & Wasson, J. H. (1998). Assessing access as a first step toward improving the quality of care for very old adults. *Journal of Ambulatory Care Management, 121*(3), 17–26.

Citizens' Health Care Working Group. (2005). *The health report to the American people.* Retrieved from http://govinfo.library.unt.edu/chc/healthreport/healthreport.php

The Commonwealth Fund Commission on a High Performance Health System. (2006a). *Framework for a high performance health system for the United States: An ambitious agenda for the next president.* Retrieved from http://www.commonwealthfund.org/usr_doc/AmbitiousAgenda_1075.pdf?section=4039

The Commonwealth Fund Commission on a High Performance Health System. (2006b). *Why not the best? Results from a national scorecard on U.S. health system performance.* Retrieved from http://www.commonwealthfund.org/usr_doc/Commission_whynotthebest_951.pdf

The Commonwealth Fund Commission on a High Performance Health System. (2008). *Why not the best? Results from the National Scorecard on U.S. Health System Performance, 2008.* New York: The Commonwealth Fund.

Conwell, L. J., & Cohen, J. W. (2005). *Characteristics of people with high medical expenses in the U.S. civilian noninstitutionalized population, 2002.* Statistical Brief #73. Agency for Healthcare Research and Quality, Rockville, MD. Retrieved from http://www.meps.ahrq.gov/PrintProducts/PrintProdLookup.asp?ProductType=StatisticalBrief

Cutler, D. M., & McClellan, M. (2001). Is technological change in medicine worth it? *Health Affairs, 20*(1), 11–29.

Davis, K., Schoen, C., Guterman, S., & Shih, T. (2007). *Slowing the growth of U.S. health care expenditures: What are the options?* Retrieved from http://www.commonwealthfund.org/publications/publications_show.htm?doc_id=449510

DeNavas-Walt, C., Proctor, B. D., & Smith, J. C. (2010). U.S. Census Bureau, Current Population Reports, P60-238. *Income, poverty, and health insurance coverage in the United States: 2009.* Washington, DC: U.S. Government Printing Office.

Docteur, E., Suppanz, I. I., & Woo, J. (2003). *The U.S. health system: An assessment and prospective directions for reform.* Paris: Organisation for Economic Co-operation and Development.

Health Care and Education Reconciliation Act of 2010, Pub. L. 111–152, 124 stat. 1029.

HealthReform.gov. (2009). *Health disparities: A case for closing the gap.* Retrieved from http://www.healthreform.gov/reports/healthdisparities/index.html

Institute of Medicine. (1999). *To err is human: Building a safer health system.* Washington, DC: National Academy Press.

Institute of Medicine, Committee on the Consequences of Uninsurance. (2004). *Insuring America's health: Principles and recommendations.* Washington, DC: National Academies Press.

Kaiser Family Foundation. (2004). *The uninsured: A primer, key facts about Americans without health insurance.* Retrieved from http://www.kff.org/uninsured

Kaiser Family Foundation. (2009). *Medicaid and the uninsured.* Washington, DC: Kaiser Family Foundation.

Kane, C. (2004). *The practice arrangements of patient care physicians.* American Medical Association, Physician Marketplace Report no. 2004-02.

Keehan, S. P., Lazenby, H. C., Zezza, M. A., & Catlin, A. C. (2004). *Health care financing review.* 1:1. Web Exclusive. Retrieved from http://www.cms.hhs.gov/NationalHealthExpendData/downloads/keehan-age-estimates.pdf

Klevins, R. M., Edwards, J. R., Richards, C. L., Horan, T. C., Gaynes, R. P., Pollock, D. A., & Cardo, D. M. (2007). Estimated healthcare-associated infections and deaths in U.S. hospitals, 2002. *Public Health Reports, 122*(2), 160–166.

Kofman, M., & Pollitz, K. (2006). *Health insurance regulation by states and the federal government: A review of current approaches and proposals for change.* Washington, DC: Health Policy Institute, Georgetown University.

Macinko, J., Starfield, B., & Shi, L. (2003). The contribution of primary care systems to health outcomes within Organization for Economic Co-operation and Development (OECD) Countries, 1970–1998. *Health Services Research, 38*(3), 831–865.

Mangione-Smith, R., DeCristofaro, A. H., Setodji, C. M., Keesey, J., Klein, D. J., Adams, J. L., & McGlynn, E. A. (2007). The quality of ambulatory care delivered to children in the United States. *New England Journal of Medicine, 357*(15), 1515–1523.

McGlynn, E. A., Asch, S. M., Adams, J., Keesey, J., Hicks, J., DeCristofaro, A., & Kerr, E. A. (2003). The quality of health care delivered to adults in the United States. *New England Journal of Medicine, 348*(26), 2635–2645.

McWilliams, J. M., Meara, E., Zaslavsky, A. M., & Ayanian, J. Z. (2007). Use of health services by previously uninsured Medicare beneficiaries. New *England Journal of Medicine, 357*(2), 143–153.

Nabili, S. (2010). *What is a hospitalist?* Retrieved from http://www.medicinenet.com/script/main/art .asp?articlekey=93946

National Practitioner Data Bank–Healthcare Integrity and Protection Data Bank. (2008). *Why the NPDB was created.* Retrieved from http://www.npdb-hipdb.hrsa .gov/npdb.html

National Practitioner Data Bank–Healthcare Integrity and Protection Data Bank. (2009). *Healthcare Integrity and Protection Data Bank.* Retrieved from http://www .npdb-hipdb.hrsa.gov/hipdb.html

National Practitioner Data Bank–Health Integrity and Protection Data Bank. (2010). *Public Use Data File.* Retrieved from http://www.npdb-hipdb.hrsa.gov /publicdata.html

Organisation for Economic Co-operation and Development. (2005). *OECD health data 2006: Most frequently requested data.* Retrieved from http://www.oecd.org /document/16/0,2340.en_2649_37407_2085200_1 _1_1_37407.00.html

Organisation for Economic Co-operation and Development. (2009). *Health at a glance: 2009 OECD indicators.* Retrieved from http://www.oecd.org/health /healthataglance

Patient Protection and Affordable Care Act of 2010, Pub. L. 111–148, 124 stat. 119.

Physicians for a National Health Program. (1999). *How much does single payer national health care cost?* Retrieved

from http://thirdworldtraveler.com/Health /HowMuchSPCost.html

Schoen, C., Davis, D., How, S. K. H., & Schoenbaum, S. C. (2006). U.S. health system performance: A national scorecard. *Health Affairs, 25*(6), W457–475 (September 20, 2006), doi:10.1377/hlthaff.25.w457

Schoen, C., Doty, M. M., Collins, S. R., & Holmgren, A. L. (2005). Insured but not protected: How many adults are underinsured? *Health Affairs,* (Suppl Web Exclusive), W5–289.

Schoen, C., Osborn, R., Doty, M. M., Bishop, M., Peugh, J., & Murukutla, N. (2007). Toward higher-performance health systems: Adults' health care experiences in seven countries, 2007. *Health Affairs, 26*(6), W717–W734.

University of Maine. (2001). *The U.S. health care system: Best in the world, or just the most expensive?* Retrieved from http://dll.umaine.edu/ble/U.S.%20HCweb.pdf

U.S. Bureau of the Census. (2008). *Income, poverty, and health insurance coverage in the United States: 2007.* Washington, DC: U.S. Department of Commerce, Bureau of the Census.

U.S. Central Intelligence Agency. (2010). *The world factbook.* Retrieved from http://www.cia.gov/library /publications/the-world-factbook

U.S. Department of Health and Human Services. (2000). *Healthy people 2010: Understanding and improving health.* Washington, DC: USDHHS.

U.S. Department of Health and Human Services. (2009). *Healthy people 2020 framework.* Retrieved from http:// healthypeople.gov/hp2020/Objectives/framework. aspx

Vanlandingham, B., Powe, N. R., Marone, B., Diener-West, M., & Rubin, H. R. (2005). The shortage of on-call specialist physician coverage in U.S. hospitals. Presented at the Academy Health Meeting, Boston, MA.

Woolhandler, S., & Himmelstein, D. U. (1997). Costs of care and administration at for-profit and other hospitals in the United States. *New England Journal of Medicine, 336*(11), 769–774.

World Health Organization. (2000). *The world health report—health systems: Improving performance.* Retrieved from http://www.who.int/whr/2000/en/index.html

Chapter 3

Health Fraud

Chapter Objectives

The student will:

- Explain health fraud and cite some ways that it is perpetrated.
- List ways to check on the authenticity of a product or service.
- Explain quackery and how it is practiced.
- Explain how health care fraud drives up the cost of health care.
- List ways to prevent health care fraud.
- Discuss weight loss fraud.
- Explain steps to ensure that a fitness program is right for you.
- Identify clues to fraud involving chronic conditions such as HIV/AIDS, diabetes, cancer, and arthritis.
- Explain various scams related to sexual enhancement, genetic tests, aging, and influenza.

Identifying Health Fraud

Fraud is an intentional act perpetrated to be deceptive in order to gain something of value. It is usually an act of greed. The U.S. Food and Drug Administration (FDA; Kurtzweil, 1999) defines the term **health fraud** as "articles of unproven effectiveness that are promoted to improve health, well being, or appearance." Health fraud is often practiced through the delivery of some kind of service or treatment. Health fraud marketers are quite sophisticated about promoting their products, often using gimmicks and catchy phrases to gain consumers' attention and trust. Frauds often use **half-truths**, deceptive statements that contain some element of truth but are partly false. Other half-truths may be completely true as far as they go, but omit important information. For example, a marketer may claim to have never heard from a dissatisfied customer but omits the fact that he never publishes any contact information so that customers may report their dissatisfaction.

We should be wary of products promoted through **testimonials**, sometimes presented as case histories. Often, these statements are fiction. Even if a testimonial is true, it does not mean that the statements it contains apply to every user. It is very difficult to prove or even find evidence of the truth of a testimonial. It is even more difficult to determine if the reported cure resulted from the treatment, the **placebo effect**, or the body's ability to heal itself. Scientific study is the best way to determine if something works, not a single example.

Consumers should be suspicious of products that claim to cure a wide range of unrelated diseases, especially serious conditions. No product can treat every disease and condition, and few can treat more than one. Many serious conditions have no cures, only therapies to help manage them.

Another frequent claim is that a product can bring quick relief or a quick cure, especially if the condition is serious. For example, the phrase "eliminates skin cancer in days" implies that the treatment works quickly. However, the phrase "in days" does not specify if it is ten days or one thousand. Such vague language is another tip-off of fraudulent advertising. Even proven treatments often do not cure serious diseases quickly.

The word "natural" is often used to market food products and nutrition supplements. It is a good attention-grabber and suggests to many people that the product is safer and more wholesome than other products. The FDA has not defined the word "natural," although it is broadly applied to foods to imply that they are minimally processed and free of synthetic preservatives, antibiotics, growth hormones, and artificial sweeteners, colors, or flavorings. Most foods labeled as natural are not subject to government controls other than regulations and health codes that apply to all foods (Food Marketing Institute, 2008).

The term "all natural" is also used and misused to sell treatments, especially herbs. While it is true that many approved medications are based on natural ingredients, "all natural" and "natural" do not really mean safe, and they certainly do not mean the product is effective. Naturally occurring substances can cause serious discomfort, illness, or even death. They can interact with medications and supplements in unpredictable ways. Some products described as natural may be exposed to bacteria or contaminated with pesticides and herbicides.

The phrases "revolutionary innovation," "miracle cure," "exclusive product," "new discovery," "secret ingredient," "ancient remedy," or "magical" should arouse suspicion. If the product was really an effective cure for a serious condition, it would be widely reported in the media and marketed with FDA approval to give it credibility. This type of credibility would boost sales far beyond what could be gained through extravagant, unverified claims. Similarly, products purported to be "ancient remedies" or based on "folklore" or "tradition" are usually fraudulent. These claims suggest that if the product or some

form of it has been around for a long time, it must be effective. This is simply not true. Additionally, some herbs reportedly used in ancient times for medicinal purposes carry risks identified in recent years (Kurtzweil, 1999).

Many fraudulent treatments are offered to Americans from outside the United States. Some unethical promoters arrange charter flights for sick people to European, Latin American, or Caribbean clinics for exotic, expensive, but unproven cures. Desperate patients with terminal illnesses are usually the targets of these ploys.

If a product comes with a money-back guarantee, it should be viewed very skeptically. Guarantees are almost never given by legitimate pharmaceutical companies, because medicines do not work the same way on every individual. Marketers of fraudulent products rarely are available, having closed their Web site or post office box by the time customers press for refunds.

Unproven weight loss products are often marketed as "easy" or "rapid" with promises of dramatic weight loss while eating whatever you want and with no physical activity. For most people, the only way to lose weight is to consume fewer calories and increase activity. A reasonable and healthy weight loss is about one to two pounds a week. Promises of the loss of huge amounts of weight should be red flags because rapid weight loss is usually followed by rapid weight gain. See Chapter 8 on weight loss.

Fraudulent promoters often use meaningless but impressive-sounding jargon. One marketer stated in a promotion that "One of the many natural ingredients is inolitol hexanicontinate." Another claimed to promote "thermogenesis, which converts stored fats into soluble lipids." Sometimes, the terms are lifted from a study published in a reputable scientific journal, even though the study may have been on another subject altogether. Unfortunately, few consumers actually read the original study. Unscrupulous promoters may simply coin words or phrases, or use names for ingredients that appear in similar products.

Frauds frequently make claims of a conspiracy theory. This is a form of ad hominem attack in which, armed with little or no evidence of his claim, the fraud attacks those who disagree with him, often labeling them "unprofessional," "incompetent," or "biased." The consistent theme running through the variations of these claims is that the medical community, the pharmaceutical industry, the Food and Drug Administration, or all of them conspire to keep the fraud's products or services off the market. They claim that by suppressing the products and services, physicians and drug companies are eliminating competition for financial gain. These claims are bogus. Physicians rarely give much thought to many of the products that health frauds may be selling. They are also prone to look askance at treatment methods that have no scientific basis or documentation of effectiveness. Pharmaceutical companies are in business to make a profit. If a product was effective, it is absurd to think that drug companies would shun it. As for the FDA, the Dietary Supplement and Health Education Act has handcuffed the agency's ability to regulate, let alone eliminate, untested products that are treated as dietary supplements. Marketers often escape government scrutiny by labeling their products as supplements (see Chapter 7).

Another method used by health frauds to defend themselves is the false analogy. For example, by claiming that sharks have cartilage rather than a skeletal system and that they never get cancer, it has been claimed that human consumption of shark cartilage will prevent cancer. Another example is the claim that a certain fungus may cause flower bulbs to become dormant. The next step in the analogy is to suggest that the same fungus can make human skin cells dormant, thus slowing aging. Both analogies are based on logical fallacies, ways to confuse people while hiding an argument that is supported by no data or science.

Perhaps one of the most incredible claims for effectiveness is based on the so-called Doctrine of Signatures, the ancient belief that the form and shape of a drug source determine its therapeutic value. Mistress Moss, a well-known colonial herbalist, advocated for the doctrine. She believed that when you go to different climates, you encounter different diseases and different plants to treat the ailments. These plants had to have an appearance relevant to the disease. If you have heart problems, you use a plant with heart-shaped leaves or red roots. If you have arthritis, you use a plant with swollen joints. This doctrine is alleged to be the basis for three of the most popular aphrodisiacs sold in parts of Asia and sometimes exported elsewhere. Because of their phallic shape, deer antlers, ginseng root, and rhinoceros horn are highly valued as agents of virility. Any subsequent increase in libido or sexual potency is most likely related to the placebo effect. Modern-day paraherbalists have reached into historical misunderstandings and superstition for "signature" products. For example, eyebright, a flower with white to bluish corona and a bright yellow spot near its center, resembles a human eye with its pupil. Medieval herbalists believed that the plant was effective against eye disease, a basis for today's fraud to grow and market eyebright.

A good rule to follow about health care products is: If it sounds too good to be true, it probably is.

There are many ways to check on the authenticity and value of a product. For example, it is a good idea to:

- Talk to a physician, pharmacist, or other health care professional.
- Check with the Better Business Bureau or state attorney general's office to see if other consumers have filed complaints about the product.
- Check with the appropriate health professional nonprofit group such as the American Heart Association, American Diabetes Association, Arthritis Foundation, or Epilepsy Foundation of America.
- Contact the FDA office closest to you. The FDA can tell you if the agency has taken action against the product or the marketer.
- Understand that newspapers, magazines, and radio and television stations do not have to verify that the ads they run carry truthful information.

Health Quackery

Quackery is a pejorative term describing health practices or remedies that have no compelling scientific basis. Recall that fraud is an intentional act perpetrated to be deceptive. Quackery, although usually a form of health fraud, may or may not be intentional. It is the promotion of methods that are known to be useless or that are unproven and likely to be useless. Quacks, sometimes called charlatans, are the individuals who practice quackery, pretending to have medical skills they do not have. There are a number of forms of quackery practiced in a number of ways, often by highly skilled manipulators of people and information. This might include questionable ideas, untrue statements, or worthless products.

The origins of medicine and quackery may have coincided. Hippocrates, often called the father of medicine, observed in 400 B.C. that there are four bodily fluids—blood, phlegm, yellow bile, and black bile—and that illness resulted from an imbalance in the fluids or "humors." Building on Hippocrates, Galen believed that blood was formed by life-giving spirits in the liver and channeled to the heart. Blood was used up after reaching other parts of the body, and the spirits in the liver made a fresh supply. Galen's beliefs persisted for 1,400 years, leading to the notion that restoring health required getting the humors back in balance by purging or vomiting, starving, and bloodletting. Purging was usually induced with doses of mercury, calomel, or other chemicals or poisons.

Bloodletting took on a particular popularity and persisted through colonial times and the early nineteenth century. George Washington died in 1799 of a throat infection after his physicians bled him. He may have been drained of as much as several pints of blood in a day. This practice was considered "heroic" because the doctor was ready to kill the patient in order to cure him.

Today, quacks have more ways than ever to peddle their potions. In addition to television, radio, magazines, newspapers, **infomercials**, mail, and word of mouth, they now use the Internet. It is as if the Web was made for people to market "miracle cures" and remedies of all kinds. E-mail boxes are frequently stuffed with ads for all manner of treatments.

Many quacks believe in their products, honestly thinking that the worthless product or service they are promoting is effective. In some cases, users of products who are convinced that they work become word-of-mouth promoters and, unintentionally, quacks. For example, quackery may involve telling people that something, such as a preservative in food, is bad for them. This may be followed by a pitch to sell "natural food" that the quack actually believes is healthier.

QUACKERY THROUGH THE YEARS

The history of quackery is intriguing. Many examples show the gullibility of customers as well as a twisted view of science. A few examples are:

- American colonists maintained a loyalty to British brands. Attempting to satisfy their customers, colonial druggists simply refilled British drug bottles with local ingredients, including alcohol, opium, and cocaine in various forms. One product, named Venice Treacle, contained over 60 ingredients, including flesh of viper. Both the British and the colonists believed in an inverse relationship between taste and effectiveness. Cotton Mather recommended a remedy that was mostly cow urine and dung, certain to taste horrible.
- Benjamin Franklin's confirmation of electricity with his famous kite and key experiment led to a surge in the use of electricity in healing. Austrian doctor Franz Mesmer set up an extravagant establishment in Paris. Mesmer directed patients to hold hands around a

wooden tub of liquid, iron filings, and glass powder from which projected metal rods.
A glass armonica played soothing, celestial tones in the background. Dressed in a purple
robe, Mesmer would enter and touch the patients with a wand, enhancing the magnetic
potency of the "universal fluid" and transporting them into a trance from which they
awakened whole and cured. In 1784, a French court appointed a commission to study
Mesmer. The commission, of which Franklin was a member, reported that they could
find neither electrical or animal magnetism current in Mesmer's tub. Mesmer retreated
to England.

- Electropathy was very popular in the second half of the nineteenth century. It was touted
  as a cure for most diseases, including mental illness. The patient held a metal cylinder
  that was really an electrode while the healer applied a second electrode to the targeted
  body part. The electrodes connected to an electric source such as a battery or magneto.

- In 1813, Samuel Thomson, a self-taught healer who ridiculed educated physicians,
  received a patent for his herbal program. Thomson believed that disease was caused
  by a clogged system that could be cured by purging and sweating, the foundation of his
  program. His method was very popular in America.

- Throughout the second half of the nineteenth century and even into the twentieth,
  so-called snake oil solutions were pitched as medicine. Snake oil salesmen often arrived
  in wagons and preceded their shows with entertainment of various kinds. Most used a
  fire-and-brimstone sermon to bring the crowd to a fever pitch. Most of these products
  were heavy on alcohol, although some contained other ingredients. William Radam's
  Microbe Killer contained sulfuric acid, nitrate of soda, black oxide of manganese,
  sandalwood, chloride of potash, wine, pink dye, and red wine.

- At about the same time, "Dr." Sibley marketed his Re-animating Solar Tincture,
  claiming that it would "restore life in the event of sudden death."

- The Battle Creek Sanitarium was one of the most well-known health resorts in the world
  during the early twentieth century. Dr. John Harvey Kellogg, the chief of staff, was
  credited with developing Kellogg's Corn Flakes in the sanitarium's diet program. He also
  developed the vibratory chair. Looking much like the electric chair used for executions,
  the chair vibrated and shook violently and was very uncomfortable. Kellogg claimed that
  a few minutes in the chair would stimulate intestinal peristalsis, and longer treatments
  would cure headaches and back pain and would increase the supply of healthy oxygen to
  the body. One wonders if there is unhealthy oxygen in Battle Creek.

- The Prostate Gland Warmer was marketed in 1918 to "stimulate the abdominal
  brain!" by inserting it into the rectum. The device consisted of a 4.25-inch probe and a
  blue lightbulb in a socket with a long cord. When plugged in, the light came on. No
  "abdominal brain" was ever located.

- During the 1920s, Dr. John R. Brinkley gained fame for restoring the sex drive in
  men in his Kansas clinic. Brinkley's method was to insert a bit of goat testicle into the
  patient's scrotum. His degree, purchased from Eclectic Medical University for $500, was
  as worthless as his transplant surgery.

- During the 1930s, Crazy Crystals were marketed in the United States as a cure for
  many diseases. Supposedly, the crystals were removed from natural spring water. The
  real ingredient was Glauber's Salt, or sodium sulfate. Other brands included Texas

(continues)

Wonder Crystals and Sleepy Salts. The user was supposed to mix the crystals with water and drink one to eight glasses a day, depending on the problem and the recommended "cure." In 1940, the Federal Trade Commission found that the products contained no therapeutic value except as a laxative.

Sources: Cox, J. (Spring 2004). That quacking sound in colonial America. *Colonial Williamsburg Journal*. Retrieved from http://history.org/Foundation/journal/Spring04/quackery.cfm

Drugstore Museum. (2003). *Tonics, nostrums and snake oil*. Retrieved from http://www.drugstoremuseum.com/sections/level_info2.php?level_id=40&level=2

Museum of Quackery. (2000). *The Museum of Questionable Medical Devices Online*. Retrieved from http://www.museumofquackery.com/devices

Quackery. (2009). Retrieved from http://www.reference.com/browse/quack+salver

Schwarcz, J. (2002). *The goat gland doctor: The story of John R. Brinkley*. Retrieved from http://www.quackwatch.org/11Ind/brinkley.html

Young, J. H. (1972). *The toadstool millionaires: A social history of patent medicines in America before federal regulation*. Princeton, NJ: Princeton University Press.

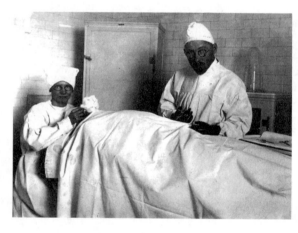

Dr. John Brinkley, seen here with his wife Minnie at their hospital in Milford, Kansas, is an example of a medical quack. Brinkley pursued several questionable procedures. His most famous was the surgical implantation of goat testicular tissue in the scrotums of human males to improve the patients' sex lives.

Some recent examples of quackery include:

- Breast enhancement products have flooded the market. For about $80, consumers can purchase packaged herbs, none of which actually increase breast size. A distributor for Volum-Bust Crème promises, "In two weeks you will have bigger, firmer breasts" and charges almost $34 for 1.7 ounces of product. Cleavage 4 contains aloe vera, tea, honey, and natural oils and claims to produce an increase "of ½ to 2 cup sizes (bra sizes) in 8 weeks." With its companion Cleavage 6 Breast Enhancement capsules, about an ounce costs nearly $80. The Breast Pump Enlarger was marketed for $10 in 1976. Four million women purchased the device. Covering her breasts with the cups—all in large size—the woman would pump a pedal with her foot. The pedal was connected to the cups by plastic tubing. The only enlargement in breast size was because of bruising.

- A device called the "Stimulator" was marketed with claims that it could relieve headache, back pain, arthritis, stress, menstrual cramps, earaches, nosebleeds, flu, and other ailments. It is essentially an electric gas barbecue grill igniter with added finger grips.

- "E-Water" and "Green Drink" were marketed by John E. Curran as a cure for cancer from his Northeastern Institute for Advanced Natural Healing and the Rhode Island Health Aid in Cranston, both in the state of Rhode Island. In August 2006, a federal judge sentenced Curran to 12.5 years in prison for fraud and money laundering related to his institute and phony products.

- DMSO is an industrial solvent. It has been reported that industrial-grade DMSO, devoid of drug labeling, is being used for self-treatment of arthritis and other disease conditions. The industrial-grade product is not of the quality used for drug purposes and is not made under conditions that are necessary for the production of human drugs and protection of users. Further, since DMSO is a "carrier" chemical, it could deliver harmful substances into the bloodstream, if they are present in impure DMSO, through use on the skin.
- ACU-DOTS Magnetic Analgesic Patches were marketed with the promise of temporary relief of minor aches and pains in the muscles and joints. The notion behind the patches is that the magnets attract iron in blood, increasing circulation and relieving pain. The idea fails because the iron in blood is not a metal; it is a mineral and is not attracted to metals.
- Iridology is the belief that the parts of the body are represented in corresponding parts of the iris of the eye. Practitioners claim that they can diagnose disease and even trace the health history of an individual by the texture, color, and location of pigments in the iris. Health imbalances are usually treated with vitamins, minerals, or herbs.
- Quacks practice virtually all over the globe. Zhang Wuben of the People's Republic of China masqueraded as a traditional Chinese medicine practitioner who came from a family of respected traditional practitioners. By portraying himself as a nutritionist rather than a physician, Zhang escaped legal liability. He represented that his formula of raw eggplant and mung beans was a general cure-all, and he wrote a best-selling book on his treatment.

It was later revealed that his medical degree was faked, his family were not as he described them, and his only education was a brief correspondence course. Nevertheless, his practice continued (Jacobs, 2010).

Those with e-mail accounts are frequently targeted with mass mailings, or spam, that promote modern forms of quackery that allegedly provide weight loss with no dietary changes and no need for physical activity. Advertisements for sexual enhancement products and unlicensed outlets for medications often flood e-mail boxes.

It is not unusual for therapies to appear to work even when they have no scientific reason to work. Beyerstein (1997) identified reasons that people may erroneously think that an ineffective therapy works. Many diseases are self-limiting— i.e., they run their course and the person gets well, largely because of the effects of the immune system. Many diseases are cyclical, meaning that sometimes the patient suffers different levels of discomfort. Arthritis is an example of a cyclical condition. Sometimes, patients may experience reduced pain and discomfort, while the underlying disease condition is not affected. The placebo effect may lead the patient to think that the therapy is effective. Beyerstein refers to "hedging their bets"—i.e., if the patient uses a scientifically verified treatment and an **alternative treatment,** he or she may assign a disproportionate share of the credit to the alternative treatment. There is always the possibility that the original diagnosis or prognosis was incorrect, leading to the conclusion that an alternative treatment cured the patient. Sometimes, a psychological improvement, a mood elevation, can be prompted by a forceful practitioner, leading to perceived improvement in the physical condition even when the practitioner's treatment was worthless. At other times, people want to avoid the embarrassment of admitting they wasted time and money on a bogus treatment. This can be psychologically upsetting, causing the patient to search for some redeeming value to the treatment. Individuals may be selective in the recall of their condition, possibly a manifestation of vigorously defending their beliefs and expectations despite the available evidence to the contrary.

Older people seem to be more vulnerable to quacks than others. A government study found that most victims of health care fraud are older than age 65 (National Institute on Aging, 2008).

The ability to persuade and dupe their customers, not the quality of their services and products, is what sustains quacks. They promise hope to the hopeless and cures to the incurable. To all, they promise longer and healthier lives. These are strong emotional motivators, and they often succeed to the tune of billions of wasted dollars per year.

Insurance or Health Care Fraud

Health care fraud is an intentional deception or misrepresentation that an individual or entity makes knowing that the misrepresentation could result in some unauthorized benefit to the individual, to the entity, or to some third party, according to the National Health Care Anti-Fraud Association (NHCAA; 2008). This definition is different from the FDA definition of "health fraud" primarily because it applies to the intentional bilking of insurers. Fraud increases the cost of health care for everyone. The NHCAA conservatively estimates that more than $60 billion (other estimates go as high as $170 billion) is lost to fraud each year in the United States. When loss occurs, the insurer must make up the losses somehow. The primary ways for private companies to do this are to increase **premiums**, **deductibles**, or **copayments**. With government programs, Medicare and Medicaid, these costs become the burden of all taxpayers.

Some examples of insurance fraud are:

- Billing the insurer for services or items not delivered, so-called phantom billing
- Billing for services or equipment that are different from and more expensive than what was delivered
- Billing multiple times for the same service

- Accepting compensation for making a referral
- "Unbundling," or billing separately for procedures that normally are covered by a single fee
- Dispensing generic drugs and charging for brand-name drugs
- Upcoding, or charging for a more complex service than was actually provided
- Miscoding, using a code number that does not apply to the specific service
- Deliberately performing medically unnecessary services for financial gain
- Ordering unnecessary tests and accepting payment for them
- Using another person's insurance card to get medical care, supplies, or equipment

To prevent health care fraud:

- Be careful about giving your insurance identification number over the telephone; do not give it to people you do not know.
- Some health providers ask for your Social Security number. To protect yourself from identity theft, try to get them to accept another form of identification because all information goes into a computer database that could be hacked or accessed by a disgruntled employee.
- Read your insurance policy and benefits statements.
- Allow only appropriate medical professionals to review your medical record or recommend services.
- Carefully review explanations of benefits that you receive from your plan. If you do not understand them or disagree with them, call the plan customer service number.
- Do not encourage your health care provider to make erroneous entries on certificates, bills, or records in order to get your insurer to pay for an item or service.
- Avoid providers who tell you that an item or service is not covered but they know how to bill your private insurer or Medicaid to get it paid.

- Do not attempt to maintain a family member, such as a divorced spouse or an aged-out child, on your policy if the person is no longer eligible.
- If you suspect that a provider has charged you for services you did not receive, billed you more than once for the same service, or misrepresented any information, call the provider and ask for information. If the provider does not resolve the matter, call your insurer and explain the situation. You can also contact your state insurance fraud program. If the problem is still not resolved, call the Health Care Fraud Hotline of the U.S. Office of Personnel Management, especially for Medicare and Medicaid issues. See the box titled "Reporting Health Fraud" on page 62 for more information.

Individuals may be prosecuted for fraud and insurance claims can be rejected if fraud can be demonstrated.

Medicare and Medicaid fraud is an insidious type of insurance fraud. This type of fraud is especially contemptible for two reasons. First, it takes advantage of elderly persons and uses them to dupe the Medicare system into paying for services not provided. Second, since Medicare is a federal program and Medicaid is a state/federal program, fraud robs all taxpayers of their hard-earned contributions to the program. Most instances of Medicare fraud consist of somebody claiming to provide services to program enrollees without really delivering them, providing services that the patient does not need, or exaggerating the services provided. Medicaid fraud often consists of individuals using another person's card or a person living in one state using an address in another state because of eligibility requirements. The Medicare or Medicaid programs expend billions of dollars cumulatively each year by providing payment for falsified or otherwise illegal claims. Eventually, this forces the government to increase Medicare premiums or taxes. In the case of Medicaid, states may change eligibility requirements or reduce the number of people covered in order to make up for the shortfall in revenue.

Some examples of Medicare and Medicaid fraud are providers who:

- Clip your toenails at a health fair and bill for "foot surgery"
- Offer a free Medicare Approved Arthritis Kit that may consists of a back brace, knee brace, elbow brace, ankle brace, and heating pad for which they bill Medicare for over $1,000 and have invested less than $100
- Pressure patients into obtaining a medical device or transportation device such as a wheelchair or scooter that they really do not need
- Offer home health care for which the patient does not qualify
- Provide ambulance service to take patients to the doctor, physical therapist, or dialysis for free but then charge the program for a non-emergency trip

Some tips you can use to avoid Medicare and Medicaid fraud are:

- Keep your Medicare or Medicaid number secret. Do not give it to anyone except a trusted physician or other approved provider.
- Keep your medical records private. Do not allow anyone, except appropriate medical professionals, to review your records.
- Ask only for services you need. Do not ask your doctor, pharmacist, or other health professional to provide unnecessary services.
- Beware of free services. Nothing is really free; someone is paying for it. Be skeptical of Medicare or Medicaid services or screenings that are advertised as free, especially if you are asked for your Medicare card number.
- Avoid providers who tell you that an item or service is not covered but they know how to bill Medicare or Medicaid to get it paid. If it is not covered, it is fraud to attempt to obtain payment.
- Request proof that the provider is endorsed by the federal government or Medicare before seeking services.

- Report suspected fraud to the Medicare or Medicaid fraud unit or to the Office of the Inspector General at 1-800-447-8477. Under the False Claims Act, those who witness fraudulent attempts to submit false claims for payment of government funds may file suit under the act. Once the suit is filed, the case is sealed while the government investigates and takes over as the plaintiff. The whistleblower may receive 10 to 30 percent of the money that is recovered.

The office of the U.S. Attorney General and the Department of Health and Human Services have targeted Medicare and Medicaid fraud. Between May 2009 and August 2010, the joint effort produced 580 criminal convictions and recovered more than $2.5 billion in fraudulent earnings.

Weight Loss Fraud

Weight loss fraud is big business. To emphasize this, between 2003 and 2006, member organizations of the Mexico, United States, Canada Health Fraud Working Group took more than 700 compliance actions against companies pushing bogus weight loss schemes (U.S. Food and Drug Administration [U.S. FDA], 2006b).

Many people become desperate when they cannot lose weight. Reasons for lack of success include ignorance of the relationship between calorie intake and calorie expenditure, poor eating and activity habits, genetics, and social and cultural environments. Desperation leads them to try anything that is offered, even if the method is intuitively without merit. They become easy prey to unscrupulous vendors of worthless or over-hyped weight loss products. These may include pills, compression wraps, plastic or nylon clothing, drinks, stimulants, exercise contraptions, or memberships to clubs. The FDA has warned consumers against using some weight loss products, including Emagrece Sim Dietary Supplement, also known as the Brazilian Diet Pill, and Herbathin Dietary Supplement. These products contain drug products that can lead to serious side effects or

injury. Unfortunately, even when products are taken off the market, they often reappear with different names or others quickly replace them on shelves and in advertising space.

The Acu-Stop 2000 is an example of weight loss quackery. The user is supposed to insert this rubber device into the ear and massage it for several minutes to activate pressure points that control appetite. Made for 17 cents, the device sold for $39.95 before being banned in 1995.

Weight loss products are often marketed on television, including in infomercials, and in magazines. Sellers use testimonials and before-and-after photos to hype their effectiveness. However, these products have seldom been shown to be effective in clinical trials.

Fitness Fraud

The fitness industry is rife with fraudulent products and services. Some fitness centers seem to be more interested in signing up members for expensive extensions of their contracts than with helping them improve their health. Prospective members should talk with current members to evaluate the services, equipment, facilities, and the amount of harassment and pressure exerted to buy more. Since centers have been known to go out of business on short notice, it is advisable to go with an established company, possibly one that is part of a national or regional chain. Visit the facility more than once at different times of the day to determine how crowded it may be and how attentive the staff are. Read the contract thoroughly and consult an attorney if you do not understand a portion of it. Get details on warranties, guarantees, and return policies. Consider the parts you do not like negotiable and get them amended in writing. Do not put your faith or money in verbal promises.

Some advertisers offer exercise equipment with the claim that their products provide a quick, easy way to get into good physical condition, keep fit, and lose weight. In truth, there is no such thing as a no-work, no-sweat, easy way to a healthy, toned body. Before you purchase the next home fitness fad, follow the advice of the Federal Trade Commission (2003a,b):

- Ignore claims that an exercise machine or device can provide long-lasting, easy, "no sweat" results in a short time. You cannot get the benefits of exercise unless you exercise. The more activity you have, the more calories you will burn and the more muscle tone you will develop. If your goal is to build muscle mass, the best way is with weight-bearing activities that force you to use those muscles against resistance.
- Question claims that a product can burn fat off a particular area of the body—for example, the stomach, hips, or buttocks. Achieving a major change in your appearance requires sensible eating and regular exercise that works the whole body. In general, you burn more calories by working the whole body or major body parts than you would by working only one body part. While it may be possible to tone a specific area, such as the abdominal muscles, loss of body fat is not specific to a certain area.
- Read the advertisement's fine print. The advertised results may be based on more than just using the machine; they also may be based on restricting calories.
- Be skeptical of testimonials and before-and-after pictures from "satisfied customers." Their experiences may not be typical. Just because one person had success with the equipment does not mean you will, too. Before-and-after photos may be impressive, but they do not show the long-term effects, the "after that" effects. Celebrity endorsements are virtually worthless to the consumer.
- Get details on warranties, guarantees, and return policies. A "30-day-money-back guarantee" may not sound as good if you have to pay shipping on the equipment you want to return.
- Do the calculations when you read statements like "three easy payments of ..." or "only $49.95 a month." The advertised cost may not include sales tax or shipping, delivery, handling, and setup fees. Find out the details before you order.
- Check out the company's customer and support services. Call the advertised toll-free numbers to get an idea of how easy it is to reach a company representative and how helpful he or she is.

It is wise to check out the product with an independent evaluator, such as *Consumer Reports.* The Better Business Bureau in your area or in the location of the company can tell you the company's record of complaints.

It is important to select equipment that fits you and your lifestyle. Regardless of the effectiveness of the equipment, most people will not use it much if it is uncomfortable. Before making your final decision, consider two questions: (1) Will the equipment help you achieve your desired goal—whether it is to build strength, increase flexibility, or improve endurance? (2) Will you stick to the program or continue to use the equipment? A good way to begin to answer the second question is to try out various pieces of equipment at a local gym, recreation center, or retailer to find the equipment that feels comfortable to you.

HIV/AIDS Fraud

Currently, there is no cure for HIV, the virus that causes AIDS. Because of the seriousness of the disease, many people are willing to try almost anything. Some unproven treatments may be harmless, except to the bank account, while others can be dangerous. Look skeptically at products or services that are:

- Said to prevent or cure HIV or AIDS
- Marketed using personal success stories
- Marketed using terms such as "foolproof," "suppressed treatments," or "amazing breakthrough"
- Claimed to be discovered and tested in another country or are available only outside the United States

- Claimed to be available only for a short time or from a single source
- Available only by paying to participate in testing an experimental treatment

Some bogus HIV/AIDS remedies that have been promoted include processed blue-green algae, a food preservative called BHT, herbal capsules, and bottles of "T cells." Another scam involves withdrawing a portion of the patient's blood, exposing it to hydrogen peroxide, and injecting it back into the body. The Antidote, a remedy purportedly derived from the blood of crocodiles, was promoted as a drug to treat AIDS and other life-threatening diseases.

Insurance companies will pay only for treatments that have been demonstrated as effective. If someone tries to tell you differently, check with your insurer or walk away. Unproven treatments often result in delaying the use of treatments that really are effective, giving the illness time to progress.

If you are ever pressured to make a decision about an HIV therapy before you are prepared to do so, it is usually best to decline. Reputable physicians do not usually exert pressure to make a decision.

Diabetes Fraud

The Mexico, United States, Canada Health Fraud Working Group (MUCH) has focused enforcement and consumer education efforts on fraudulent products to treat diabetes. In October 2000, MUCH member agencies announced that they had taken nearly 200 compliance actions against companies promoting bogus products that provided false hope to people with diabetes. In 2006, the FDA listed 23 firms to which it had sent warning letters for marketing unproven dietary supplements for diabetes treatment (U.S. FDA, 2006a). Some of the unproven claims to treat diabetes were that the treatments would:

- Drop your blood sugar 50 points in 30 days
- Eliminate insulin resistance

- Prevent the development of type 2 diabetes
- Reduce or eliminate the need for diabetes drugs and/or insulin
- Prevent diabetes-related eye disease
- Act as the natural alternative to the diabetes drug metformin

A recent scam involved claims that stem cells can be turned into beta cells that cure diabetes. While stem cells hold much promise, their use for diabetes treatment appears to be years away.

While these and other claims are attractive, they are almost never realized.

Arthritis Remedy Fraud

Arthritis is a chronic condition and the symptoms often come and go. This makes arthritis sufferers favorite targets of quacks and scammers because the disease provides the opportunity for the **regression fallacy** (failure to recognize that most medical conditions fluctuate with no treatment) to convince the customer that the product was helpful.

The variety of treatments for arthritis is huge. Herbs, oils, radiation, spinal manipulation, massage, and special diets are only a few. Magnets and copper bracelets have been sold as arthritis-curing devices. Many of these products are physically harmless but expensive, and their use may also delay getting real treatment.

While there is no cure for arthritis, there are some excellent anti-inflammatory and analgesic drugs available to help with the symptoms. Rest, heat, and physical activity help many arthritis sufferers.

Victimizing Cancer Victims

Sometimes it seems that the more frightening the condition, the more susceptible the patient to fraud and the more aggressive the quack in selling his or her products. The word "cancer" is so terrifying to many people that they are easily duped by anything offering a ray of hope. People have traveled to all parts of the world, particularly

South America, Asia, and Europe, to find a cure, only to have their hopes dashed and their bank accounts plundered. A few examples of these frauds demonstrate their power to vulnerable patients.

Powdered shark cartilage has been marketed as a cancer cure and preventative in "health food stores." I. William Lane, PhD, boosted this fallacy in a book titled *Sharks Don't Get Cancer* and in an appearance on CBS's *60 Minutes* program. After studies showed no benefit to using shark cartilage for this purpose, federal agencies took action against three companies, including Lane Labs—USA. Lane was forced to sign a consent decree to stop marketing his product for cancer therapy and to pay $550,000 in penalties (Federal Trade Commission, 2000).

Dr. Stanislaw R. Burzynski claimed that substances called "antineoplastons" could "normalize" cancer cells that are constantly being produced within the body. He was able to bolster his claim by publishing papers stating that antineoplastons extracted from urine or synthesized in his laboratory have proven effective against cancer in laboratory experiments and by appearing on television talk shows. An analysis published in the *Journal of the American Medical Association* concluded that none of Burzynski's "antineoplastons" had been proven to normalize tumor cells (Green, 1992).

Nobel Prize winner Linus Pauling, PhD, began touting vitamin C as a cure for cancer in the 1970s. He published several articles based on studies that were later shown to have serious flaws. No clinical studies to date have shown that vitamin C is effective as a cure for cancer.

One of the most famous quack remedies for cancer was laetrile, or vitamin B-17. Laetrile is produced from the apricot seed, which contains high levels of cyanide. Other versions of the promotion were said to contain ingredients from other fruits such as apple seeds as well as from almonds and other nuts. Laetrile was first marketed as a cure for cancer. Later it was said to control cancer and then was alleged to be effective in combination with other remedies of questionable value. No clinical studies demonstrated safety and effectiveness of laetrile as a treatment for cancer. It may still be available in a few places in the United States but is sold more often in Mexico.

Sexual Enhancement Products

With the introduction of Viagra in 1998 and the subsequent availability of other FDA-approved prescription drugs for erectile dysfunction (ED) like Cialis and Evitra, advertising for sexual enhancement products has become commonplace. Other products that are not scientifically validated and billed as providing "natural male enhancement" have appeared as well. The marketing of herbs for sexual enhancement has seen resurgence. Middle-aged and older men have flocked to these products, hoping to regain the sex lives they enjoyed in their youth. Even young men with no evidence of ED have tried them. As usually happens, more and more untested and fraudulent products have been quickly and aggressively marketed. Men who are experiencing symptoms of ED should see their physician, not chiropractors, pseudoscientists, herbalists, homeopaths, naturopaths, or any other nonmedical practitioner, for diagnosis and treatment.

In 2006, the FDA (U.S. FDA, 2006b) warned consumers not to use several drugs that were promoted or sold on the Internet as dietary supplements for treating ED and for enhancing sexual performance. The products are Zimaxx, Libidus, Neophase, Nasutra, Vigor-25, Actra-Rx, and 4EVERON. According to the FDA, rather than being dietary supplements, they are really drugs, some of which can interact with prescription or nonprescription medications and cause dangerous effects such as lowered blood pressure.

Many products have claimed to increase penis or breast size. Aside from breast augmentation through surgery, they are worthless. Except for the fact that many consumers were duped out of their money, one example of these promotions provides a little humor. Several years ago, several people ordered a device to increase either penis or breast size. They received a magnifying glass.

Influenza Scams

There have been cases involving contaminated, counterfeit, and ineffective influenza products. The FDA, working with U.S. Customs and Border Protection, intercepted products claiming to be a generic version of the influenza drug Tamiflu. These products really contained vitamin C and other substances not shown to be effective in treating or preventing influenza. In at least one case, the packaging was consistent with authentic flu vaccine but contained only saline solution. Individuals have been jailed for running unauthorized influenza vaccine clinics.

In 2005 and 2006, the FDA issued warning letters to marketers of useless influenza products to prevent multiple forms of influenza, including avian influenza. The issue in these cases was that they claimed that the products "kill the virus." While there are vaccines to protect against seasonal influenza, there are no vaccines for treating avian influenza in people. The FDA's Center for Devices and Radiological Health issued eight warning letters to firms that sold masks on the Internet that they claimed would prevent or cure avian influenza.

Aging Scams

If we live long enough, we will all grow old. The signs of aging accumulate constantly. Many folks find these natural indications to be unacceptable and become prey to sales pitches for pills, lotions, baths, or other treatments to slow or reverse the aging process. Many commercial products claim in their advertisements to reduce wrinkles, and hair coloring is a popular way to darken graying hair. Botox, made from the botulism toxin, temporarily smoothes out wrinkles. Aging is natural and normal, and while a product may temporarily smooth wrinkles, no treatments have yet been proven to slow the aging process. Eating a healthy diet, getting regular exercise, and not smoking are the best ways to prevent some of the diseases and conditions that occur more often with age.

A good way to identify an anti-aging fraud is a claim that aging is caused by or can be reversed by a single hormone. Human growth hormone (HGH) is an example of a product that has been marketed to slow aging. HGH is produced naturally in the body and reaches its peak in the 20s and then declines at a rate of about 14 percent per decade. HGH is a powerful chemical and should be administered only under medical advice. In fact, it is against federal law to administer HGH for anti-aging purposes.

Noni is one of many names for a fruit that grows on small trees in the Pacific Islands. The noni tree yields a fruit that is high in vitamins and minerals. Because its taste is disagreeable, it is usually processed into juice, significantly lessening its nutritional value. The juice has been touted in "health food" stores as an anti-aging supplement. The claims have not been scientifically demonstrated, and the Food and Drug Administration has sent warning letters to noni juice marketers about making unjustified claims. Noni juice is only one of many products promoted for anti-aging properties.

Home Genetic Tests

In 2006, the FDA, the Federal Trade Commission (FTC), and the Centers for Disease Control and Prevention (CDC) alerted consumers about direct-to-consumer marketing of genetic tests. These tests were marketed to examine genes and DNA to identify particular diseases and disorders. Some companies claim their tests can screen for diseases and disorders, such as heart disease, cancer, diabetes, or Alzheimer's. Some claim to be able to evaluate individual health risks, while others use the results to suggest treatments. Some genetic testing products are marketed with the claim that they can assess a person's ability to withstand certain environmental exposures, like particular toxins or cigarette smoke. The consumer should be skeptical of these claims. There is a lack of scientific studies that prove these tests give accurate results (FTC, 2006).

Some companies may also claim that a person can protect against serious disease by choosing special foods and nutritional supplements. Consequently, the results of their at-home genetics tests often include dietary advice that rarely goes beyond the standard sensible dietary recommendations. Some use the results as marketing tools, offering "customized" dietary supplements. The FDA and CDC say they know of no valid scientific studies showing that genetic tests can be used safely or effectively to recommend nutritional choices.

Recently, some companies have claimed their at-home tests can give information about how a person's body will respond to a certain treatment, and how well people will respond to a particular drug. This claim originated from current medical research that shows differences in drug effectiveness based on genetic makeup. While these tests may provide some information your doctor needs or uses to make treatment decisions for a specific condition, they are not a substitute for a physician's judgment and clinical experience.

Home genetics tests are not a substitute for a medical checkup. According to the FDA, which regulates the manufacturers of genetic tests, and the CDC, which promotes health and quality of life, some of these tests lack scientific validity, and others provide medical results that are meaningful only in the context of a full medical evaluation. The FDA and CDC say that because of the complexities involved in the testing and interpreting the results, genetic tests should be performed in a specialized laboratory and the results should be interpreted by a doctor or trained counselor who understands the value of genetic testing for a particular situation (FTC, 2006).

Even the most sophisticated genetics tests sample only a few of the more than 20,000 genes in the human body. According to the FTC (2006),

A positive result means that the testing laboratory found unusual characteristics or changes in the genes it tested. Depending on the purpose of the test, a positive result may confirm a diagnosis, identify an increased risk of developing a disease, or indicate that a person is a carrier for a particular disease. It does not necessarily mean that a disease will develop, or if it does, that the disease will be progressive or severe. A negative result means that the laboratory found no unusual characteristics or changes in the genes it tested. This could mean that a person doesn't have a particular disease, doesn't have an increased risk of developing the disease, or isn't a carrier of the disease. Or it could mean that the test missed the specific genetic changes associated with a particular disease. In short, the FDA and CDC say that genetic testing provides only one piece of information about a person's susceptibility to disease. Other factors, like family background, medical history, and environment, also contribute to the likelihood of getting a particular disease. In most cases, genetic testing makes the most sense when it is part of a physical exam that includes a patient's family background and medical history.

This lack of "black-and-white" results emphasizes the inability of the average person to interpret the results and reinforces the importance of professional counseling and interpretation.

Home tests are not as sensitive or as accurate as those in these specialized labs. One of the real risks is that a person may receive an incorrect result from a home genetics test and conclude that he or she is doomed to a life of suffering or even death at a young age. It is easy to imagine a person deciding not to have children to avoid passing on the alleged genetic risk, making arrangements for his or her imminent death, or even becoming depressed to the point of suicide.

Consumers should keep in mind that, while most other home-use medical tests undergo FDA review to provide a reasonable assurance of their safety and effectiveness, no at-home genetic tests have been reviewed by the FDA, and the FDA has not evaluated the accuracy of their claims. In 2010, drug retailer Walgreens retreated from a plan to carry genetic test kits. The FDA announced an investigation of the test manufacturer, Pathway Genomics, for marketing a medical product without the agency's approval.

Yet another problem with the use of home genetics tests is the fact that some companies post the results online. If the Web site is not secure, your information may be seen by others. Before you do business with any company online, check the privacy policy to see how they may use your personal information and whether they share customer information with marketers.

Combating Health Fraud

Consumers can fight health fraud by being informed. Statements that suggest a product is a quick and effective cure-all or diagnostic tool for a variety of ailments should be viewed with skepticism. Promotions using undocumented case histories or testimonials are always suspect to the wise consumer. Promotions that claim to be a "scientific break-through," an "ancient remedy," or a "miraculous cure" are probably not worth your time. Consumers should be cynical of products said to contain a "secret ingredient." Why would a marketer keep an ingredient secret if it were really effective? Promises of money-back guarantees are often empty; do not expect your money back if you are not satisfied.

The consumer should know the name, address, and telephone number of the business. While e-mail addresses can be useful, beware of sellers who provide only an e-mail address or Web site URL. Often, Internet bandits try to hide their real names and addresses. If you are even mildly suspicious, ask for references and check them.

Be especially careful about purchasing over the World Wide Web. Spammers send out millions of e-mails, hoping to lure a few people into a **pyramid scheme**, obtain credit card information, or gather personal information. Personal information can easily be used to steal your identity. Protect credit card information by using only Web companies that you know, and never give personal information over the Internet. See Chapter 1 for further information about Internet shopping.

Good consumers report fraudulent practices. The Federal Trade Commission regulates advertising and investigates possible fraudulent advertising. The Food and Drug Administration has the power to penalize companies that sell bogus products. The U.S. Postal Service can arrest and charge people who commit health fraud using the mail. State and local attorneys general investigate and prosecute fraud. However, none of these agencies can do their work adequately without information from the public. By reporting health fraud and quackery, individuals protect others.

REPORTING HEALTH FRAUD

Medicare and Medicaid

You may contact the Office of Inspector General on a hotline that offers a confidential means for reporting information. The hotline may be contacted as follows:

Phone: 1-800-447-8477
Fax: 1-800-223-2164 (10 pages maximum)
E-mail: HHSTips@oig.hhs.gov
Mail: Office of the Inspector General
        HHS TIPS Hotline
        P.O. Box 23489
        Washington, DC 20026

Since Medicaid is a state and federal program, it is recommended that you contact a state office as well as the Inspector General's hotline. A list of state contacts can be found at http://www.cms.gov/apps/contacts.

Mail Fraud

If you think you have been a victim of mail fraud, you may fill out a complaint at https://postalinspectors.uspis.gov/forms/MailFraudComplaint.aspx.

Food and Drug Administration

Report suspected criminal activity related to an FDA-regulated product at http://www.accessdata .fda.gov/scripts/email/oc/oci/contact.cfm.

Report unlawful sales of medical products on the Internet at http://www.accessdata.fda.gov /scripts/email/oc/buyonline/buyonlineform.cfm or

Phone: 1-800-332-1088
Fax: 1-800-332-1078
Mail: MedWatch
        5600 Fishers Lane
        Rockville, MD 20857

Report e-mails promoting medical products you think might be illegal to webcomplaints@ora .fda.gov.

Insurance Fraud

If you suspect that a provider has charged you for services you did not receive, billed you more than once for the same service, or misrepresented any information, or if you suspect other insurance fraud, report it to the office of your state insurance commissioner. If the problem is not resolved, report it to the Health Care Fraud Hotline of the U.S. Office of Personnel Management at 1-202-418-3300.

Other Issues

The Consumer Affairs division of your state attorney general's office will take complaints and reports.

SUMMARY

Unscrupulous individuals often attempt to take advantage of others for profit. This usually takes the form of fraud, including health fraud and insurance fraud.

Products and services of little value are sold by using testimonials, half-truths, and spurious claims. Purveyors of quackery are especially skilled at duping unwary customers. Consumers would be wise to check the authenticity and value of health-related products and report to authorities instances when they suspect fraud.

When the fraud involves insurance, it results in shared loss. Customers of private insurers see their costs go up, and government-sponsored insurance must raise premiums and copayments or increase taxes to cover losses. There are a number of practices used to defraud insurers; patients can assist in identifying these practices and reporting their use.

Weight loss, fitness, HIV/AIDS, arthritis, cancer, sexual problems, influenza, diabetes, and aging are among the most prominent target areas of scammers and crooks. Consumers should be skeptical about claims made by those who would try to profit from the misfortune of others.

KEY TERMS

Alternative treatment: treatment methods that have not been verified by unbiased clinical trials

Copayment: a flat fee paid by an insured person to supplement insurance costs every time he or she receives a medical service

Deductible: a fixed amount of medical expenses one must pay before health insurance starts to pay for services

Fraud: an intentional act perpetrated to be deceptive in order to gain something of value

Half-truths: deceptive statements that contain some element of truth but are partly false

Health care fraud: an intentional deception or misrepresentation that an individual or entity makes knowing that the misrepresentation could result in some unauthorized benefit to the individual, or to the entity, or to some third party

Health fraud: services or articles of unproven effectiveness that are promoted to improve health, well-being, or appearance

Infomercial: a broadcast advertisement filling an entire program slot

Placebo effect: a positive response to a product, device, or procedure that cannot be accounted for by pharmacologic or other direct physical action

Premiums: the amount a person and/or employer pays for insurance coverage

Pyramid scheme: a fraudulent scheme in which people are recruited to make payments to others above them in a hierarchy while expecting to receive payments from people recruited below them

Quackery: promotion of health practices or remedies that have no compelling scientific basis

Regression fallacy: failure to recognize that health conditions change without treatment and ascribing changes in conditions to some therapy

Testimonial: a written or spoken statement by a person purported to have used a product or service extolling the virtues of the product or service

STUDY QUESTIONS

1. Why should consumers give little credence to testimonials?
2. How is the word "natural" misused in marketing?
3. Why should consumers view money-back guarantees for health products with skepticism?
4. How can consumers check on the authenticity of a product?
5. How is quackery practiced?
6. What are some reasons that people think ineffective therapies work?
7. How is health care fraud committed?
8. How does health care fraud affect the cost of health care?
9. How can individuals prevent health care fraud?
10. How can people identify fitness programs and equipment that best fit their needs?
11. What would lead you to believe that an HIV/AIDS, cancer, diabetes, or arthritis treatment is fraudulent?

REFERENCES

Beyerstein, B. L. (1997). *Why bogus therapies seem to work.* Retrieved from http://www.csicop.org/si/show/why_bogus_therapies_seem_to_work

Federal Trade Commission. (2000, June 29). "Operation Cure.all" nets shark cartilage promoters: Two companies charged with making false and unsubstantiated claims for their shark cartilage and skin cream as cancer treatments. FTC news release.

Federal Trade Commission. (2003a). *Avoiding the muscle hustle: Tips for buying exercise equipment.* Retrieved from http://www.ftc.gov/bcp/conline/pubs/alerts/musclealrt.htm

Federal Trade Commission. (2003b). *Pump fiction: Tips for buying exercise equipment.* Retrieved from http://www.ftc.gov/bcp/edu/pubs/consumer/products/pro10.shtm

Federal Trade Commission. (2006). *At-home genetics tests: A healthy dose of skepticism may be the best prescription.* Retrieved from http://www.ftc.gov/bcp/edu/pubs/consumer/health/hea02.shtm

Food Marketing Institute. (2008). *Natural and organic foods: Executive summary.* Retrieved from http://www.fda.gov/ohrms/dockets/dockets/06p0094/06p-0094-cp00001-05-Tab-04-Food-Marketing-Institute-vol1.pdf

Green, S. (1992). "Antineoplastons": An unproved cancer therapy. *Journal of the American Medical Association, 267*(21), 2924–2928.

Jacobs, A. (2010, October 6). Rampant fraud threat to China's brisk ascent. *New York Times.*

Kurtzweil, P. (1999). How to spot health fraud. *FDA Consumer Magazine.* Retrieved from http://www.fda.gov/fdac/features/1999/699_fraud.html

National Health Care Anti-Fraud Association. (2008). *The problem of health care fraud.* Retrieved from http://www.nhcaa.org/eweb/DynamicPage.aspx?webcode=anti_fraud_resource_centr&wpscode=TheProblemOfHCFraud

National Institute on Aging, U.S. Department of Health and Human Services. (2008). *Health quackery: Spotting health scams.* Retrieved from http://www.nia.nih.gov/HealthInformation/Publications/quackery.htm

U.S. Food and Drug Administration. (2006a). *List of firms receiving warning letters for marketing unproven dietary supplements for diabetes with illegal drug claims.* Retrieved from http://www.cfsan.fda.gov/~dms/dialist.html

U.S. Food and Drug Administration. (2006b). *Cracking down on health fraud.* Retrieved from http://www.fda.gov/fdac/features/2006/606_fraud.htm

Health Insurance

Chapter 4

Chapter Objectives

The student will:

- Explain how group health insurance reduces insurance costs.
- Discuss factors that affect access to health insurance, costs, and the type of plan chosen by an individual or family.
- Explain traditional indemnity insurance.
- Explain the different models of health maintenance organizations.
- Compare and contrast health maintenance organizations, preferred provider organizations, and point-of-service plans.
- Explain COBRA.
- Explain Medicare, Medicaid, and SCHIPs.
- Compare and contrast the various types of supplemental insurance.
- Contrast health savings accounts, health reimbursement accounts, and flexible savings accounts.
- Explain the substantive changes in health insurance that will take place as a result of the Health Care and Education Reform Act and the Patient Protection and Affordable Care Act.

Health insurance began in earnest in the United States during the 1930s with Blue Cross offering prepaid hospitalization. Soon, physicians formed Blue Shield. Advances in health care and their higher costs served as the impetus to the development of health insurance. Commercial insurance companies, observing the success of Blue Cross and Blue Shield, soon began offering **group plans** for health insurance. With the costs associated with health care consistently rising, the role of health insurance has steadily grown. Recall from Chapter 2 that about 70 percent of payments for health care are currently made through some type of insurance.

Health insurance is an evolving entity. Until the early 1970s, most people had traditional **indemnity insurance**. These are now usually called **fee-for-service** plans. With the passage of the Health Maintenance Organization (HMO) Act (1973), the way that health care is delivered and health care providers are compensated changed dramatically. A marketplace of varying insurance products emerged following the passage of the act. While a number of options for health care are available, no single type is better for all people. Individuals in the market for insurance should look at their families' needs and preferences and the costs associated with various options.

The U.S. Census Bureau (DeNavas-Walt, Proctor, & Smith, 2010) estimated that 55.8 percent of Americans get health insurance through their employers, down from 58.5 percent in 2008. Others get it through various organizations, such as their professional organization. These are referred to as group plans because people in a designated group, usually a set of employees

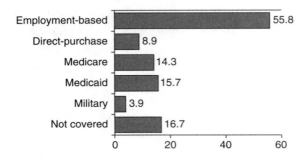

**FIGURE 4.1 PERCENT COVERAGE BY TYPE OF
HEALTH INSURANCE, 2009**

Source: DeNavas-Walt, C., Proctor, B, D., & Smith,
J. C. (2010). Income, poverty, and health insurance
coverage in the United States: 2009. Washington, DC:
U.S. Census Bureau.

Note: Estimates by type are not mutually exclusive; people
can be covered by more than one type of health insurance
during the year. Military care includes Tricare, Civilian and
Medical Program of the Department of Veterans Affairs
(CHAMPVA), and care provided by the Department of
Veterans Affairs and the military.

Health Reform — 2010

In March 2010, President Obama signed the
Health Care and Education Reconciliation Act.
This act made some changes to the Patient
Protection and Affordable Care Act that had
been signed into law a few days before. While
touted as health care reform, the law is largely
a reform of health insurance. This legislation
was the culmination of decades of attempts to
change the way health care is delivered and paid
for in the United States. The box demonstrates
the history of changes and attempts to change
health insurance.

Almost 50.7 million Americans were with-
out health insurance in 2009 (DeNavas-Walt,
Proctor, & Smith, 2010), prior to passage of the
HCERA/PPACA. According to the Congressional

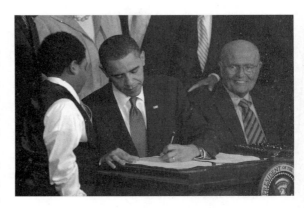

President Barack Obama signing historic health care
reform legislation in 2010.

of a particular employer, can purchase health
insurance at lower **premiums**, or payments, for
the coverage than individuals or families could
negotiate. The group plans bring down costs
because more people share the risk, thus lowering
premiums. This, in turn, reduces the costs for the
average individual or family.

People who are unemployed or whose employers
do not provide group health insurance must often
purchase insurance on the open market. This is usually quite expensive. See Figure 4.1 for information
about the health insurance status of Americans.

HISTORY OF HEALTH CARE REFORM

The landmark Patient Protection and Affordable Care Act, signed into law in March 2010,
capped a long and arduous process to reform the health care and health insurance systems in the
United States. Several attempts preceded the passage of the act.

- During the early 1900s, the Progressive Era, President Theodore Roosevelt supported
  health insurance, but most of the initiative for reform took place outside of government.
- In 1912, after campaigning on a promise of national health insurance, Theodore
  Roosevelt was defeated in the presidential election.
- In 1929, Baylor Hospital in Dallas created what is thought to be the first example of
  modern health insurance by providing prepaid coverage for members of a teachers union.

- In 1931, Dr. Michael Abraham Shadid of Enid, Oklahoma, formed a comprehensive health care service in which members paid a flat fee that is independent of the amount of care they receive. This is believed to be the first health maintenance organization.
- In 1932, the Wilbur Commission recommended that group medical practices and group repayment systems be expanded to assist the millions of people who did not have access to adequate health care.
- In 1938, early insurance plans, while omitting coverage for those older than age 66 and the unemployed, advertised premiums of "under 3 cents a day for hospital care."
- In 1939, the National Health Act gave general support for a national health program to be funded by federal grants to the states. However, the 1938 election had brought a revival of conservatism that doomed most social policy change.
- In 1943, the Wagner-Murray-Dingell Bill was first introduced. It called for compulsory national health insurance and a payroll tax. Opposition was strong. It was compared to communism and, despite being introduced in every session for 14 years, the bill never passed.
- In 1945, newly elected President Harry S. Truman released a 10-year plan that included compulsory coverage, more hospital construction, and doubling the number of physicians and nurses. Due to opposition from the American Medical Association and references to "socialized medicine" at a time when anticommunism sentiment was high, at the beginning of the Cold War, the plan went nowhere in Congress.
- In 1946, Congress passed the Hospital Survey and Construction Act, better known as the Hill-Burton Act, which provided for construction of large health care delivery facilities, especially in rural areas. The act provided the basis for hospital regulation. It also required hospitals to provide charity care and forbade discrimination on the basis of race, religion, or nationality.
- By 1951, 77 million Americans had purchased accident or sickness insurance.
- In 1954, the Internal Revenue Act provided exemptions from income taxes for certain employee benefits, including pensions and health insurance.
- In 1960, Congress passed the Kerr-Mills Act, giving states federal grants to cover health care costs for the elderly poor. By 1963, Kerr-Mills had proved ineffective when only 28 states had chosen to participate and many of them had not budgeted sufficiently.
- In a televised 1962 address, President John F. Kennedy promoted health insurance for Social Security recipients, an idea that made little headway in Congress due to the lobbying of the medical community.
- On July 31, 1965, President Lyndon B. Johnson signed into law a bill that established Titles XVIII and XIX of the Social Security Act, the Medicare and Medicaid programs to provide health care for those older than 65, the blind, the disabled, and the poor.
- During the presidential campaign in 1971, competing health care plans were introduced by President Richard M. Nixon and Senator Edward M. Kennedy. This was the beginning of Kennedy's decades-long attempt to reform the health care system.
- In 1972, President Nixon signed the Social Security Amendments. The amendments established professional standards review organizations (PSROs) to review Medicare patient care for evaluation purposes.
- In 1973, President Nixon signed the Health Maintenance Organization Act into law. The act provided for $375 million to fund demonstration projects.

(continues)

- In 1974, Congress exempted large corporations' self-insurance programs from state regulation by passing the Employee Retirement Income Security Act (ERISA).
- In 1975, the National Health Planning and Resources Development Act was signed by President Gerald R. Ford, mandating the establishment of health systems agencies (HSAs) across the country. The major intent of the law was to provide local direction and control of health care planning.
- With the passage of Medicare and Medicaid to provide an organized system of funding, HSAs to control planning, HMOs to deliver services, and PSROs to provide evaluation, the major elements of a national health care system were in place. However, no unifying legislation was ever passed.
- In 1976, President Jimmy Carter called for a comprehensive national health insurance system with mandatory and universal coverage. Recession relegated health insurance to a very low legislative priority level.
- In 1986, Congress passed the Consolidated Omnibus Budget Reconciliation Act (COBRA), which contained a provision that allows employees to continue their group health insurance plans for up to 18 months after losing their jobs. COBRA contained the Emergency Medical Treatment and Labor Act, which required hospitals participating in Medicare and operating active emergency rooms to provide appropriate medical screenings and stabilizing treatments.
- In 1988, President Ronald Reagan signed into law the Medicare Catastrophic Coverage Act. The law set ceilings on Medicare patients' payments for hospitalization, physician fees, and prescription drugs, but it required the entire funding to come from Medicare beneficiaries in the form of surcharges. A retrenchment of this magnitude is unprecedented in postwar social welfare policy. Though the bill was repealed in 1989, the experience also appears to have soured Congress toward enacting further increases in Medicare benefits for elderly and disabled beneficiaries (Rice, Desmond, & Gabel, 1990).
- In 1993, President Bill Clinton appointed his wife, Hillary Rodham Clinton, to head a task force to develop a plan to provide universal health care coverage in which insurance companies would compete in a highly regulated market. The resulting legislation, the Health Security Act, was defeated in Congress the next year.
- In 1996, the Health Insurance Portability and Accountability Act was passed. HIPAA prohibits employment discrimination based on health status, sets standards for the privacy of medical records, and protects people in group health insurance plans from being excluded based on preexisting conditions.
- In 1997, President Clinton signed into law Title XXI of the Social Security Act, the State Children's Health Insurance Program (SCHIP), which provides health insurance to millions of children.
- In 2003, President George W. Bush signed the Medicare Modernization Act. The act established prescription medication coverage (Part D) for Medicare beneficiaries.
- In November 2008, Barack Obama was elected president. The hallmark of his campaign was a pledge to reform the health care system, including a "public option," a government option for providing health insurance.
- In March 2010, Congress passed and President Obama signed into law the Patient Protection and Affordable Care Act.

Budget Office, when the provisions of the legislation are implemented, 32.5 million will have
gained coverage. About 92 percent of the population that is not eligible for Medicare will be
able to get coverage, compared with 81 percent
before implementation. By 2019, enrollment
in Medicaid and the State Children's Health
Insurance Program will reach 82.2 million (Sisko
et al., 2010). Many of the provisions of the law

will not go into effect until 2014 or later. It is
important to note that before the total implementation of the law, certain provisions may be
changed or eliminated by Congress or challenged
in court by individuals, businesses, and states.
Many of the provisions will go into effect within
months of signing and others take effect in 2011.
See the box below for some of these "immediate"
changes.

"IMMEDIATE" EFFECTS OF THE PATIENT PROTECTION AND AFFORDABLE CARE ACT OF 2010

- Small businesses may receive tax credits of up to 35 percent of premiums to make cover-age more affordable. (Beginning in 2014, the small business tax credits will increase to 50 percent of premiums.)
- New health plans in all markets and grandfathered plans are prohibited from denying coverage to children with preexisting conditions. (Starting in 2014, the prohibition will be extended to all persons.)
- A temporary subsidized high-risk pool provides access to affordable insurance for those who are uninsured because of a preexisting condition.
- Insurance companies are prohibited from dropping coverage of people who get sick and need the benefits.
- A $250 rebate is provided to Medicare prescription drug beneficiaries who hit the "donut hole" (see discussion of Medicare later in the chapter) in 2010. After that, they will receive a pharmaceutical manufacturers' discount of 50 percent on brand-name drugs, increasing to a 75 percent discount on brand-name and generic drugs. The "donut hole" will be closed completely by 2020.
- New health plans and certain grandfathered plans are required to allow people younger than 26 to remain on their parents' policy.
- A temporary insurance program helps offset the costs of premiums for employers and retirees for health benefits for retirees ages 55–54.
- Health insurance companies are banned from placing lifetime caps on coverage.
- The use of annual limits is restricted to ensure access to needed care in all new plans and grandfathered group health plans. The Secretary of Health and Human Services will define the restrictions. (Beginning in 2014, annual limits will be prohibited for all new plans and grandfathered group health plans.)
- Health insurance companies are banned from establishing eligibility rules for coverage that have the effect of discriminating in favor of those earning higher wages.
- A grant program supports states in requiring health insurance companies to submit justifi-cation for all requested premium increases. Insurance companies with excess or unjustified premium exchanges may not be able to participate in health insurance exchanges.

Sources: The White House. (2010). *Key provisions of health reform that take effect immediately.* Retrieved from http://www.whitehouse.gov/healthreform/immediate-benefits.

Democratic Policy Committee. (2010). *The Patient Protection and Affordable Care Act: Implementation timeline.* Retrieved from http://dpc.senate.gov/healthreformbill65.pdf

Exchanges

One of the primary features of the HCERA/ PPACA is the provision that requires the development of health insurance **exchanges** by 2014. The purpose of exchanges is to provide help to people who work for small businesses that cannot afford to contract for a group plan and for individuals who might purchase insurance on their own. Under the legislation, each state sets up its own health insurance exchange. Each exchange is a marketplace of plans, making it possible for consumers to compare the plans for cost and coverage options.

People who cannot afford the insurance offered on the exchange can get subsidies to cover part of the cost. Subsidies will be available for families with incomes up to 400 percent of the federal poverty level. Families with incomes up to 133 percent of the poverty level will be eligible for Medicaid, a federal-state program for low-income citizens. Childless adults, formerly excluded from Medicaid, may enroll beginning in 2014. There are caps on out-of-pocket expenses. The caps are $11,900 per year per family and $5,900 per year for individuals; these amounts are likely to change over time.

Another feature of the legislation is the requirement that every citizen buy insurance, either through an exchange or through employers. Failure to do so would result in a fine payable to the Internal Revenue Service. There is some doubt that the fines will be high enough to motivate all people to purchase health insurance.

The cost of group health insurance has been prohibitive for many small businesses. The HCERA/PPACA offers tax credits of up to 35 percent of the cost of insurance premiums to small businesses if they offer insurance for employees. Beginning in 2014, the tax credit jumps to 50 percent of premiums.

The Congressional Budget Office (2010) estimates that 24 million people will purchase coverage through exchanges. Sisko et al. (2010) estimate that by 2019, 30.6 million people will be enrolled in exchanges. Another 16 million will enroll in Medicaid.

Fairness in Coverage: Toward Universality

Before implementation of the HCERA/PPACA, insurance companies could refuse coverage based on a person's medical history. They also charged vastly higher prices to people with **preexisting conditions**. Some insurers even deny coverage to victims of domestic violence. Soon after passage of the law, insurance companies were forbidden from denying coverage to children with preexisting conditions. The law also provides immediate relief for uninsured Americans with preexisting conditions who are on the verge of bankruptcy due to their health care costs. In 2014, insurance companies will be barred from denying coverage to people with preexisting conditions. Until then, those people will have access to a temporary "high-risk pool" of insurance plans, although the coverage is not as comprehensive.

Before passage of HCERA/PPACA, insurance companies usually set age limits on children of insured parents. Often, these young adults could not be covered under their parents' plans unless they were enrolled in college full-time and were still subject to age limitations. The new law requires that young people be allowed to stay on their parents' insurance until age 26. This applies to all new plans and some existing plans.

Employers with more than 50 workers are required to offer insurance. Failure to do so will

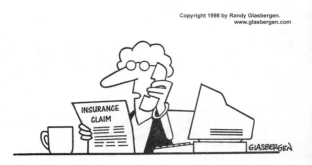

Copyright 1998 by Randy Glasbergen.
www.glasbergen.com

"Breakable bones, a tendency to bleed when cut, vulnerability to germs and viruses. These are all preexisting conditions."

Source: © Randy Glasbergen, used with permission from www.glasbergen.com.

result in a fine of $2,000 per employee if any of their employees get the federal subsidies to buy their own coverage. Since this amount is far less than the premium an employer would pay, it is questionable that it will serve as incentive for large companies to provide group insurance. For most people who get their health insurance through their work, there will be very little change.

The HCERA/PPACA mandates that U.S. citizens and legal residents be covered by some form of health insurance. Those without coverage will pay a tax penalty that will top out at 2.5 percent of household income. These penalties, coupled with those placed on employers, and the incentives, are efforts to reach universal coverage.

Before implementation of the HCERA/PPACA, insurance companies were free to drop people from coverage once they got sick. This practice is called **rescission** and the HCERA/PPACA bans the practice. Lifetime limits on the amount of medical care the insurer would pay are also forbidden. Annual limits are also tightly restricted under the law. These provisions take place immediately.

The HCERA/PPACA provides help for early retirees. For retired persons ages 55–64, there is a temporary reinsurance program to offset the cost of expensive premiums for employers and retirees. After 2014, when the exchanges are established, the reinsurance program will disappear.

It makes little difference that a person has health insurance if he or she does not have access to primary health care. Currently, 65 million Americans live in communities where they cannot easily access a primary care provider.

The HCERA/PPACA invests in scholarship and loan repayment programs through the National Health Service Corps to expand the health care workforce. It includes incentives for primary care practitioners to practice in underserved areas. **Primary care physicians** and general surgeons who practice in health professional shortage areas can receive a 10 percent bonus payment.

Cutting Costs

The HCERA/PPACA requires new private insurance plans to cover preventive health services, including vaccinations, with no **copayments** or **deductibles**. It also eliminates copayments for preventive services and deductibles under Medicare. The law provides new, free annual wellness visits that include physical examinations. It also helps provide individuals with the information they need to make healthy decisions, improves education on disease prevention and public health, and invests in a national prevention and public health strategy. By emphasizing preventive services and diagnosing health problems early, the use of expensive treatments should be reduced over the years, thus cutting overall costs.

States will require health insurance companies to submit justification for all requested premium increases. Insurance companies with excessive or unjustified premiums may not be allowed to participate in the health insurance exchanges.

One of the many reasons for the rapid growth of health care spending is misuse and fraud. The HCERA/PPACA provides several tools to reduce fraud (see box).

HOW THE PATIENT PROTECTION AND AFFORDABLE CARE ACT FIGHTS FRAUD

The Affordable Care Act will improve and expand consumer protections, strengthen Medicare, and reduce health care costs. One important way it achieves these goals is by improving government-wide efforts to fight fraud and waste. The new law contains some critical new tools to improve and enhance the administration's efforts to prevent, detect, and take strong enforcement action against fraud in Medicare, Medicaid, and the Children's Health Insurance Program, as well as private insurance. The new law contains:

(continues)

Tough new rules and sentences for criminals: The Affordable Care Act directs the Sentencing Commission to increase the federal sentencing guidelines for health care fraud offenses by 20 to 50 percent for crimes that involve more than $1,000,000 in losses. The law makes obstructing a fraud investigation a crime and makes it easier for the government to recapture any funds acquired through fraudulent practices. And the law makes it easier for the Department of Justice (DOJ) to investigate potential fraud or wrongdoing at facilities like nursing homes.

Enhanced screening and other enrollment requirements: The Affordable Care Act provides critical tools for fraud prevention, including new authorities for stepped-up oversight of providers and suppliers participating or enrolling in Medicare, Medicaid, and CHIP such as mandatory licensure checks. Based on the level of risk of fraud, waste, and abuse, providers could be subject to fingerprinting, site visits, and criminal background checks before they begin billing Medicare, Medicaid, or CHIP. The act also allows the Secretary of Health and Human Services to prohibit new providers from joining the program when necessary to prevent or combat fraud, waste or abuse. The law also allows the secretary to withhold payment to any Medicare or Medicaid providers if a credible allegation of fraud has been made and an investigation is pending.

New resources to fight fraud: The Affordable Care Act provides an additional $350 million over the next 10 years to help fight fraud through the Health Care Fraud and Abuse Control account from fiscal years 2011 through 2020. The act also allows these funds to support the hiring of new officials and agents that can help prevent and identify fraud.

Sharing data to fight fraud: Building on the Obama administration initiatives, the law requires the secretary to expand the Centers for Medicare and Medicaid Services' integrated data repository to include information from Medicaid, the Veterans Administration, the Department of Defense, Social Security Disability Insurance, and the Indian Health Service, and it enhances data-matching agreements among federal agencies. These agreements will make it easier for the federal government to share data, identify criminals, and prevent fraud. The DOJ and the Office of Inspector General (OIG) both receive clearer rights to access Centers for Medicare and Medicaid Services claims and payment databases. The secretary also now has authority to require states to report additional Medicaid data elements with respect to program integrity, program oversight, and administration.

New tools to prevent fraud: The Affordable Care Act requires providers and suppliers to establish plans detailing how they will follow the rules and prevent fraud as a condition of enrollment in Medicare, Medicaid, or CHIP. Other prevention provisions focus on high fraud-risk providers and suppliers including durable medical equipment suppliers, home health agencies, and community mental health centers (CMHCs). For example, CMHCs will now be required to serve at least 40 percent non-Medicare beneficiaries to crack down on centers that bill Medicare but are not legitimate CMHCs.

The bill also strengthens the government's authority to require surety bonds as a condition of doing business with Medicare. To crack down on fraud in orders and referrals, providers and suppliers who order or refer certain items or services for Medicare beneficiaries will be required to enroll in Medicare and maintain documentation on orders and referrals.

Expanded overpayment recovery efforts: The secretary of HHS is provided new authorities to identify and recover overpayments to Medicaid, Medicare Advantage, and Part D (the Medicare drug benefit) through expansion of the Recovery Audit Contractors program. Providers, suppliers, Medicare Advantage plans, and Part D plans must self-report and return Medicare and Medicaid overpayments within 60 days of identification.

Enhanced penalties to deter fraud and abuse: The Affordable Care Act provides the OIG with the authority to impose stronger civil and monetary penalties on those found to have committed fraud. The secretary also is provided new authority to prevent providers from participating in Medicare or Medicaid. For example, the secretary may exclude providers and suppliers for providing false information on an application to enroll or participate in a federal health care program. Individuals who order or prescribe an item or service while being excluded from a federal health care program, individuals who make false statements on applications or contracts to participate in a federal health care program, and providers who identify a Medicare overpayment and do not return it are also subject to strict new fines and penalties under the new law. Finally, the law ensures that states may terminate a provider under Medicaid if a provider is terminated under Medicare or another state Medicaid program.

Greater oversight of private insurance abuses: The new law provides enhanced tools and authorities to address abuses of multiple employer welfare arrangements and protect employers and employees from insurance scams. It also gives new powers to the secretary and inspector general to investigate and audit the health insurance exchanges. This, plus the new rules to ensure accountability in the insurance industry, will protect consumers and increase the affordability of health care.

Source: U.S. Department of Health and Human Services. (2010). *The Affordable Care Act: New tools to fight fraud, strengthen medicare and protect taxpayer dollars.* Retrieved from http://www.healthreform.gov/affordablecareact_summary.html

The HCERA/PPACA is estimated to cost about $940 billion over 10 years. However, it is estimated to reduce the federal deficit by about $138 billion over the first 10 years and $1.2 trillion in the second 10 years (Elmendorf, 2010). In addition, the law adds at least nine years to the solvency of the Medicare Hospital Insurance Trust Fund.

Selecting a Health Insurance Plan

Before choosing a health insurance plan, whether through employer-sponsored programs, exchanges, or individual purchase, consumers should consider their own needs, values, and risk tolerance. They should consider whether family members suffer from chronic health conditions or disabilities. These are things that insurance companies call preexisting conditions, and they may affect the size of the premium or, in some cases, access to coverage at all. Discrimination on the basis of preexisting conditions will be outlawed under HCERA/PPACA. Consider whether you or members of your family work or otherwise engage in activities that would put you at risk for serious

injury or if you travel a lot. You should think about changes that may occur in the near future, such as having children or retiring. You should also decide how comprehensive you need your coverage to be. Many people find it important to be able to choose their doctors and health care facilities; these issues may affect the type of insurance you choose.

The process of selecting an insurance plan requires consumers to think about the coverage that they require. Some plans provide coverage for dental care, vision care, mental health counseling and treatment, and substance abuse treatment. Many provide for some alternative therapies, such as acupuncture and chiropractic. Consumers should consider the potential for needing home health care, nursing home coverage, or hospice care. Most people find it important to have insurance that covers basic health screenings such as Pap smears and mammograms. If you are of reproductive age, coverage for obstetrical and family planning services may be an important consideration for you. Recognizing your future needs can help you select your plan.

The financial components of the decision are very important. Consumers should think about how much they can spend on health insurance and how much they can afford to spend if their health insurance does not pay completely for services. It is important to know the limits of coverage options in case of a serious injury or major illness and if there are annual or lifetime limits. It is also important to understand how comfortable you are with filing claims, keeping records, and dealing with claims offices about financial issues.

When more than one family member is eligible to purchase health insurance, say from two group plans from two employers, they should discuss with their insurance coordinators the policies' **coordination of benefits**. This is a clause in an insurance policy that restricts the total amount paid out by each insurer when there are multiple policies.

Once the individual understands his or her needs and preferences and resolves financial questions, he or she can begin comparing health insurance plans. Employers who offer group plans usually provide a side-by-side comparison of the features of the plans. Exchanges are expected to do so. However, people purchasing policies on their own will have to do more in-depth analysis of the components of various plans.

Traditional Health Insurance

For many years, the indemnity or fee-for-service plan was the norm. For most people, it was the only option. Policy holders pay a monthly premium with rates that vary depending on factors such as whether coverage is for an individual, couple, or family with children, or if any of the insured has a preexisting medical condition.

In indemnity plans, you pay the doctor or hospital and then submit a claim for reimbursement. You must pay a fixed amount of your medical expenses before your health insurance starts to pay. This amount is called the deductible. Usually, there is a fixed amount that you pay each year before reaching your deductible. Fee-for-service coverage means that there is a charge for each individual service that is provided.

Under this type of coverage, the subscriber (patient) has complete autonomy in choosing doctors, hospitals, and other health care providers, so long as they accept the insurance. Patients even refer themselves to specialists without getting permission, and the insurance company does not get to decide whether the visit is necessary. There are some exceptions. For instance, a person who is not incapacitated may need approval from the insurer to visit an emergency room; otherwise, the insurer may not pay the bill.

In addition to the deductible, there may be **coinsurance**, the amount you are required to pay for medical care after you have met the deductible. For example, the insurance company may pay 80 percent of the claim while the subscriber pays 20 percent. For this reason, fee-for-service plans can result in high out-of-pocket expenses. Fee-for-service plans often include a maximum for out-of-pocket expenses, after which the insurance company will pay 100 percent of all costs. The maximum can be quite high. In addition, indemnity plans often have **lifetime limits** on benefits paid. For example, a plan may contain a lifetime limit of $1,000,000 for any covered individual. Under fee-for-service plans, insurers will only pay for "**reasonable, usual, and customary charges**." A charge is considered reasonable, usual, and customary if it conforms to the general prevailing cost of that service within your geographic area. Unfortunately for the consumer, it is the insurance company that computes this standard. Once it computes the reasonable, usual, and customary charges, the insurance company will determine how much it is willing to pay for the service. The individual must pay the difference if the provider charges more.

Traditionally, fee-for-service plans have not paid for preventive care such as annual checkups, pelvic exams, and health screening. However, some insurers are including them because accumulated evidence supports the concept that preventive care can prevent costly illnesses later, thus saving money in the long run.

Major medical plans have been a mainstay for young people who are not covered by a group plan. Under a major medical plan, the deductible is very high. This means that the insurance company incurs no cost unless the covered individual has a major health problem, such as a serious injury or cancer. After the deductible is met, the insurer usually pays 80 percent of costs and the insured pays the remainder. Young people often choose this type of plan because they are usually healthy and the premiums are relatively low.

Somewhat similar to the major medical plan, **catastrophic insurance** is a type of fee-for-service health insurance policy that is designed to give protection against momentous, tragic health occurrences. It is sometimes referred to as a **high-deductible health plan** because low monthly premiums are traded for a significantly higher deductible. This means that with this plan, routine doctor visits may not be covered or may be covered at lower rates and prescription costs are more expensive, but monthly premiums are lower, so the subscriber takes on more out-of-pocket expenses in exchange for lower premiums. If you are healthy and need few medical services, you save money, but if something catastrophic happens, you have coverage.

For some people, major medical and high-deductible health insurance plans may make sense. These are usually young, healthy people who do not have high medical bills. When combined with health savings accounts, discussed later in this chapter, high-deductible plans can allow families who are healthy to put money aside with tax benefits.

There are two basic types of catastrophic plan: comprehensive and supplemental. A comprehensive plan offers coverage comparable to more traditional health care plans. There is a high deductible and monthly fees are still relatively low, but they are higher than those in supplemental catastrophic plans. The advantage of a comprehensive plan is that you can be covered for emergency services, but at a lower monthly premium than a traditional plan. A supplemental plan acts as a complement to other insurance plans you might have. Medical appliances, nursing care, and psychiatric care might be included in the supplementary plan. In both types of catastrophic

insurance plans, once your deductible is met, the insurance company covers the major medical expenses it deems necessary, like hospital stays, surgeries, lab tests, and intensive care. Like in other insurance plans, elective procedures are not covered (Jeffries, 2010).

A person shopping for a fee-for-service health insurance plan should obtain the following information:

- Monthly premium and total yearly cost
- What is covered (e.g., prescription drugs, home care)
- Limits on coverage of hospital or home care days
- Coverage of preexisting conditions
- Amount of coinsurance and deductible
- Maximum out-of-pocket expense in a year
- Whether there is a lifetime maximum cap that the insurer will pay and, if so, what it is

Indemnity plans are regulated by state insurance commissions. The commission or the state health department can provide information about available plans.

Managed Care

Managed care is not a new concept. It has been around since the 1930s. The Health Maintenance Organization Act of 1973 provided a major impetus for managed care because it provided funding for health maintenance organizations, one of three types of managed care.

All managed care plans involve an agreement between the insurer and a network of health care providers. Policy holders are encouraged to use the providers in the network by the fact that the insurer will pay only for services delivered within the network or it will pay only a percentage of the cost of the care if received outside the network.

Health Maintenance Organizations

Health maintenance organizations come in two basic models—the closed or staff model and the open or individual practice association

(IPA) model. In the staff model, the HMO has central medical offices and clinics that, in some cases, it owns. The HMO employs the providers. In other words, the doctors and nurses work for the HMO as full- or part-time employees. Closed models are more likely to be associated with group plans than with individuals. In the IPA model, the HMO establishes a network of individual or group practices, including physicians and other providers, and hospitals, laboratories, and other facilities. The IPA results in fewer centralized locations for patients to seek medical care.

In HMOs, each patient has a primary care physician, usually the family physician, internist, pediatrician, or gynecologist. The PCP coordinates patient care. In order to see a specialist, you must get a referral from your PCP and you must see only the physicians approved by the HMO. In most cases, the PCP must get approval from the HMO before making the referral, so there is a risk that you may be denied medical care that you need. If you decide to see an out-of-network physician or go to a facility that is not in the network, the HMO will not pay for the charges. In emergency situations, if you are conscious and can pick up the phone, you generally must get clearance before you can visit an emergency room.

Many HMOs charge a copayment, a flat fee every time you receive a medical service. For example, you may make a copayment of $10 every time you see your PCP and $20 each time you visit a specialist. However, copayments and premiums are generally lower than those of traditional insurance and there is no deductible. In most cases, there is no lifetime limit of coverage. Another benefit of an HMO plan is the minimal paperwork they require.

Some HMOs have generated controversy, as in plans wherein doctors receive financial incentives for reducing the amount of medical services provided to patients. One method of doing this has been to pay doctors a fixed monthly fee for each patient, regardless of the treatment they need or receive.

Preferred Provider Organizations

Preferred provider organizations (PPOs) are similar to HMOs in many ways. While there is a network of providers, like in the HMO, the insured person may see any doctor. PPOs make arrangements for lower fees with a network of providers and give financial incentives to policy holders if they stay within the network. For example, a visit to an in-network provider might result in a copay of $10. However, if you go to an out-of-network provider, you would pay the entire bill up front and then submit the bill to your insurance company. The insurer might pay for an 80 percent reimbursement. In addition, you may have to meet a deductible before the insurer will pay anything. Exclusive provider organizations are PPOs that will pay nothing if you choose to visit a provider who is not in the network.

PPO subscribers may be allowed to refer themselves to an in-network specialist without getting advance approval. Many PPOs do not pay for preventive services.

PPOs are preferable for people who like the freedom to choose their own physicians and not be constrained by the limitations of a network.

Point of Service

Point-of-service (POS) plans have similarities to both HMOs and PPOs. Like the HMO, they use the PCP to coordinate patient care and to act as the gatekeeper to receiving care from a specialist. Like PPOs and HMOs, the POS has a network of doctors from which to choose.

If a patient goes out of the network, he or she may still receive some coverage. If a PCP refers the patient to a specialist who is not in the network, the plan usually covers most or all of the charges. Self-referral can be done, but it results in much cost and a good deal of paperwork.

POS plans usually cover preventive care services. They often cover workshops on nutrition and smoking cessation programs and may even provide discounts at health clubs.

In choosing from managed care plans, the consumer should attempt to ascertain the following information:

- The monthly premiums and total yearly costs
- Copayments
- Limits on surgery, mental health care, prescription drugs, home care, or other support
- The doctors and other health care professionals in the network
- The facilities and their proximity to home and workplace
- The ease of getting appointments and how far in advance routine visits must be scheduled
- The services offered, including preventive services
- Costs of using out-of-network providers
- The process for resolving member complaints

- The process used to review the qualifications of doctors before they are added to the plan
- The process of review of the performance of providers, including hospitals
- Accreditations, if any

Managed care plans are regulated by federal and state agencies. The office of the insurance commissioner in your state can usually provide information about the plans.

COBRA

Congress passed the landmark Consolidated Omnibus Budget Reconciliation Act health benefit provisions in 1986. According to the U.S. Department of Labor (2009), "COBRA provides certain former employees, retirees, spouses, former spouses, and dependent children the right to temporary continuation of health coverage at group rates. This coverage, however, is only

TABLE 4.1 COMPARISON OF DIFFERENT TYPES OF MANAGED CARE

Feature	HMO	PPO	POS
Patient chooses PCP as gatekeeper to coordinate care	Yes	No	Yes for services in the network but not for services outside the network
Referral needed to see specialist	Yes	Not if the specialist is in the network	Yes
Coverage for out-of-network providers	Usually not	Yes, but reimbursement is less in some	Yes, but there may be a deductible and a high copayment; no if referred by the PCP
Copayments	Yes	Yes	Minimal
Deductible	No	Some may have limited deductibles	Not for services in the network
Emergency treatment coverage	Yes, but there is a defined approval procedure, including notification of the HMO as soon as possible	Yes, but benefits may be reduced if member sees a doctor outside the network	Yes
Preventive care	Yes	Yes	Yes

available when coverage is lost due to certain specific events. Group health coverage for COBRA participants is usually more expensive than health coverage for active employees, since usually the employer pays a part of the premium for active employees while COBRA participants generally pay the entire premium themselves. It is ordinarily less expensive, though, than individual health coverage."

Private-sector group plans of employers with 20 or more employees and employees of state and local governments are subject to COBRA. An individual is considered qualified for COBRA coverage if he or she was covered by a group health plan on the day before termination and is an employee, the employee's spouse, or an employee's dependent child. Most people who purchase COBRA insurance do so when they voluntarily or involuntarily terminate employment from a job that offered group health insurance or if their hours are reduced significantly.

COBRA benefits are usually the same as the beneficiary had before the termination of employment. Qualified beneficiaries must be allowed to make the same choices given to non-COBRA beneficiaries under the plan, such as during periods of open enrollment by the plan. With some exceptions, COBRA beneficiaries generally are eligible for group coverage during a maximum of 18 months for events due to employment termination or reduction of hours of work. Certain events during the initial period of coverage may permit a beneficiary to receive a maximum of 36 months of coverage.

While COBRA was spurred by federal law, the cost of it is borne by the beneficiary. If a person is covered by a group plan at work, the employee pays a portion of the monthly premium and the employer pays a much larger share. When a person becomes a COBRA beneficiary, he or she must pay the total premium—both the employer's and the employee's share—plus a 2 percent administrative fee. This total premium is often more than an unemployed person can afford, making the optional program out of the reach of many people.

Government-Sponsored Health Insurance

Medicare

Medicare is a federal health insurance program, introduced in 1965 as an amendment to the Social Security Act, for people older than 65, others with certain disabilities, and all people with end-stage renal disease. The Medicare program is the second-largest social insurance program in the United States, with 45.2 million beneficiaries and total expenditures of $468 billion in 2008 (Centers for Medicare and Medicaid Services, 2009). Medicare is funded by payroll deductions and premiums charged to subscribers. Most Medicare benefits will be unchanged under HCERA/PPACA.

The Medicare program has several components.

- Medicare Part A, or Hospital Insurance, helps pay for hospital, home health, skilled nursing facility, and hospice care for the aged and disabled. Most people pay no premium for Part A because they or a spouse already paid for it through their payroll taxes while working.
- Medicare Part B, one of the Supplemental Medical Insurance portions, helps pay for physician, outpatient hospital, home health, and other services for the aged and disabled who have voluntarily enrolled. It also covers some other medical services that Part A does not, such as some of the services of physical and occupational therapists, and some home health care. Part B helps pay for these covered services and supplies when they are medically necessary. Most people pay a monthly premium for Part B.
- Part C, or Medicare Advantage Plan, serves as an alternative to traditional Part A and Part B coverage. People reaching the age of 65 will automatically be enrolled in Part A with the option of enrolling in Parts B and D. However, beneficiaries can choose to enroll in

and receive care from private Medicare Advantage and certain other health insurance plans that contract with Medicare. Part C combines Parts A and B coverage but is provided by private insurance companies. Beneficiaries have the option of adding Part D if coverage is not already included. Medicare Advantage Plans include HMO, PPO, private fee-for-service plans, and Medicare special needs plans.

- Part D, another portion of the Supplemental Medical Insurance, provides subsidized access to prescription drug insurance coverage on a voluntary basis for all beneficiaries and premium and cost-sharing subsidies for low-income enrollees. Part D coverage is not provided within the traditional Medicare program. Instead, beneficiaries must affirmatively enroll in one of many hundreds of Part D plans offered by private companies.

One of the interesting facets of Part D is the coverage gap known as the "donut hole." Part D subscribers pay a deductible and a copayment for prescription medications until the cost reaches $2,830 in any year. Once the subscriber reaches $2,830 in total drug costs, he or she must pay the full cost of prescription drugs until out-of-pocket cost reaches $4,550. After that, the insurance pays almost all of the cost of prescription drugs. The amount between $2,830 and $4,550 is the "donut hole." Under the HCERA/PPACA, Medicare beneficiaries receive a discount starting at 50 percent in 2011 on prescription drugs in the "donut hole." By 2020, the coverage gap is supposed to close completely.

Many people who are covered by Medicare also purchase so-called Medigap policies. Generally, when you buy these policies, you must have Parts A and B. Medigap policies are sold by private insurance companies, not the government, and they pay for health services not covered by Medicare and for Medicare's deductibles and coinsurance. There are as many as 10 standard plans, so it is important to shop with care to make sure you purchase a plan that fits your needs. Medigap

policies must be purchased on an individual basis and not on a family basis.

Medicaid

The Medicaid program was signed into law in 1965 as an amendment to the Social Security Act. Medicaid is a federal and state health insurance program that is available only to certain low-income individuals and families who fit into an eligibility group that is recognized by federal and state law. Each state sets its own eligibility guidelines. Many groups of people are covered by Medicaid. Generally, eligibility falls into three classifications:

1. Categorically needy, based on income and, in some cases, age
2. Medically needy
3. Special groups, including Medicare beneficiaries and working disabled individuals

Even within these groups, though, certain requirements must be met. These may include age, pregnancy, disability, or blindness; income and resources (like bank accounts, real property, or other items that can be sold for cash); and whether the applicant is a U.S. citizen or a lawfully admitted immigrant. The rules for counting income and resources vary from state to state and from group to group; there are special rules for those who live in nursing homes and for disabled children living at home. Adults who do not have children living with them and who are not disabled or elderly cannot qualify for Medicaid no matter how limited their resources unless their state has been granted a waiver to allow them to enroll in the program. States may also issue waivers for other people. The HCERA/PPACA requires states to include low-income childless adults in 2014. The number of Medicaid beneficiaries will swell from its current 59 million; the number covered by Medicaid in 2009 was about 47.8 million, or 15.7 percent of the U.S. population (DeNavas-Walt, Proctor, & Smith, 2010).

The Medicaid program is funded through federal and state monies. States have different federal matching rates to fund the services provided under their Medicaid programs. For this reason, Medicaid is considered a joint federal-state program. States have the flexibility to increase income limits to allow more people to qualify for Medicaid in the same general categories of people, including low-income children, parents, pregnant women with incomes above the mandatory cutoff levels; the blind, elderly, and disabled with incomes above the Supplementary Security Income (SSI) but below 100 percent of the poverty level; nursing home residents with incomes above the SSI but below 300 percent of the poverty level; people with disabilities who work and have incomes above the SSI limit; and medically needy people who require institutional care but who have incomes that are too high to qualify for SSI (FamiliesUSA, 2010). From 2014 to 2016, under HCERA/PPACA, the federal government will pay 100 percent of costs for covering newly eligible individuals.

Under federal law, states must provide a minimum benefit package in Medicaid. These mandatory benefits include physician services, hospital services, family planning, health center services, and nursing facility services. The benefit package for children is more comprehensive than the one for adults because federal law requires states to provide coverage for certain health screenings and services that are medically necessary under the Early and Periodic Screening Diagnostic and Treatment (EPSDT) benefit. States may also provide "optional" services if approved by the federal government. For example, dental care, eyeglasses, mental health care, prescription drugs, and home health care may be approved as optional services.

State Children's Health Insurance Program

Most states offer a Children's Health Insurance Program (SCHIP), which is available to people younger than age 19. Eligible children have families whose incomes exceed the eligibility level for Medicaid but are not enough to buy private insurance. In most states, families whose earnings are below 200 percent of the federal poverty line may enroll their children in SCHIP. Families have to pay a small premium or copayment, depending on their income.

SCHIP covers immunizations and care for healthy babies and children at no cost. However, states are free to cover or not cover other health services.

It is estimated that in 2008, 7.3 million children were uninsured on an average day. Sixty-five percent (4.7 million) were eligible for Medicaid and SCHIP (Kenney, Lynch, Cook, & Phong, 2010), but their parents had not enrolled them.

Supplemental Plans

There are a number of different types of insurance offered in addition to regular insurance. They are designed to cover expenses not covered by primary health insurance. They are not designed to substitute for main, or comprehensive, insurance. In some cases, these plans are money makers for the insurer and provide little coverage for the insured.

One of the most questionable types of supplemental insurance is disease coverage insurance. For example, a company may offer special cancer coverage or AIDS coverage. Usually these plans offer limited benefits. For example, they may offer an unsubstantial lump sum if you or a family member is diagnosed with cancer or they may cover certain, specific care costs. Most people who have health insurance do not need special disease policies because their main insurance covers their needs regardless of disease. It would be better for most people to consider buying a comprehensive health insurance plan rather than a disease-specific plan.

Many group health insurance plans do not cover vision or dental care. Often, the employer offers a supplemental vision or dental policy. These policies may have high premiums and limited benefits. For instance, it is not unusual to have a maximum annual benefit of only $1,500 for dental coverage.

Some companies offer coverage only for injuries suffered in accidents. They may cover hospital and medical care following an accident. Just as with disease coverage, it is often duplicative. Some of these policies also cover death, dismemberment, and disability.

Disability insurance replaces income you lose if you cannot work due to an injury or long-term illness. A typical benefit is about 60 percent of the income at the time of the disability. These benefits can be used for utilities, groceries, or housing costs. Because primary health insurance covers rehabilitation costs following a major health event, disability insurance usually does not.

Hospital confinement indemnity coverage takes care of a fixed amount for each day that a person is hospitalized. The amount is seldom the total amount charged by the hospital, but it is a supplement to primary insurance. The intent is to cover deductibles, coinsurance, and other out-of-pocket expenses not covered by the comprehensive medical insurance.

Long-term care policies cover a wide range of medical, personal, and social services you might need if you have a chronic illness or disability. Long-term coverage includes adult day care, nursing home care, or care received in the individual's home or other setting. If you are considering purchasing a long-term care plan, it is important to know the **elimination period**. This is the period of time between the beginning of a disability and the time you are eligible for benefits. This may be, for instance, the number of days you must need nursing home care before your policy begins to pay. Consumers should expect that the shorter the elimination period, the higher the premium.

Travel health insurance offers coverage for medical expenses while traveling abroad. While this type of supplemental insurance is not expensive, travelers should check their primary insurance to see if a travel policy would be a duplication of coverage.

When considering purchasing some forms of supplemental insurance, there are a number of important considerations. For instance, how will benefits be coordinated with your principal insurance company? Are the benefits worth the cost of the premiums?

Tax-Advantaged Options

Congress has legislated some arrangements that give citizens a tax break to help pay for medical expenses. While not strictly insurance, these arrangements can be used to supplement insurance or to work with health insurance plans.

Health Savings Accounts

A health savings account (HSA) has some of the features of an individual retirement account (IRA). The individual can set up an HSA, or employers can assist employees in establishing the account. In the HSA, you make contributions with pre-tax dollars that you then use to pay for medical expenses. For instance, you may use your contributions to pay your insurance deductible. You may not use the account to pay insurance premiums, although it may be used to fund long-term care insurance or retirement after age 65. A main condition of HSAs is that they must be paired with a qualified, high-deductible health insurance plan. The most attractive feature of the HSA is that you can use the money in the account tax-free to pay for qualified medical expenses.

The funds in the account can be invested, similar to an IRA, so that they grow tax free, although regular income tax applies when the accumulated funds are withdrawn at age 65 or after. The funds carry over from year to year if not used and may accumulate substantially. However, you will pay a penalty if you withdraw money for nonqualified medical expenses prior to age 65.

Health Reimbursement Arrangements

Health reimbursement arrangements (HRAs) are employer-sponsored accords that allow employers to help reimburse employees for medical expenses. HRAs are often combined with high-deductible insurance to protect against catastrophic loss.

Unlike the HSA, the HRA is owned by the employer, so any carryover of funds is at the discretion of the employer. Tax savings accrue for both the employer and the employee when the funds are spent on qualified medical expenses.

Flexible Spending Accounts

With flexible spending accounts (FSAs), the employee determines how much money to withhold from each paycheck and the employer executes this decision. Money can be used to pay for any medical, dental, or vision expenses that are not covered by insurance. Some medically needed over-the-counter medications are included. The funds in the FSA cannot be used to pay insurance premiums.

The employee must accurately estimate the amount of funds his or her family will need in the coming year because any unused funds are forfeited. However, both the employee and the employer enjoy tax savings on funds spent on qualified medical expenses.

Getting the Most from Your Health Insurance

Health insurance is expensive and the cost will probably continue to climb. Therefore, it is important to get the most bang for your insurance buck. The first step is to be informed. Read your health insurance policy. If there are parts you do not understand, ask your insurance agent or benefits officer at work. Pay close attention to the benefits, coverage, and limits. Keep in mind that sales materials and plan summaries are not designed to fully educate the individual. Some insurance plans have regular newsletters that can keep you current on important policies that affect your coverage. Some have toll-free phone services in case covered individuals need information. Others provide much information on their Web sites.

Obtain basic information about accessing health care. For example, if your primary care physician is not available, whom do you see? How do you arrange for and get approval for care when you are away from home or even traveling abroad? Learn your rights to obtain emergency care.

Insurance plans define "emergency" differently. Some allow only a few hours to obtain approval, even if you are seriously injured. "Urgent care" is for problems that are not true emergencies but still require quick medical attention. These include ear infections, serious sprains, or sore throats accompanied by fever. Some policies cover care at a walk-in medical facility and some will not; it is helpful to know your coverage ahead of time. Find out where you obtain lab tests and diagnostic tests such as x-rays. You should inquire as to second opinions. Are they covered under your plan? Are they required, encouraged, or discouraged?

Wise consumers establish a close relationship with their PCP. The more the doctor thinks you want to be a partner in your health care, the more likely he or she is to cultivate that kind of relationship and to fight insurance bureaucrats for approval of procedures. Ask your doctor about regular screenings and about the benefits and risks of various treatments and tests. Know the policies contained in your plan.

Keep records. Store all receipts for medical services and all correspondence from your insurer in a safe, readily accessible place. Keep records of all correspondence with the company, including claims forms, copies of bills, and records of payment. Log all calls with the company by date and time, the person with whom you spoke, and the contents of the conversation. Record your health concerns and keep a log of your symptoms. Keep records of immunizations, illnesses, treatments, and emergency room and hospital visits. Keep a list of your medications. Maintain these records for all family members.

Know what your rights are if something goes wrong. There should be a formal process to complain about service or treatment. Many plans have an appeals process if you disagree with the plan's decisions. If you are in a managed care plan, you may be able to switch plans only during a specific open enrollment period. There may also be limitations on when you can change your PCP. Knowledge of these policies can save a great deal of angst.

SUMMARY

There are a number of types of health insurance that are available to most Americans. Indemnity and fee-for-service plans are the oldest types of plan. Most people get their health insurance through their jobs, in group plans. Many of the plans offered by employers are some variation on managed care, including health maintenance organizations, preferred provider organizations, and point-of-service plans. COBRA plans are available for those who leave jobs in which they have group health insurance.

The Health Care and Education Reconciliation Act and the Patient Protection and Affordable Care Act, both passed in 2010, provide for more people to be covered by health insurance by requiring that most Americans purchase coverage. It provides incentives to do so and penalties for individuals who do not purchase insurance and for large employers that do not offer group coverage. The law provides for the establishment of marketplaces of health insurance plans, called exchanges, for those who do not have insurance options through work. There are also consumer protections built into the legislation, including the elimination of discrimination based on preexisting conditions.

There are government health insurance plans. Medicare is a multi-part health insurance program for people over age 65, others with disabilities, and people with end-stage renal disease. Medicaid is federal-state insurance for people of limited income. The State Children's Health Insurance Program is available for people younger than 19 whose families' incomes exceed the eligibility level for Medicaid but are not enough to buy private insurance.

Various supplemental plans are available. Some may cover care for specific disease, others for vision or dental care. There are supplemental policies for long-term care, travel, and other specific situations.

There are several programs that take advantage of favorable tax law. These include health savings accounts, health reimbursement arrangements, and flexible spending accounts.

Before purchasing insurance, wise consumers determine their needs. Consumers should also compare plans for coverage and costs. It is critical to understand the policy and know your rights.

KEY TERMS

Catastrophic insurance: a type of fee-for-service health insurance policy that is designed to give protection against momentous tragic health occurrences

Coinsurance: the amount the subscriber is required to pay for medical care after the deductible has been met

Coordination of benefits: a clause in an insurance policy that restricts the total amount paid out by each insurer when there are multiple policies

Copayment: a flat fee that is charged every time you receive a medical service

Deductible: a fixed amount of medical expenses the subscriber must pay before health insurance starts to pay

Elimination period: the period of time between the beginning of a disability and the time you are eligible for benefits

Exchange: a marketplace of health insurance plans from which consumers may choose

Fee-for-service: a type of insurance in which the subscriber pays for a service, submits a claim to the insurance company, and, if the service is covered in the policy, receives reimbursement

Group plans: insurance plans, usually offered by employers or large organizations such as professional associations or unions, that allow employees or members to purchase insurance and that keeps premiums down because of the large pool of persons covered

High-deductible health plan: a catastrophic insurance plan

Indemnity insurance: a type of health insurance that requires the subscriber to pay certain charges, such as copayments and deductibles, and which allows the insured to choose his or her health care provider

Lifetime limits: the maximum amount an insurance policy will pay for health services for the life of an individual

Major medical plan: an insurance plan that covers major hospital and medical expenses

Managed care: a system of health care delivery with the goal of reducing costs and use

Preexisting condition: a health problem that existed before the individual's health insurance goes into effect

Preferred provider organization: a type of managed care organization of health care providers and hospitals that have contracted with an insurer or a third-party administrator to provide health care at reduced rates to the insurer's or administrator's clients

Premium: the amount a person and/or his or her employer pays for insurance

Primary care physician: the physician who handles most of your care and who makes referrals to specialists

Reasonable, usual, and customary charge: a calculation by an insurer of what it believes is the appropriate fee to pay for a specific health care product or service in a specified geographic area

Rescission: a practice used by insurance companies to drop people from coverage once they get sick

STUDY QUESTIONS

1. How do group health insurance plans result in reduced premiums for subscribers?
2. What are some variables that influence a family's choice of insurance plans?
3. What are the characteristics of indemnity plans?
4. What are the differences in staff model health maintenance organizations and individual practice associations?
5. How do HMOs, PPOs, and POSs differ?
6. Who is eligible for COBRA?
7. What are Parts A, B, C, and D of Medicare?
8. Compare Medicaid and Medicare.
9. When considering purchasing a supplemental health insurance policy, what are some issues to take into account?
10. How will the HCERA/PPACA increase the percentage of people covered by health insurance? What are other important features of the legislation?

REFERENCES

Centers for Medicare and Medicaid Services. (2009). *Overview trustees report*. Retrieved from http://www.cms.hhs.gov/ReportsTrustFunds/

Congressional Budget Office. (2010). *Health care*. Retrieved from http://www.cbo.gov/publications/collections/health.cfm

DeNavas-Walt, C., Proctor, B. D., & Smith, J. C. (2010). U.S. Census Bureau, Current Population Reports, P60-238. *Income, poverty, and health insurance coverage in the United States: 2009*. Washington, DC: U.S. Government Printing Office.

Elmendorf, D. W. (2010, March 18). Personal communication to Speaker of the United States House of Representatives Nancy Pelosi.

Families USA. (2010). *About Medicaid*. Retrieved from http://www.familiesusa.org/issues/medicaid/about-medicaid.html

Health Care and Education Reconciliation Act of 2010, Pub. L. 111–152, 124 stat. 1029.

Health Maintenance Organization Act of 1973, 42 U.S.C. § 300e.

Jeffries, M. (2010). *How catastrophic insurance works*. Retrieved from http://health.howstuffworks.com/insurance/catastrophic-insurance.htm

Kenney, G. M., Lynch, V., Cook, A., & Phong, S. (2010). Who and where are the children yet to enroll in Medicaid and the Children's Health Insurance Program? *Health Affairs*. doi: 10.1377/hlthaff.2010.0747

Patient Protection and Affordable Care Act of 2010, Pub. L. 111–148, 124 stat. 119.

Rice, T., Desmond, K., & Gabel, J. (1990). The Medicare Catastrophic Coverage Act: A post-mortem. *Health Affairs*, 9(3), 75–87. doi: 10.1377/hlthaff.9.3.75

Sisko, A. M., Truffer, C. J., Keehan, S. P., Poisal, J. A., Clemens, M. K., & Madison, A. J. (2010). National health spending projections: The estimated impact of reform through 2019. *Health Affairs*. doi: 10.1377/hlthaff.2010.0788

U.S. Department of Labor. (2009). *FAQs for employees about COBRA continuation health coverage*. Retrieved from http://www.dol.gov/ebsa/faqs/faq_consumer_cobra.HTML

Chapter 5

Medications

Chapter Objectives

The student will:

- Define "effectiveness," "safety," and "adverse effects" as the terms are applied to medications.
- Discuss reasons for increased spending for prescription drugs.
- List guidelines for safe use of prescription and nonprescription drugs.
- Explain the three kinds of names given to a prescription drug.
- Compare generic and brand name drugs.
- Explain "chemical equivalence," "bioequivalence," and "bioavailability" as the terms are applied to prescription drugs.
- Discuss issues related to online pharmacies.
- Discuss orphan drugs and government efforts to support their development.
- Describe how over-the-counter drugs differ from prescription drugs.
- List several over-the-counter analgesics.
- Explain "behind-the-counter" drugs and the arguments on both sides of the issue.

The purchase and use of medications are crucial to the life and health of many consumers. People use medications for a variety of reasons. Given the widespread use of medications among Americans, it is wise to become familiar with the background of drugs and with concepts for safe use.

High costs have made prescription medications difficult to obtain for many Americans on fixed incomes and/or without health insurance. The per capita expenditure on pharmaceuticals is higher in the United States than in any other industrialized country. Figure 5.1 demonstrates relative expenditures among several nations.

The choice to use medications is a complex one. Consumers should endeavor to gain information regarding the effectiveness of medications. **Effectiveness** means there is a reasonable expectation that, in a significant proportion of the target population, the pharmacological effect, when used under adequate directions for use and warnings against unsafe use, will serve a clinically significant function in the diagnosis, cure, mitigation, treatment, or prevention of disease in humans (U.S. Food and Drug Administration [U.S. FDA], 2008).

Consumers should also attempt to know the relative safety of a drug. **Safety** is defined as the relative freedom from harmful effect to persons affected, directly or indirectly, by a product when prudently administered, taking into consideration the character of the product in relation to the condition of the recipient at the time (U.S. FDA, 2008).

Besides consulting your physician or pharmacist, there are a number of excellent publications that provide information about safety and effectiveness of medications. For example, the

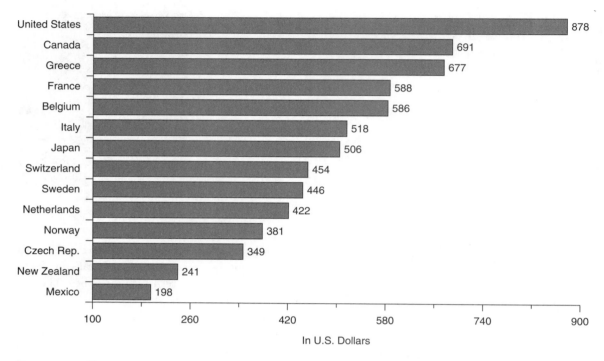

Nation	Expenditure (U.S. Dollars)
United States	878
Canada	691
Greece	677
France	588
Belgium	586
Italy	518
Japan	506
Switzerland	454
Sweden	446
Netherlands	422
Norway	381
Czech Rep.	349
New Zealand	241
Mexico	198

In U.S. Dollars

FIGURE 5.1 EXPENDITURES ON PRESCRIBED PHARMACEUTICALS PER CAPITA: SELECTED NATIONS, 2007

Source: Data based on Organisation for Economic Co-operation and Development. (2009). Health at a glance 2009: OECD indicators. Retrieved from http://dx.doi.10.1787/health_glance-2009-en

Physicians' Desk Reference, The Merck Manual of Diagnosis and Therapy, and *Worst Pills, Best Pills,* a publication of Public Citizen's Health Research Group, are three references that provide useful information about medications.

Prescription Drugs

Prescription drugs are those that require a written order, called a prescription, that gives the user the legal right to purchase and use the drug. The Food and Drug Administration decides whether a drug is so potentially dangerous that a licensed physician must supervise its use. Some states allow other nonphysician professionals, including nurse practitioners, physician assistants, and psychologists, to supervise prescription drug use under limited circumstances. A prescription is normally in written form. Drugs that have less potential for abuse or addiction may be prescribed by a physician by telephone call to a pharmacist.

Also, with expanding technology, many physicians can now transmit prescriptions electronically to pharmacists.

According to *Forbes* magazine (Herbert, 2010), the most frequently prescribed prescription drug

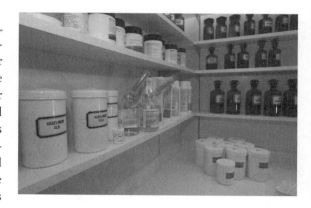

Modern pharmacies handle an array of prescription drugs, requiring superbly educated professionals and extensive electronic records keeping.

in 2009 was Vicodin, a combination of hydro-codone, a narcotic, and acetaminophen. Vicodin is a painkiller prescribed over 128 million times in 2009 even as an FDA panel recommended banning it. The next most frequently prescribed drugs were:

- Simvastatin, aka Zocor, prescribed over 83 million times to lower cholesterol
- Lisinopril, aka Prinivil and Zestril, prescribed over 81 million times to lower blood pressure
- Levothyroxine sodium, aka Synthroid and Levoxyl, prescribed over 66 million times for thyroid disorders
- Azithromycin, aka Zithromax, prescribed almost 54 million times as an antibiotic

According to IMS Health (2010), spending for prescription drugs in the United States was over $300 billion in 2009, over 5 percent more than in 2008. That is almost eight times more than the amount spent in 1990. Three main factors drive changes in prescription drug spending: changes in number of prescriptions dispensed, price changes, and changes in the types of drugs used. From 1994 to 2005, the number of prescriptions purchased increased 71 percent, while the U.S. population increased only 9 percent. Retail prescription prices increased an average of 7.5 percent a year from 1994 to 2006, almost triple the rate of inflation. Prescription drug spending is affected when new drugs enter the market and when existing drugs lose patent protection. New drugs usually increase overall drug spending as they replace older medications.

Americans are using more prescription medications. According to the National Center for Health Statistics (Gu, Dillon, & Burt, 2010), 48 percent of Americans took at least one prescription drug in the past month, compared with 44 percent 10 years earlier. The use of two or more drugs increased from 25 to 31 percent, and the use of five or more drugs increased from 6 to 11 percent. In 2007–08, one out of every five children used at least one prescription drug in the past month.

The U.S. Department of Health and Human Services (Poisal et al., 2007) projects drug spend-

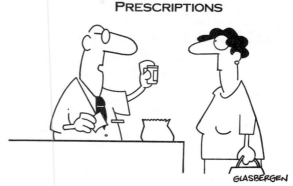

PRESCRIPTIONS

"This is one of those new miracle drugs. If you can afford it, it's a miracle."

Source: © Randy Glasbergen, used with permission from www.glasbergen.com.

ing to increase from $200.7 billion in 2005 to $497.5 billion in 2016, an increase of 148 percent in 11 years. Drug spending as a percentage of overall health care spending is projected to rise from 10 percent in 2005 to 12 percent in 2016.

The price of prescription drugs has caused many Americans, especially older people, to look for alternatives to traditional neighborhood pharmacies, including neighboring countries and the Internet. These choices may carry risks.

The U.S. Food and Drug Administration approves prescription medications for specific purposes. This approval is based on a series of studies usually done by or sponsored by the pharmaceutical company that wishes to market the drug. The fact that pharmaceutical companies test or fund the testing of the products from which they stand to profit alarms some people. The approval process for new prescription drugs is described in the box on page 90 titled "New Prescription Drug Approval."

All medications can cause **adverse effects**, also known as **side effects**. Indeed, in 2005 there were almost 90,000 serious adverse drug events reported in the United States, a 2.6-fold increase from 1998. Of those reported events, there were over 15,100 fatal adverse drug events, a 2.7-fold increase over 1998 (Moore, Cohen, & Furberg, 2007). Consumers should be aware of the possible

NEW PRESCRIPTION DRUG APPROVAL

It takes about 12 years on average and over $350 million to get a new prescription drug to the pharmacy shelf. This process includes research and development of the compound and testing for safety and effectiveness. Only about 1 in 1,000 compounds that enter laboratory testing ever make it to human testing. This partially explains the high cost of prescription drugs to the consumer. The process in gaining approval is the following:

- The compound is screened in small animals for potential action.
- It is tested for toxicity in small and large animals.
- It is tested for adverse effects and absorption in animals.
- If the previous tests are satisfactory to the sponsoring company, it will submit to the FDA an Investigational New Drug Application for testing on humans. If the application is approved, testing on 20 to 80 healthy human volunteers is conducted to determine toxicity, absorption, and metabolism (bioavailability and excretion). This process usually takes about a year.
- In the second phase of human tests, 100 to 300 volunteers who have the condition that the drug is expected to treat will receive the drug to test its effectiveness. This process usually takes about two years.
- In the third phase of human tests, 1,000 to 3,000 patients in clinics and hospitals receive the compound and are monitored carefully to determine effectiveness and to identify adverse effects. This process takes about three years.

All trials involving the drug are conducted by the pharmaceutical company, not the FDA. Plans for trials involving humans must be approved by the FDA.

If all these tests are promising, the company submits a New Drug Application (NDA) with full information on manufacturing specifications, stability and bioavailablility data, method of analysis of each of the dosage forms the sponsor intends to market, packaging and labeling for both physician and consumer, and the results of any additional toxicological studies not already submitted in the Investigational New Drug Application. A panel of experts is appointed to evaluate the testing data. Since the application can exceed 100,000 pages, this process can take up to two and a half years. The panel will make a recommendation to the commissioner of the FDA, who will then make the final decision on approval of the product. If approved, the company must submit regular postmarketing reports to the FDA, with the emphasis on adverse reports. At any time during the development and testing phases, the pharmaceutical company can apply for a patent for the compound. This will protect the compound from being marketed by another company for 20 years from the date of the patent.

adverse effects and make adjustments, such as curtailing driving until they are sure that there are no adverse effects or they have been able to cope with them successfully. A few guidelines for using prescription drugs appear in the box on page 91 titled "Guidelines for Using Prescription Drugs Safely."

The labels of prescription medications contain useful information—name of the drug, how much to take, how often to take it, and the expiration date. They do not tell you what the drug does, its side effects, or warnings. For this information, you must read the package insert.

Prescription drugs are chemicals, some derived from nature, some from laboratory chemicals, and some from a combination of the two. The complete chemical description of the molecule making up the drug is its **chemical name**. Drugs are marketed by their **brand names**, a simple name

GUIDELINES FOR USING PRESCRIPTION DRUGS SAFELY

1. When a physician prescribes a medication, tell him or her all of the other drugs you are taking, as well as about allergies and past problems with medications.
2. If you visit a physician for the first time, take all of your medications (prescription, nonprescription, dietary supplements, etc.) so that a list can be entered in your chart.
3. Ask for information from the pharmacist. Pharmacists are experts on medications.
4. Read the label and package insert several times before use. Observe precautions.
5. Use nondrug approaches when possible. Examples include socializing with others or hobbies to cope with loneliness and isolation, and physical activity and dietary changes to control weight.
6. Follow prescription directions, including dosage and frequency.
7. Consult with your physician and use care when discontinuing a prescription medication.
8. Consult with your physician immediately if you are experiencing any unforeseen drug reactions or interactions. Consider that any new symptom you develop after starting a drug for the first time may be related to the drug.
9. Never share prescriptions with someone else.
10. Do not move medications from the original container to other containers.
11. Use pill boxes carefully.
12. Take plentiful supplies in original containers on trips.
13. Never take medications in the dark.
14. Carefully discard medications after the expiration date.
15. Store medications in a secure location, out of the reach of children.
16. Clean out medicine storage areas regularly.
17. Do not store medications in bathrooms or in other humid or hot areas.
18. Close bottles properly after each use.

applied by the manufacturer and approved by the FDA. The brand name usually describes the function in some way. The brand name is copyrighted and protected by law indefinitely. Pharmaceutical companies obtain patents on new drugs; patents last for 20 years. During that time, only the patent-holding company can legally produce and market the drug. After the patent expires, other companies can manufacture and market the drug. These companies must use the **generic name**, a shorter, simpler version of the chemical name. The generic name cannot be copyrighted. Generic names are the official—i.e., legal—names of drugs and are listed in the *United States Pharmacopeia.* The *USP* is an official public standards-setting authority for all prescription and over-the-counter medicines and other health care products manufactured or sold in the United States.

Generic Prescription Drugs

Prescription drugs are identified by a brand name and a chemical name. When the patent expires on a prescription drug, the same chemical may be manufactured and sold by another company. That product is sold under the shortened version of the chemical name and is called a generic drug. Generics are attractive to consumers because they are much less expensive than brand name drugs. Approximately three-fourths of FDA-approved drugs have generic counterparts (Kaiser Family Foundation, 2007).

In 1984, generic drugs accounted for less than 19 percent of all prescriptions filled. Excluding mail orders, 64.5 percent of prescriptions dispensed in 2008 were generic medications (National Association of Chain Drug Stores,

2008). Sales of generic prescriptions in the United States rose to $54.1 billion in 2006 (Generic Pharmaceutical Association, 2006), or about 20 percent of all prescription drug revenue.

Major pharmaceutical companies have tried to convince the public that their products are produced to higher standards than generics. This claim implies that name brand drugs are safer and more effective than those produced by generic companies. However, brand name pharmaceutical firms make copies of their own or other brand name drugs but sell them without the brand name, effectively making them generics. These products account for about half of all generic drug production. In truth, the quality of prescription drugs, generic or brand name, depends on the vigilance of the Food and Drug Administration. The FDA regulates both brand name and generic drugs and is required by law to hold them to the same standards for quality and purity, manufacturing facilities, and content. Consider the following facts (U.S. FDA, 2009a):

- The firm seeking to sell a generic drug must show that its drug delivers the same amount of active ingredient in the same time frame as the original product.
- The FDA requires generics to have the same quality, strength, purity, and stability as brand name drugs.
- The FDA requires all drugs to be safe and effective and that their benefits outweigh their risks.
- The FDA will not permit drugs to be made in substandard facilities. The agency

conducts about 3,500 inspections a year to ensure standards are met.

- The FDA monitors reports of adverse drug reactions and has found no difference in the rates between generics and brand name drugs.

Applicants for generic drugs must demonstrate that their product is the **chemical equivalent** of the brand name drug—i.e., that it contains essentially identical amounts of identical ingredients in identical doses. A generic drug must also be the **bioequivalent** of the brand name drug—i.e., it performs in the same manner as the original drug. However, generics are not required to undergo the same extensive clinical trials that have already been applied in the development of the pioneer or brand name drug. Generics also must be shown to have the same **bioavailability** as the pioneer drug. This means that the generic must deliver the same amount of the active ingredients into the bloodstream in the same amount of time as the original drug. The *Electronic Orange Book* (U.S. FDA, 2007a) contains much current information about generic drugs, both prescription and nonprescription.

In recent years, the serious problem of abuse of prescription drugs has spread to children and teenagers. Where use of marijuana, cigarettes, and alcohol were once youths' first drug experiences, many young people now use prescription drugs early in life. The ready availability of these products makes it easy for teens to obtain and abuse prescription medications. See the box titled "Abuse of Prescription Drugs by Teens."

ABUSE OF PRESCRIPTION DRUGS BY TEENS

The abuse of prescription drugs by teens has become a major concern for parents and government officials. The following are indicative of the scale of the problem:

- In 2008, 1.5 percent of 12- and 13-year-olds used prescription-type drugs nonmedically.
- Among 14- and 15-year-olds, 3.0 percent used prescription-type drugs nonmedically in 2008.
- Among 16- and 17-year-olds, 4.0 percent used prescription-type drugs nonmedically in 2008.

- In 2009, 20.2 percent of students had taken prescription drugs (e.g., Oxycontin, Percocet, Vicodin, Adderall, Ritalin, or Xanax) without a doctor's prescription one or more times during their life.

The prevalence of having ever taken prescription drugs without a doctor's prescription in 2009 was higher among white (23.0 percent) than black (11.8 percent) or Hispanic (17.2 percent) teens. The prevalence of having ever taken a prescription drug without a prescription was 15.1 percent among 9th-grade students, 18.2 percent among 10th graders, 22.7 percent among 11th graders, and 25.8 percent among 12th-grade students. Teens in western and southeastern states are more likely to abuse prescription pain relievers than those in other sections of the United States.

The nonmedical use of psychotherapeutic prescription drugs is a growing concern because it seems that young people are less worried about the dangers of using these drugs outside of medical regimen, probably because they are widely used for legitimate purposes. In addition, direct-to-consumer advertising implies widespread use and low risk.

About 47 percent of teens who use prescription drugs say they get them for free from a relative or friend. Ten percent say they buy pain relievers from a friend or relative, and another 10 percent say they take the drugs without asking. Thirty-nine percent of 14- to 20-year-olds say it is easy to get prescription drugs online or by phone.

Sources: Teenage Research Unlimited. (2006). *Research findings: Underage alcohol access & consumption, Internet, phone and mail.* Retrieved from http://www.wswa.org/public/media/tru-research/TRUSurvey080206.pdf

U.S. Centers for Disease Control and Prevention. (2010). Youth Risk Behavior Surveillance—2009. *Morbidity and Mortality Weekly, 55*(SS-5).

U.S. Department of Health and Human Services, Substance Abuse and Mental Health Services Administration. (2009). *Results from the 2008 National Survey on Drug Use and Health: National findings.* Retrieved from http://www.oas.samhsa.gov/NSDUH/2k8NSDUH/2k8results.cfm#2.2

U.S. Department of Health and Human Services, Substance Abuse and Mental Health Services Administration. (2006). *The 2005 National Survey on Drug Use and Health.* Retrieved from http://www.oas.samhsa.gov/NSDUN/2k5NSDUH/2k5results.htm

Internet Prescriptions

Many reputable pharmacies provide Internet service with mail delivery. Some insurers contract with pharmacies to provide online service. Pharmacies are regulated by state laws. They are required to be licensed in the states in which their headquarters are physically located. Most states also require licenses for out-of-state pharmacies that ship medications to their residents. Federal agencies, such as the Food and Drug Administration, also regulate the sale of drugs. Generally, if your insurance company recommends or requires an online service, it is trustworthy.

A growing number of online pharmacies are not providing the medications ordered and purchased with credit cards, or sell counterfeit medications with no guarantee that they contain the ingredients expected. Many of these fraudulent pharmacies operate outside the United States and are not licensed by U.S. authorities, so American customers have little protection or recourse. Check with the National Association of Boards of Pharmacy to determine if a site is licensed and in good standing. The association's Web site is http://www.nabp.net, and the telephone number is 1-847-698-6227.

Some medicines sold online are fake, counterfeit, or "copycat" medicines. Some are too strong or too weak. Some have dangerous ingredients or have expired, meaning the last date they should be used has passed. Some have not been tested for safety and effectiveness, and many are not manufactured according to U.S. safety standards. Many are not labeled, stored, or shipped correctly.

In a report by the General Accounting Office (2004), 68 pharmacy Web sites were tested. The office paid for but never received six drug orders. Twenty-four U.S. and all 21 foreign Internet pharmacies, other than the Canadian pharmacies, issued medications based on their own medical questionnaires or had no prescription requirements. All of the Canadian pharmacies required the patient to provide a prescription. None of the 21 samples from foreign countries other than Canada included dispensing pharmacy labels that provided instructions for use, and only about one-third included warning information. Thirteen of the 21 samples displayed other problems associated with the handling of drugs. Many of the drug samples from other foreign pharmacies (10 of 21 samples) were unapproved for the U.S. market because, for example, the labeling or the facilities in which they were manufactured had not been approved by the FDA. In addition, some medications were counterfeit, contained lesser amounts of the active ingredient than prescribed, or had significantly different chemical compositions from those of the products that were ordered. About one-fifth of the Internet pharmacies that sent samples were found to be under investigation by the FDA or the Drug Enforcement Administration (DEA).

The situation is so bad that some Internet pharmacies, rather than requiring a prescription or an examination, have the customer fill out a questionnaire online before shipment of the drug. This is no way to do a diagnosis. Others do not even go as far as requiring a questionnaire, dispensing drugs to anyone with a credit card. The National Center on Addiction and Substance Abuse at Columbia University searched the Internet during a one-month period in 2008 and found 365 Web sites advertising or offering controlled prescription drugs for sale. Only two of the sites were

certified by the National Association of Boards of Pharmacy as Verified Internet Pharmacy Practice Sites. Of the 159 sites where the customer places an order and pays to purchase the drugs, 42 percent explicitly stated that no prescription was needed, 45 percent offered "online consultation," and 13 percent made no mention of a prescription. Only 15 percent of all sites offering controlled prescription drugs for sale required that a prescription be faxed or mailed or that the patient's doctor be contacted for the prescription; half of these sites simply required a patient to fax a prescription, allowing opportunities for prescription tampering or multiple use.

Physicians sometimes lend their names to these enterprises without much fear of discipline. The FDA and the DEA have investigated several Internet companies for mail fraud, smuggling drugs, selling adulterated or counterfeit drugs, lack of doctor-patient relationship, and selling controlled substances without a prescription.

The National Association of Boards of Pharmacy (NABP, 2004), which represents boards of pharmacy in all 50 states and the District of Columbia, offers the following advice when considering online orders for medication:

- Suspect e-pharmacies will dispense prescription medications without requiring you to mail in a prescription, or they may not contact your doctor to obtain a valid verbal prescription.
- If the online pharmacy does not have a toll-free number posted on its site, be suspicious.
- If a site does not advertise the availability of pharmacists for medication consultation, avoid it.
- Be leery of online pharmacies that sell a limited number of medications, especially those that specialize only in medications that treat sexual dysfunction or assist in weight loss.

The NABP allows consumers to check the legitimacy of online pharmacies through its Verified Internet Pharmacy Practice Sites program.

The New Jersey Division of Consumer Affairs (2009) offered the following advice to consumers:

- Don't buy from sites that offer to provide drugs for the first time without a physical examination or that sell drugs that have not been approved by the FDA.
- Reputable online pharmacies will always ask for a prescription to be mailed or for a doctor's phone number to verify the order.
- Do not do business with sites that do not have a registered pharmacist who is available to answer your questions.
- Do not purchase prescription drugs from foreign Web sites.
- Once the drugs arrive, compare the package and bills to the medication you already have at home. Check to make sure the expiration date is not less than three months away. An expiration date that is less than three months away is a red flag that the pharmacy may not be following traditional practices.
- Check for a street address and phone number when you are online. The site should also have a detailed privacy statement.
- Talk to your health care professional before using any medications for the first time.
- Sites that dispense medications to patients who have not seen a doctor are breaking federal law, because it is illegal to obtain drugs over the Internet if you have not visited a physician.

The National Consumer League's Fraud Center (2004a) also warns about buying from sites that advertise "miracle drugs" or a "new cure" for a serious disease. These drugs are not usually approved by the FDA and could be ineffective or dangerous.

A final issue with online pharmacies that applies to other Internet businesses is that of patient privacy. Some online pharmacies do not respect or even make a commitment to protect individual privacy. To protect yourself, look for privacy and security policies that are easy to find and understand. Do not give any personal information such as Social Security number, credit card number, insurance number, or medical history, unless you are sure the Web site will keep your information safe and private. Make sure that the site will not sell your information. Reputable companies have privacy policies that they make available regularly.

Drugs from Canada

The incredible increase in drug prices has driven patients to travel to foreign countries, particularly Canada, to obtain prescription medications. The prices are frequently much lower in Canada.

The FDA and the pharmaceutical industry have complained and alleged that importing drugs from other countries is unsafe, due to possible counterfeiting, poor quality control in manufacturing, and contamination. Ironically, many medications sold in Canada are manufactured by prominent American pharmaceutical companies in the United States, shipped to Canada, and then sold to Americans at lower prices than they could find at home. Most authorities believe that most of the drugs sold by Canadian pharmacies to Americans are perfectly safe.

The federal government of the United States has banned importation of drugs from Canada by ordinary citizens. However, grassroots pressure may force the Congress to consider allowing U.S. citizens to purchase drugs from Canadian pharmacies.

While it may be argued that Canadian pharmacies provide quality medications to Americans, the same cannot be said about pharmacies in every country. The consumer should be wary about importing medications.

Counterfeit Drugs

Counterfeit drugs are products falsely sold under brand names. The packaging may be nearly identical to that of original drugs but they may not provide accurate information. Counterfeiting can include sticking fraudulent labels on expired drugs, filling vials with water, and putting adulterants like chalk into medicine packets. Many counterfeit drugs originate outside the United States, with India and China being prominent sources. The Center for Medicine in the Public Interest (Pitts, 2010) estimated that the counterfeit drug business generated $75 billion in 2010, up 92 percent from 2005.

Patients are at risk for serious health problems when using counterfeit drugs. These include side effects, allergic reactions, and worsening health because the product is ineffective. Effects can be lethal.

Counterfeit drugs are not the same as generics. Generics must meet strict standards. However, counterfeit drugs are produced in environments not regulated by the government. Their ingredients, amounts of ingredients, safety, and effectiveness may not match that of the original product. Counterfeit drugs are illegally produced for profit rather than for therapy.

In 1987, Congress passed the Prescription Drug Marketing Act, designed in part to affect the movement of counterfeit drugs. This law required the FDA to develop and implement regulations that would require the recording and tracking of the transport and sale of prescription drugs. This record would be kept in a document called a pedigree. This is important because over the years, the path that a drug takes from manufacturer to patient has become ever more circuitous and difficult to follow. The FDA delayed issuing regulations until 1999. At that point, complaints from the drug wholesaling industry intensified, leading to many delays. Finally, on December 1, 2006, the FDA rules went into effect. A pedigree is now required for prescription drug products sold, purchased, or traded by entities other than manufacturers or authorized distributors of record. In anticipation of the December 1, 2006, effective date, the FDA issued a guidance document entitled *Guidance for Industry: PDMA Requirements, Questions and Answers* and a *Compliance Policy Guide* clarifying how the FDA intended to interpret and enforce the pedigree requirements.

A secondary effect of requiring the pedigree may be a more effective tracking of drugs into and out of Canada, something that U.S.

pharmaceutical companies hope will reduce the traffic across the border.

The FDA is working with companies that make and sell drugs to identify and prevent counterfeit drugs. The agency hopes to work with other government agencies to stem the tide of counterfeit drugs by strengthening laws to license and regulate drug wholesalers and distributors, adopting safe business practices by all players in the drug distribution chain, implementing new technologies to prevent counterfeiting, developing a system for reporting counterfeit drugs to the FDA quickly, working with governments and businesses in foreign countries, and educating consumers and health professionals about the risks of counterfeit drugs and how to report and respond.

The National Consumers League (2004b) offered the following advice for avoiding counterfeit drugs:

- *Know your medications.* If you know the size, shape, color, taste, and side effects of the prescriptions you take, you will more easily identify possible counterfeits. Contact your pharmacist or doctor if you notice anything different about a medication.

- *Pay attention to packaging.* Check for altered or unsealed containers, or changes in the packaging or label. Contact your pharmacist or doctor if you notice any changes.

- *Buy prescription medications only from a safe, reputable source.* If the seller is unfamiliar to you, check with your state board of pharmacy or the National Association of Boards of Pharmacy at http://www.nabp.net or call 1-847-698-6227. These sources can tell you if the pharmacy is licensed.

- *When you buy medications online, make sure the seller is properly licensed.* Your state board of pharmacy or the National Association of Boards of Pharmacy can tell you if the online seller is licensed. You should check the state board of pharmacy where the online seller is located, and your own state board of pharmacy. Some sites display a seal, such as the NABP's VIPPS seal, as proof that the site has met state and federal requirements. Dealing with pharmacies that display the VIPPS seal, which means they are Verified Internet Pharmacy Practice Sites, or other similar certification seals provides more confidence that they and the products they sell are legitimate. See a list of VIPPS-accredited pharmacies at http://www.nabp.net/vipps/consumer/listall.asp.

- *If you believe you have bought a counterfeit drug, report it.* Contact the pharmacist who sold you the medication. Your pharmacist will know if there has been a legitimate change in the color, shape, taste, or packaging of the medication. You can also report your suspicions to the Food and Drug Administration (FDA). If you bought the drug by mail, by telephone, or in person, contact the FDA's MedWatch program at 1-800-332-1088 or at http://www.fda.gov/medwatch/. To report a counterfeit drug that you bought on the Internet, use the online form at http://www.fda.gov/oc/buyonline/buyonlineform.htm or call MedWatch. In addition, ask your doctor for medical advice if you have taken drugs you suspect are counterfeit.

Orphan Drugs

Orphan drugs are those that few people use. They usually treat rare diseases, those afflicting less than 200,000 Americans. There are about 6,000 such diseases and conditions. Because the cost of developing new drugs is so high, it is seldom profitable for pharmaceutical companies to produce orphan drugs.

In order to provide an strong incentive to companies to produce drugs for rare conditions, the U.S. Congress passed the Orphan Drug Act in 1983 as an amendment to the Federal Food, Drug and Cosmetic Act. Under the act, the Secretary of Health and Human Services may make grants to and enter into contracts with public and private entities and individuals to assist in (1) defraying the costs of qualified clinical testing expenses incurred in connection with the development of drugs for rare diseases and conditions, (2) defraying the costs of developing medical devices for rare diseases or conditions, and (3) defraying the costs of developing medical foods for rare diseases or conditions (U.S. FDA, 2007b). The law provides seven-year marketing exclusivity to sponsors of approved orphan products, a tax credit of 50 percent of the cost of conducting human clinical testing, and research grants for clinical testing of new therapies to treat orphan diseases. Exclusive marketing rights limit competition by preventing other companies from marketing the same version of the drug unless they can prove clinical superiority (U.S. Department of Health and Human Services, 2001). The act provides strong incentives to pharmaceutical companies to produce drugs that would otherwise be unprofitable.

These financial incentives have made drugs available to many suffering people who would not otherwise have received relief by stimulating the development of new medications. Between 1983 and 2010, 347 new drugs received marketing approval under the act (Hempel, 2010). Many orphan drugs, including those approved for multiple sclerosis, cystic fibrosis, and hemophilia, are considered breakthroughs.

Nonprescription Medications

Nonprescription medications are usually called "over-the-counter" or OTC drugs. These are medications that can be purchased without a prescription. The FDA has decided that these drugs are safe enough that the purchasing decision can be left entirely in the hands of the patient. Use of these products amounts to self-medication; they are usually taken without the benefit of medical advice. Officially, these are drugs that are (1) intended to treat ailments that are self-diagnosing and for which no medical monitoring is needed for safe use and (2) not habit-forming or toxic.

OTC drugs generally have these characteristics:

- Their benefits outweigh their risks
- The potential for **misuse** and **abuse** is low
- The consumer can use them for self-diagnosed conditions
- They can be adequately labeled
- Health practitioners are not needed for the safe and effective use of the product

No one knows exactly how many nonprescription drug products are marketed at any time. According to the FDA (2009b), there are about 800 significant active ingredients in more than 100,000 OTC products. Retailers' shelves contain a growing choice of nonprescription medicines to treat an expanding range of ailments. While OTC medicines usually treat symptoms rather than curing diseases, they often do more than relieve aches, pains, and itches. Some can prevent diseases like tooth decay, cure diseases like athlete's foot, and, with a doctor's guidance, help manage recurring conditions like vaginal yeast infection, migraine, and minor pain in arthritis.

Using OTC medications to relieve symptoms is usually safe, but it is also possible that, by masking symptoms, they can hide serious conditions or let minor ones develop into more critical conditions. In addition, there are over 178,000 hospitalizations in the United States because of misuse of OTC drugs (United Health Foundation, 2007). See the box on page 99 titled "Self-Medicating with Nonprescription Drugs."

The information on a nonprescription drug package is as important as the information you need to take a prescription drug safely, so do not ignore the label when taking an OTC medicine. Consumers should look for:

- Product name
- "Active ingredients," therapeutic substances in medicine
- "Purpose," the product category (such as antihistamine, antacid, or cough suppressant)
- "Uses," the symptoms or conditions the product will treat or prevent
- "Warnings," such as when not to use the product, when to stop taking it, when to see a doctor, and possible side effects
- "Directions," such as how much to take, how to take it, and how long to take it
- "Other information," such as storage information
- "Inactive ingredients," including substances such as binders, colors, or flavoring

Consumers should pay particular attention to the advice to consult a professional before taking a nonprescription medication, especially for the first time. While the FDA is charged with regulating OTC medications, there is no requirement that the manufacturers tell anyone, including the FDA, when they change ingredients or amount of ingredients, unless the ingredient is new. Your physician or pharmacist may be able to provide this information and provide consultation.

Although usually mild, interactions involving OTC drugs can produce unwanted results or make medicines less effective. It is especially important to know about drug interactions if you are taking prescription drugs and OTC drugs at the same time. Some drugs can also interact with foods and beverages, as well as with health conditions such as diabetes, kidney disease, and high blood pressure. Here are a few drug interaction cautions for some common OTC ingredients:

- Avoid alcohol if you are taking antihistamines, cough-cold products with the ingredient dextromethorphan, or drugs that treat sleeplessness.
- Do not use drugs that treat sleeplessness if you are taking prescription sedatives or tranquilizers. Alcohol can intensify the effect of sleep-promoting drugs.
- Check with your doctor before taking products containing aspirin if you are taking a prescription blood thinner or if you have diabetes or gout.
- Do not use laxatives when you have stomach pain, nausea, or vomiting.

- Unless directed by a doctor, do not use a nasal decongestant if you are taking a prescription drug for high blood pressure or depression, or if you have heart or prostate problems, thyroid disease, or diabetes.

All medications should be stored in secure places, where children cannot reach them. Protect children by never taking medications, OTC or prescription, in front of them because children imitate the behavior of adults. Never tell a child that medicine is candy. Use child-resistant containers and keep them tightly closed.

Consumers should be aware that the marketing of OTC drugs is very aggressive and is seldom very informative. We should be careful to avoid falling prey to advertising of products we really do not need. See Chapter 9 on advertising.

The wise consumer shops for economy. Many nonprescription medications come in "store brands." These products are generally as effective as the original, brand name product but are much less expensive. The consumer should read the label to make sure that the active ingredient is the same and in the same amount and that the inactive ingredients are the same. Inactive ingredients may

SELF-MEDICATING WITH NONPRESCRIPTION DRUGS

1. Before deciding to self-medicate, consult a physician or registered pharmacist if you have any doubts. Be especially careful if you are pregnant or nursing.
2. Never treat severe or persistent symptoms except on the advice of a physician. For example, treat adult diarrhea for only 24 hours, indigestion for only five days, and colds for only seven days. If symptoms do not subside, see a physician.
3. Take the medication as directed.
4. Use single-entity medications. They are usually more effective than multiple-ingredient products and are less likely to cause adverse effects.
5. Avoid taking several OTC medications simultaneously.
6. If you are prescribed medication by a physician, tell him or her about any OTC medication you are using.
7. Be wary of time-release preparations. They may not release the effective dose at one time.
8. Avoid taking two or more products that contain the same ingredients.
9. Do not crush or break pills or capsules unless instructed to do so by the label information.
10. Use "extra strength" medication carefully. It is easier to take inappropriate dosages because each pill or capsule may contain more. "Extra strength" medication may cost more per milligram than regular strength products.
11. Read and follow directions on the package and insert. Look for information on side effects and interactions with other medications.
12. Look for hidden additives in the list of ingredients, including alcohol, sugar, and salt.
13. Before surgery, tell your physician about any OTC medications you may be taking.
14. Inspect the package for tampering and broken seals.
15. Shop for OTC medications that you use frequently when you are feeling well. You are more likely to spend the time to shop for economy and to read the label carefully.
16. Store the medication in its original container.
17. Discard the product after its expiration date.

have different functions, such as those that disperse or break down the ingredients so that the body can absorb them or those that hold a pill together so that it does not turn into powder. Shopping for commonly used medications before you actually need them encourages more careful comparisons of product and price than when you are feeling poorly.

A Word About Pain Relievers

Pain relievers, or **analgesics**, when used correctly, are safe and effective. Millions of people use these medicines every day. Not using them according to the label directions can have serious consequences. You should know the active ingredients and directions of use for all your medicines. Active ingredients in OTC medicines can be the same ingredients found in prescription medicines, although usually in smaller quantities. Many OTC medicines sold for different uses have the same active ingredient. For example, a cold-and-cough remedy may have the same active ingredient as a headache remedy or a prescription pain reliever.

There are two main types of OTC pain relievers. Some contain acetaminophen and others contain nonsteroidal anti-inflammatory drugs (NSAIDs). These medicines are used to relieve the minor aches and pains associated with headaches, colds, flu, arthritis, toothaches, and menstrual cramps. They are also used to treat migraine headaches and to reduce fever.

Acetaminophen is a very common pain reliever and fever reducer. Taking too much of this active ingredient can lead to liver damage. Liver toxicity from acetaminophen poisoning is by far the most common cause of acute liver failure in the United States (Larson et al., 2005). The risk for liver damage may be increased if you drink three or more alcoholic drinks while using acetaminophen-containing medicines. The FDA is considering strengthening warning labels on some acetaminophen products and eliminating some products from the marketplace.

NSAIDs are common pain relievers and fever reducers. They also relieve inflammation, unlike acetaminophen. Examples of OTC NSAIDs are aspirin, ibuprofen, naproxen sodium, and ketoprofen. Gastric bleeding is a common side effect of these products. There are some factors that can increase your risk for stomach bleeding, including:

- Age older than 60
- Taking prescription blood thinners
- Previous stomach ulcers
- Other bleeding problems

If any of these factors apply to you, you should talk to your doctor before using NSAIDS. NSAIDs can also cause reversible damage to the kidneys. The risk of kidney damage may increase in:

- People who are older than 60
- People who have high blood pressure, heart disease, or preexisting kidney disease
- People who are taking a diuretic

The FDA recommends that you talk with your health care professional if you have questions about using an OTC medicine before using it in combination with other medicines—either OTC or prescription medicine (U.S. FDA, 2004).

Behind-the-Counter Medications

On March 9, 2006, President George W. Bush signed the Combat Methamphetamine Epidemic Act, a part of the USA Patriot Improvement and Reauthorization Act of 2005 that required that all drug products containing the ingredient pseudoephedrine, mostly cold medicines, be kept behind the pharmacy counter. Further, the law required that the products must be sold in limited quantities to consumers after they show identification and sign a logbook. This action took place because pseudoephedrine is a key ingredient in the production of methamphetamine, a powerful and highly addictive stimulant that is produced illegally. The process of producing methamphetamine has resulted in explosions that have wrecked neighborhoods and cost lives. The 2006 law affects many OTC products for children and adults, such as Tylenol Flu NightTime Gelcaps, Advil Allergy Sinus Caplets, and Sudafed Nasal Decongestant Tablets. The law also limits the amount of pseudoephedrine an individual can purchase to 3.6 grams in a single day and 9 grams in a month at a retail store. This legislation formally introduced to Americans the "behind-the-counter" (BTC) concept.

Current law allows the FDA only two choices when classifying medications—prescription or nonprescription. As Field (2005) wrote, "Some products may fall somewhere in between those that are so potentially dangerous to require physician supervision and those that are so safe that purchase and use is left to the consumer. These drugs may pose hazards that make direct patient purchase risky but that are not sufficiently grave so as to require medical supervision. Existing laws give the FDA little room to maneuver."

Numerous pharmacists believe that it is time for many prescription drugs to become BTC drugs. Likewise, they say some OTC drugs that are too dangerous for direct public sale should be moved behind the counter, where the pharmacist would be able to intervene in a purchase. Pharmacists would advise patients on the proper use and risks of the drugs. They could also refer patients to physicians when appropriate.

Proponents of the BTC class argue that pharmacists are thoroughly trained in the uses and risks of medication and, since they already provide advice and counseling to patients on both prescription and OTC medications, they are capable of doing so for BTC medication buyers.

Those who oppose the BTC concept fear that a third class of drugs might result in higher prices while limiting availability of some OTC medications. They worry that OTC drugs currently available at a range of retailers, including supermarkets and convenience stores, would be available only at pharmacies. The American Medical Association fears that some prescription drugs will be dropped to the BTC class and sold with reduced supervision, allowing for more risk to the consumer.

The BTC concept is already in use in the United Kingdom, Canada, Australia, New Zealand, and Singapore. The U.S. General Accounting Office (1995), now called the Government Accountability Office, found that safeguards against abuse in these countries are easily circumvented and that actual counseling of patients by pharmacists is infrequent and incomplete. In 1985 the concept was also tried as an experiment in Florida in which pharmacists were permitted to prescribe a limited number of drugs without physician supervision. The authority was rarely used.

In order for the BTC concept to work in the United States, pharmacists would have to be willing and active participants. They would have to respect their enhanced role as educators and counselors. Their education would have to be strengthened to include more training in patient counseling. Their willingness to counsel patients would probably depend on the availability of reimbursement for patient counseling from insurance and other sources, a factor that is now missing (Field, 2005).

Any change to the prescription-OTC classification system would require Congress to amend or change the law that established the current prescription/nonprescription classifications. It is unlikely that such a change would come quickly.

Disposing of Unused Medicines

Good consumers protect the environment when disposing of drugs, including veterinary medicines. Besides direct environmental concerns, when chemicals such as medications make their way into the soil, such as those flushed down septic systems, they may eventually get into the water supply. Some may even end up in the food supply. This can result in human consumption of small amounts of drugs. Among other problems, this may result in a gradual adaptive response to antibiotics, rendering them less effective. However, there is still serious debate in the scientific community about the risks associated with drug residues. It would be responsible for consumers to exercise care in disposing of unused or expired drugs.

The White House Office of National Drug Control Policy (ONDCP), working with the FDA, developed consumer guidance for the proper disposal of prescription drugs. Many of the recommendations also apply to nonprescription medications. The Consumer Information Center of the FDA (2009) summarized the guidelines:

- Follow any specific disposal instructions on the drug label or patient information that accompanies the medication. Do not flush prescription drugs down the toilet unless this information specifically instructs you to do so.
- If no instructions are given, throw the drugs into the household trash, but first:
  1. Take them out of their original containers and mix them with an undesirable substance, such as used coffee grounds or kitty litter. The medication will be less appealing to children and pets, and unrecognizable to people who may intentionally go through your trash.
  2. Put them in a sealable bag, empty can, or other container to prevent the medication from leaking or breaking out of a garbage bag.
- Take advantage of community drug take-back programs that allow the public to bring unused drugs to a central location for proper disposal. Call your city or county government's household trash and recycling service (see the blue pages in your telephone directory) to see if a take-back program is available in your community.

To protect your privacy, it is useful to scratch out all identifying information from the prescription label.

SUMMARY

We rely on government to ensure the safety and effectiveness of drugs that we purchase and use. Consumers should exercise caution in using medications. Consumers also have responsibility in using drugs in ways that are safe and allow them to do what they are supposed to do.

Prescription drugs are those that require physician supervision through the use of written authorization to use the drug. Over-the-counter drugs are those that do not require a prescription. A third category of drugs, behind-the-counter, currently applies to products that contain pseudoephedrine but possibly other ingredients in the future.

Generic drugs are prescription drugs manufactured by a secondary producer but to the same high standards as the original manufacturer. They save money while delivering the same quality as brand name drugs.

Consumers should use caution in purchasing drugs, especially on the Internet and in foreign countries. Sources located outside the United States are generally unregulated by American authorities and may be offering counterfeit or otherwise less effective and less safe products.

Nonprescription drugs have low potential for abuse and misuse, but they should be taken with care. They usually do not cure but may be effective at relieving symptoms. Examples of nonprescription medications are the analgesics acetaminophen and NSAIDs.

Disposal of unused drugs should be done carefully and with respect to guidelines developed by the manufacturer and the Food and Drug Administration. Improper disposal has the potential for long-term consequences to individual health and to the environment.

KEY TERMS

Abuse (of drugs): the use of a drug in a manner, in amounts, or in situations such that the use of the drug causes problems or increases the chances that problems will occur; usually excessive or persistent usage without regard to accepted medical practice

Adverse effects: effects, other than those for which the drug is being taken, that may occur as a result of its use; also called side effects

Analgesics: drugs that relieve pain without loss of consciousness

Bioavailability: amount of the active ingredients of a drug that gets into the bloodstream in a specific amount of time

Bioequivalent: describing two or more drugs that perform in the same manner; often used to describe a generic drug in comparison to its brand name counterpart

Brand name: a simple name for a drug applied by the manufacturer and approved by the Food and Drug Administration; the name used in marketing

Chemical equivalent: drugs that contain essentially identical amounts of identical ingredients in identical doses; often used to compare generic drugs with their brand name counterparts

Chemical name: the complete chemical description of the molecule making up the drug

Effectiveness: there is a reasonable expectation that, in a significant proportion of the target population, the pharmacological effect, when used under adequate directions for use and warnings against unsafe use, will serve a clinically significant function in the diagnosis, cure, mitigation, treatment, or prevention of disease

Generic name: a short, simple version of the chemical name of a drug

Misuse (of drugs): use of a drug for purposes for which it is not intended, for appropriate purposes but in improper doses, or in inappropriate combinations

Nonprescription drugs: medications that can be purchased without a prescription; also called over-the-counter drugs

Orphan drug: a drug that treats a rare condition

Prescription drugs: medications that require a written order, called a prescription, that gives the user the legal right to purchase and use the drug

Safety: the relative freedom from harmful effect to persons affected, directly or indirectly, by a product when prudently administered, taking into consideration the character of the product in relation to the condition of the recipient at the time

Side effects: effects, other than those for which the drug is being taken, that may occur as a result of its use; also called adverse effects

STUDY QUESTIONS

1. What do the terms "effective," "safety," and "adverse effects" mean with respect to drugs?
2. What are the factors that drive the increases in prescription spending?
3. List several guidelines for safe use of prescription drugs.
4. Explain the differences in the chemical name, brand name, and generic name of a prescription drug.
5. Compare generic and brand name drugs.
6. What does it mean when two drugs are chemically equivalent? Bioequivalent?
7. What is bioavailability?
8. What are some signs that indicate that you should use increased caution when using an online pharmacy?
9. What is the difference between counterfeit and generic drugs?
10. What are orphan drugs? What has the federal government done to promote their development?
11. What are over-the-counter drugs? What are their characteristics?
12. What information is found on an over-the-counter drug label?
13. List guidelines for the safe use of over-the-counter drugs.
14. What are the different over-the-counter pain relievers?
15. What are behind-the-counter drugs? Why was this designation developed? Why do some people oppose it? Why do others support it?

REFERENCES

Consumer Information Center. (2009). *How to dispose of unused medicines.* Retrieved from http://www.fda.gov/downloads/Drugs/ResourcesForYou/Consumers/BuyingUsingMedicineSafely/UnderstandingOver-the-CounterMedicines/ucm107163.pdf

Field, R. I. (2005). Support grows for a third class of "behind-the-counter" drugs." *Health Care and Law, 30*(5), 260–261.

Generic Pharmaceutical Association. (2006). *About generics: Statistics.* Retrieved from http://www.gphaonline.org/Content/NavigationMenu/AboutGenerics/Statistics.default.htm

Gu, Q., Dillon, C. F., & Burt, V. L. (2010). *Prescription drug use continues to increase: U.S. prescription drug data for 2007–2008.* NCHS Data Brief Number 42, September. Atlanta, GA: Centers for Disease Control and Prevention.

Hempel, C. (2010). *Orphan Drug Act—A colossal failure considering rare disease drug statistics.* Retrieved from http://addiandcassi.com/orphan-drug-act-a-collosal-failure-considering-rare-disease-drug-statistics/

Herbert, M. (2010). *America's most popular drugs.* Retrieved from http://www.forbes.com/2010/05/11/narcotic-painkiller-vicodin-business-healthcare-popular-drugs.htm

IMS Health. (2010). *IMS reports U.S. prescription sales grew 5.1 percent in 2009, to $300.3.* Retrieved from http://www.imshealth.com/portal/site/imshealth/menuitem.a46c6d4df3db4b3d88f611019418c22a

Kaiser Family Foundation. (2007). *Prescription drug trends.* Retrieved from http://www.kff.org/rxdrugs/upload/3057_06.pdf

Larson, A. M., Polson, J., Fontana, R. J., Davern, T. J., Lalani, E., Hynan, L. S., & Lee, W. M. (2005). Acetaminophen-induced acute liver failure: Results of a United States multicenter, prospective Study. *Hepatology, 42*(6), 1364–1372.

Moore, T. J., Cohen, M. R., & Furberg, C. D. (2007). Serious adverse drug events reported to the Food and Drug Administration, 1998–2005. *Archives of Internal Medicine, 167*(16), 1752–1759.

National Association of Boards of Pharmacy. (2004). *VIPPS.* Retrieved from http://www.nabp.net/vipps/intro.asp

National Association of Chain Drug Stores. (2008). *NACDS Foundation chain pharmacy industry profile, 2008.* Retrieved from http://www.nacds.org

National Center on Addiction and Substance Abuse at Columbia University. (2008). *"You've Got Drugs! V," Prescription Drug Pushers on the Internet.* New York: CASA.

National Consumers League. (2004a). *Tips for buying drugs safely.* Retrieved from http://fraud.org/fakedrugs/onlinerx.htm

National Consumers League. (2004b). *Tips for avoiding counterfeit drugs.* Retrieved from http://www.fraud.org/fakedrugs/tips.htm

New Jersey Division of Consumer Affairs. (2009). *Buying prescription drugs online—Is it safe?* Retrieved from http://www.state.nj.us/lps/ca/brief/online.pdf

Orphan Drug Act. (1983). Pub. L. 97-414.

Pitts, P. (2010). *Counterfeit drugs and China NEW.* Retrieved from http://cmpi.org/in-the-news/testimony/counterfeit-drugs-and-china-new/

Poisal, J. A., Truffer, C., Smith, S., Sisko, A., Cowan, C., Keehan, S., & Dickensheets, B. (2007). Health spending projections through 2016: Modest changes obscure Part D's impact. *Health Affairs.* Retrieved from http://www.cms.hhs.gov/NationalHealthExpendData/03_NationalHealthAccountsProjected.asp#TopOfPage

Prescription Drug Monitoring Act. (1987). Pub. L. 100-293, 102 stat. 95.

Rubin, R. (2005). Pharmacies offer behind the counter service. *USAToday.* Retrieved from http://www.usatoday.com/news/health/2005-02-07-pharmacists-x.htm

United Health Foundation. (2007). *Over-the-counter drugs … safe when used as directed.* Retrieved from http://www.unitedhealthfoundation.org/otc.html

U.S. Department of Health and Human Services. (2001). *The orphan drug act: Implementation and impact.* Washington, DC: U.S. Department of Health and Human Services, OEI-09-00-00380.

U.S. Food and Drug Administration. (2004). *Health hints: Use caution with pain relievers.* Retrieved from http://www.fda.gov/cder/drug/analgesics/healthHints.htm

U.S. Food and Drug Administration. (2007a). *Electronic orange book.* Retrieved from http://www.fda.gov/cder/ob

U.S. Food and Drug Administration. (2007b). *Orphan drug act (as amended).* Retrieved from http://www.fda.gov/orphan/oda.htm

U.S. Food and Drug Administration. (2008). *CFR—Code of federal regulations Title 21.* Retrieved from http://www.accessdata.fda.gov/scripts/cdrh/cfdocs/cfcfr/CFRSearch.cfm?fr=601.25

U.S. Food and Drug Administration. (2009a). *FDA ensures equivalence of generic drugs.* Retrieved from http://www.fda.gov/Drugs/EmergencyPreparedness/BioterrorismandDrugPreparedness/ucm134444.htm

U.S. Food and Drug Administration. (2009b). *Office of Nonprescription Drug Products—What we do.* Retrieved from http://www.fda.gov/AboutFDA/CentersOffices/CDER/ucm106342.htm

U.S. General Accounting Office. (1995). *Pharmacist-controlled nonprescription drugs.* Report GAO/PEMD-95-12. Washington, DC: U.S. General Accounting Office.

U.S. General Accounting Office. (2004). *Internet pharmacies: Some pose risks to consumers.* Retrieved from http://www.gao.gov/new.items/d04820.pdf

USA Patriot Improvement and Reauthorization Act of 2005. (2005). Pub. L.109–177.

Chapter 6

Complementary and Alternative Medicine

Chapter Objectives

The student will:

- Distinguish among conventional medicine, complementary therapies, and alternative therapies.
- Explain integrative therapy.
- Explain the five categories of complementary and alternative medicine.
- Discuss the reasons for the popularity of complementary and alternative medicine and the characteristics of people most likely to use them.
- Explain the tenets supporting several complementary and alternative therapies.
- List the information needed to decide on using a complementary or alternative therapy and identify sources of that information.

Conventional medicine is that which has undergone extensive testing in multiple trials and has been shown to exceed some agreed-upon standards of safety and effectiveness. It is practiced by holders of Doctor of Medicine (MD) or Doctor of Osteopathy (DO) degrees and by allied health professionals, such as physical therapists, registered nurses, and psychologists. It is also referred to as **allopathy** or allopathic medicine.

Complementary and alternative medicine (CAM), according to the National Center for Complementary and Alternative Medicine (NCCAM; 2004), is a group of diverse medical

and health care systems, practices, and products that are not currently considered to be part of conventional medicine—i.e., they have not been shown through unbiased testing to be safe and effective. What is or is not properly considered alternative or complementary changes frequently as an increasing number of treatments undergo rigorous study and are proven effective or not. Applying the term "medicine" to complementary and alternative therapies or practices is inconsistent with the belief that, before a practice can be regarded as real medicine, conventional medicine, or medical practice it must be scientifically demonstrated to be safe and effective for the purposes for which it is intended. However, we shall use the acronym CAM—complementary and alternative medicine—to be consistent with common usage. CAM has been around as long as there has been medicine. It is difficult to pinpoint any origins of CAM because humans have attempted various remedies since our appearance on the planet, and the evolution of conventional medicine and the standards for its acceptability have taken centuries.

It is important to distinguish between complementary and alternative therapy. **Complementary therapy** is used together with conventional medicine. Some complementary therapies may relieve certain symptoms as the patient undergoes conventional treatment. For example, meditation or guided imagery can reduce stress, and ginger tea may help reduce nausea. **Alternative therapy**, in contrast, is used in place of conventional medicine. Alternative therapies are either unproven due to a lack of scientific testing or they have been tested and found to be ineffective. Over 1,000 alternative therapies have been identified (Inglis & West, 1983; Segen, 1998; Raso, 1994, 1998). Alternative therapy is often described as unconventional or nontraditional. A third category, **integrative therapy**, usually combines mainstream medical therapies for which there is some high-quality scientific evidence of safety and effectiveness with alternative or even ancient therapies, frequently within a **holistic approach**, meaning a combination of mind, body, and spirit. The term "integrative therapy" is sometimes used in place of "complementary and alternative therapy" with the hope of generating more credibility.

Many CAM practitioners base their work around a few core philosophies (MayoClinic.com, 2005). Embedded in these philosophies is the concept that the CAM practitioner is a facilitator who helps the body to heal itself. Boosting the immune system is preferable to treating an infection with antibiotics. CAM emphasizes prevention, something many criticize conventional medicine for minimizing. CAM also stresses that it is the patient who actually does the healing and the practitioner only offers guidance.

Although basic philosophies are fairly easy to discern, it is important to understand that many alternative treatments have their origins in religion, folklore, chance, and experience. It is also curious that although the various methods have originated from diverse roots, they are frequently applied together. Finally, by identifying oneself as a facilitator rather than a physician and claiming that the patient and his or her body do the healing, the responsibility for failure is shifted from the practitioner.

Why the Two Sides of "Medicine"?

Before modern medicine, people who became ill or injured turned to shamans or to folk medicine. Examples of folk medicine include covering a wart with a penny and then burying the penny, and treating a cold with chicken soup. In the late 1800s, things began to change as scientific, fact-based medicine became more popular and use of folk medicine diminished. Licensing for doctors became commonplace. Medical schools became politically powerful in the licensing of practitioners. Because folk medicine was not rooted in science and reason, those who practiced only this tradition could not be licensed. CAM practitioners and conventional doctors became rivals and they remained divided for many years.

Many in the medical community consider most alternative therapies to be quackery. Medical doctors have historically viewed practitioners of alternative therapies as untrained hucksters who claimed to have the cure for everything in one bottle and who were in practice only for profit. They saw alternative practitioners as opportunists who took advantage of people in their weakest moments by selling them expensive unproven therapies. There is good reason for conventional physicians to be skeptical about CAM. Physicians' education and experience are closely linked to science—controlled, objective studies of diagnostic and treatment modalities. The articles in their professional journals are largely based on rigorous scientific research. They view diagnosis and treatment in terms of science, while many complementary and alternative methods lack the science to demonstrate their safety and effectiveness and rely extensively on **anecdotal evidence**.

Some practitioners of alternative therapies make exaggerated claims about curing diseases. Others ask patients to forgo or delay conventional treatments while using unproven therapies. These delays may result in advancement of disease and even death of the patient. Some forms of alternative therapies can themselves be harmful.

In the 1970s, interest in CAM began to increase. Initial costs of CAM can appear to be lower than medical care, a fact that attracts some patients, although total costs over time may be large. Other reasons for increased interest include the fact that modern medicine is incapable of curing everything, a willingness to try new things, and desperation on the part of seriously ill individuals who

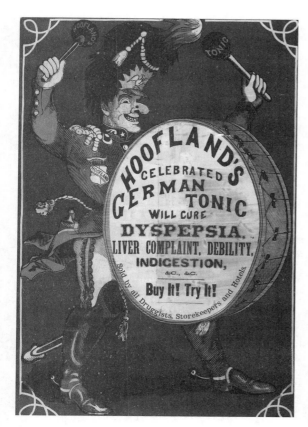

A nineteenth-century label for a treatment that would be called "alternative" today. As is common with alternative therapies, it is claimed to be effective against a variety of ailments.

were not helped by even the most modern medical techniques. As a result of this renewed interest on the part of patients, many physicians became more knowledgeable about and even accepting of CAM. While fewer recommend alternative remedies, many allopathic physicians are receptive to complementary therapies. It is not unusual for physicians to recommend dietary supplements. A few even refer patients to chiropractors for treatment of back pain. Some allopathic hospitals offer aromatherapy and massage (see the box on page 128). Most hospitals have chaplains who provide religious services to patients and their families, often in the form of prayer for the recovery of a patient.

Many practitioners of alternative therapies claim to be persecuted by the conventional medical community. Some have alleged that drug companies and universities will not conduct research on their methods because those institutions cannot profit from them. Perhaps the biggest breakthrough in the legitimization of complementary and alternative therapies was the founding of the National Center for Complementary and Alternative Medicine in the National Institutes of Health in 1998. The best way to determine effectiveness is through science, with the state-of-the-art level of evaluation through the use of random controlled trials. The NCCAM supports research into various alternative and complementary therapies. This research is still relatively scarce in comparison with studies on drugs or medical devices. In 2008, more than 7,500 CAM trials were indexed in MEDLINE, a huge database of articles published in over 5,200 biomedical journals from the United States and over 80 from other countries, with more than 1,600 involving children aged 18 years or younger (Chan, 2008). This is far less than the number of trials conducted on conventional medicine. The reasons for this discrepancy include the facts that research is expensive and most studies done on drugs and devices are conducted by wealthy pharmaceutical companies. In addition, in the typical research study, participants receiving a treatment receive consistent measured treatment for a condition. CAM practitioners, in contrast, are not as consistent in their treatments, dosages, and directions, making research more difficult.

Some scientific evidence exists for some CAM, especially complementary medicine. There are key questions yet to be answered through well-designed studies for most of them. Some of these questions include: Are these therapies safe? Do they really work for the medical conditions for which they are used? Are they superior to medical treatments already available?

Alternative practices have been described by Skrabanek and McCormick (1990) as being distinguished by two features: (1) they do not derive from a coherent or established body of evidence, and (2) they are not subjected to rigorous assessment to establish their value. Perhaps the route from alternative to complementary and possibly to conventional medicine passes through these features.

The list of what is considered to be CAM is in a constant state of change. When therapies are demonstrated through carefully controlled studies to be safe and effective, they are usually adopted into conventional health care and are, therefore, not complementary or alternative anymore.

Categories of CAM

The NCCAM (2004) classifies CAM into five categories or domains:

1. *Alternative "medical" systems (sometimes called healing systems)*. These systems are built upon complete systems of theory and practice rather than just a single practice, such as massage or use of an herb. Often, they have evolved apart from and earlier than the conventional medical approach used in the United States. Examples of systems that have developed in Western cultures include homeopathic therapy, naturopathy, and some Native American systems. Examples of systems that have developed in non-Western cultures include traditional Chinese medicine and Ayurveda. Healing systems revolve around a philosophy or lifestyle.

2. *Mind-body interventions*. Mind-body therapy uses a variety of techniques designed to enhance the mind's capacity to affect bodily function and symptoms. If your mind and body are not communicating, you could get sick. Some techniques that were considered CAM in the past have become mainstream. These include patient support groups and cognitive-behavioral therapy. Other mind-body techniques are still considered CAM, including meditation, prayer, yoga, hypnosis, biofeedback, mental healing, and therapies that use creative outlets such as art, music, or dance.

3. *Biologically based therapies*. Biologically based therapies in CAM use substances found in nature, such as herbs, foods, and vitamins. Some of these are dietary supplements, herbal products, and the use of other so-called natural but scientifically unproven therapies such as using shark cartilage to treat cancer. It should be noted that herbs as dietary supplements are not regulated as drugs, so little proof exists that these remedies can help you and there is no guarantee that they are safe.

4. *Manipulative and body-based methods*. Manipulative and body-based methods in CAM are based on manipulation and/or movement of one or more parts of the body. Some examples are chiropractic, osteopathic manipulation, reflexology, and massage.

5. *Energy therapies*. Energy therapists believe that an energy force flows through the body. If the flow of energy is blocked, they reason, you become sick. There are of two types of energy therapies:

   - *Biofield therapies* are intended to affect energy fields that purportedly surround and/or penetrate the human body. The existence of such fields has not been scientifically proven. Some forms of energy therapy manipulate biofields by applying pressure and or manipulating the body by placing the hands in, or through, these fields. Examples include qi gong, Reiki, and therapeutic touch.
   - *Bioelectromagnetic-based therapies* involve the unconventional use of electromagnetic fields, such as pulsed fields, or alternating- or direct-current fields.

Some practitioners believe that an energy force flows through the body that, if blocked or unbalanced, can result in sickness. Unblocking or balancing this force is the goal of these therapies.

Figures 6.1 and 6.2 display data from the National Health Interview Survey (Barnes, Bloom, & Nahin, 2008), indicating the choices of CAM therapies used by children and adults. The survey interviews were conducted in 29,266 homes and with 75,764 individuals.

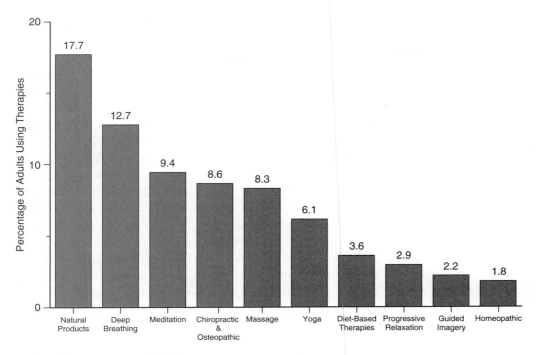

FIGURE 6.1 MOST COMMON CAM THERAPIES AMONG ADULTS, 2007

Source: Barnes, P. M., Bloom, B., & Nahin, R. (2008). Complementary and alternative health medicine use among adults and children: United States, 2007. CDC National Health Statistics Report no. 12.

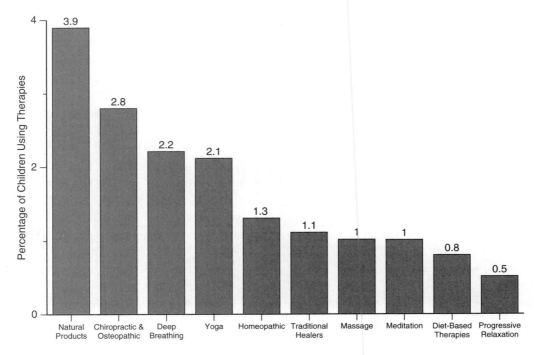

FIGURE 6.2 MOST COMMON CAM THERAPIES AMONG CHILDREN, 2007

Source: Barnes, P. M., Bloom, B., & Nahin, R. (2008). Complementary and alternative health medicine use among adults and children: United States, 2007. CDC National Health Statistics Report no. 12.

How Popular Is CAM?

In December 2008, the U.S. Centers for Disease Control and Prevention and the NCCAM released the results of the 2007 National Health Interview Survey (NHIS). The NHIS yielded information about the use of CAM during 2007. Almost 4 out of 10 adults reported using CAM therapy in the past 12 months. Approximately 1 in 9 children used CAM in the past 12 months, and children whose parents used CAM were five times as likely to use CAM as children whose parents did not use CAM. Figures 6.3 and 6.4 demonstrate the percentages of use by age and ethnicity.

The NHIS also revealed that women were more likely than men to use CAM. Use rose with educational levels. People who had been hospitalized in the past year were more likely to use CAM. Former smokers, compared with current smokers or those who have never smoked, were more likely

to have used CAM. Adult use was more prevalent in the West.

CAM is used for a variety of conditions. Figures 6.5 and 6.6 present NHIS data relative to the diseases or conditions for which CAM is used most frequently.

As Figure 6.6 shows, the most common CAM-treated condition among children was back and neck pain in 2007. Figure 6.2 shows that chiropractic and osteopathic treatment together were the second most common CAM treatment for children. Children accounted for about 14 percent of all visits to chiropractors (Kemper, Vohra, & Walls, 2008). Chiropractic treatment for children is a very controversial issue. Figure 6.6 also shows that CAM was used to treat head and chest colds is in a relatively high percentage of children. Echinacea, an herb frequently used to treat the common cold, was taken by more than 37 percent of children during the past 12 months before the survey. Clinical evidence of any benefit of

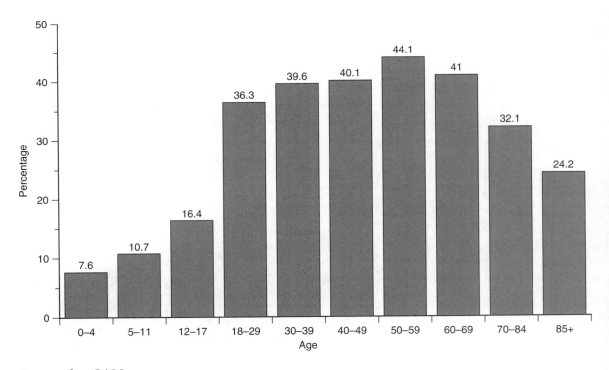

FIGURE 6.3 CAM USE BY AGE, 2007

Source: Barnes, P. M., Bloom, B., & Nahin, R. (2008). Complementary and alternative health medicine use among adults and children: United States, 2007. CDC National Health Statistics Report no. 12.

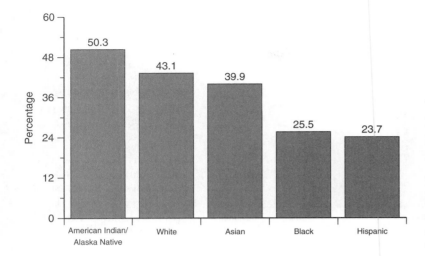

FIGURE 6.4 CAM USE BY RACE/ETHNICITY AMONG ADULTS, 2007

Source: Barnes, P. M., Bloom, B., & Nahin, R. (2008). Complementary and alternative health medicine use among adults and children: United States, 2007. CDC National Health Statistics Report no. 12.

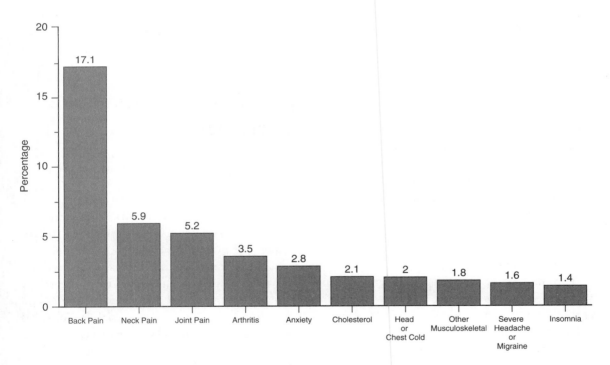

FIGURE 6.5 DISEASES/CONDITIONS FOR WHICH CAM IS MOST FREQUENTLY USED AMONG ADULTS, 2007

Source: Barnes, P. M., Bloom, B., & Nahin, R. (2008). Complementary and alternative health medicine use among adults and children: United States, 2007. CDC National Health Statistics Report no. 12.

echinacea is inconclusive, and safety has not been demonstrated.

In 2007, 38.1 million adults made an estimated 354.2 million visits to CAM practitioners. The popularity of CAM results in the spending of considerable dollars. The out-of-pocket costs for office visits were estimated at $11.9 billion, with about three-quarters of those visits and out-of-pocket costs associated with manipulative and body-based therapies. The total adult out-of-pocket

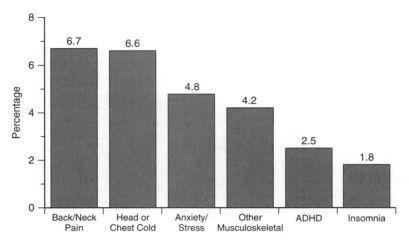

FIGURE 6.6 DISEASES/ CONDITIONS FOR WHICH CAM IS MOST FREQUENTLY USED AMONG CHILDREN, 2007

Source: Barnes, P. M., Bloom, B., & Nahin, R. (2008). Complementary and alternative health medicine use among adults and children: United States, 2007. CDC National Health Statistics Report no. 12.

expenditures were about $33.9 billion. Almost two-thirds of that total was spent on self-care. About 44 percent of all out-of-pocket costs for CAM was spent on the purchase of nonvitamin, nonmineral, natural products, a total of $14.8 billion (Nahin, Barnes, Stussman, & Bloom, 2009).

It is clear that many users of CAM are not primarily dissatisfied with conventional medical care but have a more holistic approach to health (Astin, 1998) or simply appreciate multiple treatment options. Chan (2008) made this point by suggesting that what was once identified as "alternative medicine" has become "complementary," "holistic," or "integrative." The line between CAM and allopathic medicine may be shifting in the perception of many.

The effectiveness and safety of alternative and complementary practices are controversial. Much of the evidence we have about CAM is anecdotal—that is, it is based on unscientific observation and accounts of an individual's personal experience. Anecdotal evidence, while good for stimulating more serious inquiry, offers little help to those seeking scientific evidence of the safety and efficacy of a practice. Reliance on anecdotal evidence can be dangerous. If a treatment appears safe and effective for one person, others may try it. This experience, often shared through word of mouth, may explain why laypersons find CAM so appealing. However, age, physiology, lifestyle, use of medications, and other factors may combine to make results very different. The possibility also

exists that any result noticed by an individual could be a result of the placebo effect. It is often stated with regard to CAM that more and better research is needed.

Examples of Alternative Therapies

Homeopathy

Samuel Hahnemann, a German physician who had grown disenchanted with the treatment methods of the late 1700s that included bloodletting and placing caustic or hot substances on the skin to draw out infections, developed his own theory based on three principles: the law of similars, the minimum dose, and the single remedy. Homeopathy is a controversial area of CAM because its basic principles are not consistent with established laws of science, including those pertaining to chemistry and physics.

The law of similars stated that if a large amount of a substance causes certain symptoms in a healthy person, smaller amounts of the same substance can treat those symptoms in someone who is ill. Hahnemann tested his notions on himself, friends, and family with different herbs, minerals, and other substances. He referred to these experiments as "provings."

The minimum dose, or the law of infinitesimals, holds that a substance's strength and effectiveness increases the more it is diluted. Essential to the process of increasing potency while decreasing the actual amount of the active ingredient is vigorous shaking after each dilution. Some homeopathic remedies are so diluted that no molecules of the healing substance remain and cannot be detected even with sophisticated technologies (Stehlin, 1996). Homeopaths answer this absence by claiming that it is the "essence" or "memory" of the substance that heals. In cases where ingredients were identified in homeopathic remedies, they included chamomile, marigold, daisy, onion, poison ivy, mercury, arsenic, pit viper venom, and hemlock (Stehlin, 1996).

Homeopaths historically prescribed only a single remedy to cover all symptoms that a patient is experiencing, mental as well as physical. In recent years, multi-ingredient remedies have become a recognized part of homeopathic practice. The treatment consists of highly individualized therapy based on the practitioner's assessment of the patient. The classical diagnostic method was to assess the person's genetic history, personal health history, body type, and present status of physical, emotional, and mental symptoms; many homeopaths are taking a more homogeneous approach to diagnosis.

A fourth precept embraced by Hahnemann held that chronic diseases are simply manifestations of a suppressed itch or psora, a kind of evil spirit. Even to fervent homeopaths, this claim seemed so outrageous that it has been abandoned.

Curiously, the NCCAM describes homeopathy as an alternative *medical* system. William Jarvis, president of the National Council Against Health Fraud and professor of Public Health and Preventive Medicine at Loma Linda University Schools of Public Health and Medicine, referred to homeopathy as "a fraud on the public with the government's blessing" (Jarvis, 1997).

Homeopathic remedies gained legal status through the 1938 Federal Food, Drug, and Cosmetic Act. The law recognized as drugs all substances in the *Homeopathic Pharmacopoeia of the United States,* which lists more than 1,200 substances. In 1970, the Food and Drug Administration withdrew approval of all homeopathic chemicals. One of the results of this decision was reduction of regulation. Homeopathic products are regulated in much the same manner as nonprescription drugs. Manufacturers of homeopathic drugs are excused from submitting new drug applications to the FDA. Their products are exempt from good manufacturing practice requirements related to expiration dating and from finished product testing for identity and strength. The reason for not requiring the same scrutiny as other drugs is the fact that homeopathic products contain little or no active ingredient and so, from a toxicity standpoint, regulation of the products was deemed to be unnecessary. In fact, because some homeopathic remedies contain no detectable amount of the "active" ingredient, it is impossible to determine if the ingredients and amounts are those stated on the labels. Proving them safe would be equally troublesome.

Alcohol is a chief ingredient in many homeopathic remedies. While conventional drugs for adults can contain no more than 10 percent alcohol, and the amount is even less for children's medications, some homeopathic remedies contain much higher amounts because they are exempted from alcohol limit rules.

Homeopathic products are not totally exempt from all FDA regulation. If they claim to treat a serious disease such as diabetes or cancer, they can be sold by prescription only. If they are sold for self-limiting conditions such as colds or headaches that eventually go away on their own, they can be sold without a prescription.

Some problems with homeopathic remedies include:

- Products promoted as homeopathic that contain nonhomeopathic active ingredients, such as vitamins or plants not listed in homeopathic references
- Lack of tamper-resistant packaging
- Lack of proper labeling
- Vague indications for use that could encompass serious disease conditions; for example, the phrase "treats gastrointestinal disorders" could refer to ailments ranging from stomachache to colon cancer

- Lack of requirement that homeopathic remedies meet certain legal standards for over-the-counter drugs

Homeopathy is practiced by some medical doctors, chiropractors, osteopaths, dentists, nurses, veterinarians, and laypeople. Only three states, Connecticut, Arizona, and Nevada, have a state licensing board that licenses medical doctors to practice homeopathy. In all, about 550 practitioners are licensed, about 200 of which are physicians. Arizona and Nevada have provisions for homeopathic medical assistants who work in conjunction with a licensed homeopathic medical doctor. According to the laws of particular states and Canadian provinces, some licensed practitioners may be allowed to use homeopathy in their practice. Minnesota and California allow registered practitioners of alternative medicine to practice without being licensed (The Council for Homeopathic Certification, 2004). Some states explicitly include homeopathy within the scope of practice of chiropractic, naturopathy, physical therapy, dentistry, nursing, and veterinary medicine.

Sampson (1996) concluded that no valid research has ever found a homeopathic remedy more effective than standard medication. The National Council Against Health Fraud (1994), in evaluating the research on homeopathy, stated that controlled studies involving homeopathic remedies appear to divide along political lines. While the results of most studies do not support the use of homeopathic remedies, some ostensibly well-designed trials have yielded positive findings. Some of these, however, have been done by homeopaths, and their reports contain rhetoric that reflects bias strong enough to undermine confidence in the researchers' veracity. The best of these studies should be repeated by objective investigators with independent analyses of the homeopathic formulations.

For those considering the use of homeopathic remedies, the best advice is "buyer beware." The inconsistency of the manufacturing of these remedies should be considered. If you decide to use a homeopathic remedy, it is wise to provide this information to your physician. While the extremely diluted quantities of active ingredients do not usually interact with other drugs, the lack of regulation and the presence of alcohol in most homeopathic remedies merit the attention of a physician when prescribing other medications. The time spent in pursuing homeopathic remedies can delay conventional treatment, making treatment more difficult. Finally, as with any alternative treatment, one should consider the cost and the possibility that the practitioner may be more interested in your money than your health.

Naturopathy

"Naturopathic medicine," or "natural medicine," is a distinct system of primary care—an art, science, philosophy, and practice of diagnosis, treatment, and prevention of illness. Its principles are based upon the observation of the nature of health and disease rather than clinical trials. "Naturopathy," a term coined by John Scheel in 1895, was popularized by Benedict Lust, "the father of naturopathy." It is founded on a holistic philosophy of health. Naturopathic practice combines traditional therapies with some current advances in modern medicine and is appropriate for the management of a broad range of health conditions affecting all people of all ages, according to the American Association of Naturopathic Physicians (2004). This description is disputed by many in conventional medicine; according to Barrett (2003), naturopathy is largely a pseudoscientific approach. It fails to meet the standards most people would require of the practice of medicine, including scientific evidence of effectiveness and a long period of training of practitioners based on scientific principles. The NCCAM refers to naturopathy as an alternative medical system.

Naturopathy is said to "facilitate the body's inherent healing mechanisms" (Turner, 1990) and to assist nature. Practitioners claim that diseases are the body's effort to purify itself and that cures result from increasing the patient's "vital force." By ridding the body of waste products and toxins, naturopaths profess to stimulate the body's natural healing process. The naturopathic practitioner administers one or more physiological, mechanical, nutritional, manual, plant, or animal devices or substances. The objective is to remove obstacles to the body's normal functioning and use natural forces to renew the body's recuperative abilities.

Many naturopaths believe that virtually all diseases are within their scope. The most comprehensive naturopathic publications illustrating this belief are two editions of *A Textbook of Natural Medicine* (Pizzorno & Murray, 1985–1996, 1999) and two editions of the *Encyclopedia of Natural Medicine* (Pizzorno & Murray, 1990, 1998). Barrett (2003) has stated that both books recommend questionable dietary measures, vitamins, minerals, and/or herbs for more than 70 health problems ranging from acne to AIDS. For many conditions, daily administration of 10 or more products is recommended, some in dosages high enough to cause toxicity. Arnold Relman (2001), editor-in-chief emeritus of the *New England Journal of Medicine,* in a review of the textbook concluded, "Many of the treatments recommended in the *Textbook* ... are not likely to be effective, and treatments proven to be effective are often totally ignored. This could endanger the health and safety of patients with serious diseases who relied solely on care from a naturopathic practitioner."

The notion of **vitalism**, also referred to as "vital force" or "life force," originated in ancient times and is the basis for a number of alternative therapies, including naturopathy. There is no scientific evidence supporting vitalism. In fact, science, including organic chemistry, contradicts it.

The concepts behind naturopathy were first developed in the late nineteenth century by Sebastian Kneipp, a German priest. Kneipp opened a "water cure" center after becoming convinced that he and a fellow student had cured themselves of tuberculosis by bathing in the Danube River. This type of experience and erroneous conclusion is typical of the founding of many alternative therapies. Kneipp also developed herbal methods using whole plants. Benedict Lust, also German, was treated by Kneipp in 1892 and, being much impressed by

the outcome, successfully lobbied Kneipp for a commission to establish the priest's practices in the United States. In 1895, Lust opened the Kneipp Water-Cure Institute in New York City and began forming Kneipp Societies for members who used Kneipp's water therapy or other drugless therapies (Cody, 1985).

In hearings before the U.S. Senate, the National Association of Naturopathic Physicians (1970) asserted that naturopathy regards the following conditions as the bases for ill health: (1) lowered vitality; (2) abnormal composition of blood and lymph; (3) maladjustment of muscles, ligaments, bones, and neurotropic disturbances; (4) accumulation of waste matter and poison in the system; (5) germs, bacteria, and parasites that invade the body and flourish because of toxic states that may provide optimum conditions for their flourishing; (6) consideration of hereditary influences; and (7) psychological disturbances.

Naturopaths often serve as primary caregivers and provide treatment at their offices and at spas where clients may stay for several weeks. Techniques include fasting, "natural food" diets, vitamins, herbs, homeopathic remedies, cell salts, manipulation, massage, exercise, colonic enemas, acupuncture, and applications of water, counseling, stress management, hypnotherapy, biofeedback, heat, cold, air, sunlight, and electricity. Some even offer minor surgery, such as removal of foreign bodies, warts, and cysts. Radiation may be used for diagnostic purposes. Methods are often used in combination. For instance, naturopaths may combine sensible dietary advice with recommendations for unproven treatments or products.

A distinction should be made between "naturopathic physicians" and "traditional" naturopaths. Those that claim the title "physician" ostensibly attend an accredited institution for training and combine elements of traditional naturopathy with conventional medical practices such as prescribing drugs and performing surgery. The "traditional" naturopath focuses on health and education rather than diagnosing and treating diseases.

There are a handful of institutions in the United States that offer degrees in naturopathy, including Doctor of Naturopathy (ND), Doctor of Naturopathic Medicine (NMD), and PhD in Naturopathy. There appear to be a sizable number of organizations that offer online or correspondence courses. In 1987, the U.S. Secretary of Education approved the Council on Naturopathic Medical Education (CNME) as an accrediting agency for full-time schools. This accreditation was based on such factors as record-keeping, physical assets, financial status, makeup of the governing body, and nondiscrimination policy rather than the scientific validity of what was taught (Barrett, 2003). While the recognition of CNME as an accrediting agency was not renewed in 2001 by the U.S. Department of Education (Riley, 2001), this was a brief interruption. The recognition was restored in 2003.

Naturopaths are licensed as independent practitioners in 13 states and the District of Columbia and in five Canadian provinces. It is unknown how many practitioners—chiropractors, acupuncturists, homeopaths—practice naturopathy without being licensed to do so. Naturopathic services are not covered by Medicare or most insurance policies. However, the American Association of Naturopathic Physicians and some of the naturopathic schools have formed the Alliance for the State Licensing of Naturopathic Physicians to press for licensure in the remaining states. Many practitioners see licensure as a means to distinguish between naturopathic physicians and "traditional" naturopaths. The American Naturopathic Medical Association has opposed licensing efforts because its members would not be able to meet the educational requirements that would probably be included in the laws.

In opposing naturopathic licensing in Massachusetts, that state's medical society stated (Atwood, 2004) that naturopathy is both potentially and actually injurious when practiced according to the accepted standards of the profession; unscientific naturopathic beliefs pose irrational challenges to proven public health measures; and irrational, unscientific beliefs and practices, which are standards in the field, abound in naturopathy. The Massachusetts Medical Society also stated that naturopathic training programs are baseless and practitioners are incapable of self-regulation commensurate with public safety.

Ayurveda

Ayurveda, which originated in India, is a system dating back more than 5,000 years. The name is derived from two Sanskrit words, *ayu,* meaning life, and *veda*—meaning knowledge or science. Literally, *ayurveda* means "the science of life." However, it is hardly scientific, being "validated" by observation, inquiry, direct examination, and knowledge derived from ancient texts (Ayurvedic Foundations, 2003).

Ayurveda uses what its practitioners call a constitutional model with the aim to provide guidance regarding food and lifestyle so that healthy people can stay healthy and people with health challenges can improve their health. It is a combination of senses, mind, body, and soul that is said to provide comprehensive knowledge about spiritual, mental, and emotional health (Jiva Institute, 2004).

Practitioners of Ayurveda believe that the mind and the body work together to regulate our physiology and, in order for them to work together, we must use our senses as information gatherers and keep them clear. For example, when the mind perceives that a specific food is entering the gastrointestinal tract, it directs the body to act accordingly by releasing various digestive enzymes. The maintenance of clarity of the senses is illustrated by the contention that if we enjoy too much of a single taste, the ability to perceive that taste is diminished.

Believers view a person as made up of five primary elements: ether (space), air, fire, water, and earth. The composition of elements is what makes individuals unique. The elements have influence on people when they are present in the environment, such as the air or weather. Three "doshas" hold primary influence in Ayurveda.

- *Vata dosha* is formed by ether and air. It governs movement and directs nerve impulses, circulation, respiration, and elimination. It is also responsible for positive characteristics like creativity and flexibility and negative aspects like fear and anxiety.

- *Pitta dosha* is the combination of fire and water. It is the process of transformation or metabolism. Converting foods into nutrients is an example of *pitta* function. The *pitta dosha* is also responsible for metabolism in the organ and tissue systems and for cellular metabolism. Emotionally, it is connected to courage, ambition, anger, and pride.
- *Kapha dosha* is the combination of water and earth. This dosha is responsible for growth. It governs emotions such as love and devotion, greed, and jealousy.

According to Ayurveda, we are all made up of unique proportions of the three doshas, called the *prakriti,* or constitution, and because of this, Ayurveda sees each person as a special mixture that accounts for our diversity.

Ayurvedic writings contain lengthy lists of alleged physical and mental characteristics associated with each body type defined by the doshas. Deepak Chopra, an endocrinologist who became quite wealthy writing books and selling ayurvedic products, stated in one of his videos that *vata* individuals are "usually lightly built with excellent agility" and "love excitement and change" (Chopra, 1994).

The doshas are essential in the practice of Ayurveda. When any of them becomes "accumulated," or there is disharmony among the doshas, Ayurveda suggests specific lifestyle and nutritional guidelines to assist the person in reducing the dosha that has become excessive. Sometimes herbal supplements are given to speed the healing. If toxins are present in the body, a cleansing process known as *pancha karma* is recommended to eliminate the toxins.

In addition to the doshas, there are other elements. The *dhatus* are the basic tissues that maintain and nourish the body, including plasma, blood, muscle, fat, bone, marrow, and reproductive fluid. *Mala* are waste materials produced as a result of metabolic activities in the body. The main mala are urine, feces, and sweat. *Srota* are channels that are responsible for transportation of food, dhatus, malas, and doshas. *Agni* means fire. According to Ayurveda, there are 13 types of agni in the body. They carry out different metabolic activities and are comparable to different types of enzymes responsible for digestion and metabolic activity in the body.

Ayurveda is more a way of life than a treatment. It is about preventing disease and enhancing health, longevity, and vitality. The *Vedas,* the ancient classics and Indian books of knowledge, provided guidance on all aspects of life, including engineering, town planning, philosophy, spirituality (Jiva Institute, 2004), methods of cooking, dietary regimen, proper attire, seasonal conduct, rules of sleeping, and environment.

Ayurvedic practitioners are trained in the United States to be clinical ayurvedic specialists (CASs). The CAS is trained to understand the client physically, emotionally, and spiritually. From this understanding, the practitioner identifies the client's constitution and the nature of any imbalances, and then designs a treatment using diet, herbs, colors, aromas, sound, yoga, and meditation. The CAS is part healer, part counselor, part coach, and part guide (California College of Ayurveda, 2004).

There is a National Ayurvedic Medical Association (NAMA) that operates in the United States. Its mission is to preserve, protect, improve, and promote the philosophy, knowledge, science, and practice of Ayurveda (NAMA, 2004). There are about eight schools that train people to use ayurvedic techniques.

There is no state or national licensing for ayurvedic practitioners, and it is not regulated or licensed by government. Standards of competency are set by the individual schools.

Chopra is America's most prominent spokesman for Ayurveda. He founded the American Association for Ayurvedic Medicine and Maharishi Ayurveda Products International, which sells instructional materials and herbal products. He has since broken his relationship with these organizations. An article in *Forbes* (Moukheiber, 1994) called him "the latest in a line of gurus who have prospered by blending pop science, pop psychology, and pop Hinduism."

Reiki

Reiki is a Japanese word meaning "Universal Life Force Energy." Characterized by the NCCAM as an "energy therapy," Reiki is a system for channeling energy to someone for the purpose of healing. It has been practiced for 2,500 years and was rediscovered by Dr. Mikao Usui, a Christian minister, in the mid-1800s.

In Reiki, "healing" is more than removing symptoms. It is to recover a greater experience of unity with the divine harmony and our true selves. Healing is seen as returning to a state of alignment with your Higher Self or true way of being (Herron, 2004b). There is, according to Herron (2004a), a vast energy field that is both more complicated and more simple than we can observe through the five senses. This energy field is said to permeate all things physical. Herron admits that no proof of the Universal Life Force Energy has been found.

Reiki, according to its adherents, creates healing by applying Universal Life Force Energy, by directing the energy that makes up the universe to the people, places, and things where there is a difference between the current form and the ideal form. They believe that beneficial effects are obtained from a "universal life energy" that practitioners channel to patients, providing strength, harmony, and balance to the body and mind. For example, if a bone is broken, the application of the Universal Life Force Energy would replace the current broken form with a strong, whole pattern.

In its simplest form, the practitioner places his or her hands on the recipient in positions taught to the practitioner. The placing of the hands supposedly allows the flow of Reiki energy through the practitioner, who is said to be only a conduit for the energy. The energy purportedly knows where to go and what to do once it gets there, treating health problems and enabling patients to

feel enlightened, with improved mental clarity, well-being, and spirituality. A first-degree Reiki practitioner learns to treat through a series of 12 to 15 hand positions placed on the body and held for two to five minutes. A second-degree Reiki practitioner "learns to send Reiki over distance through the use of special symbols which involve the opening up to the experience of the energy and listening to one's inner voice" (Bullock, 1997).

Reiki adherents believe that the world we see is only a small fragment of all that exists. This small fragment is that which our physical bodies can detect and transmit or describe to our consciousness. Reiki practitioners believe that Reiki can operate without the restraints of space. A second-degree Reiki practitioner is thought to be able to bring healing to a recipient regardless of distance. Remote healing relies on the practitioner's ability to visualize sending energy to the recipient. As Herron (2004b) wrote, "The only limit is the healer's imagination. For the healer's intent is primary in bring [*sic*] forth the Reiki energy."

Sometimes Reiki does not work to the satisfaction of the practitioner. This is explained away as the lack of willingness on the part of recipients to cast off old habits and patterns, to accept change and to accept healing.

Jarvis (1999) stated that Reiki is only a variation of other healing superstitions and that Reiki literature instructs practitioners in how to avoid regulation and accountability. Reiki has been studied for some health conditions, but it has not been studied through enough well-designed clinical trials to lend confidence in its use with serious medical conditions. There is some evidence of usefulness in relieving stress, depression, and pain relief, especially if used with more proven medical treatments as a complementary treatment. Many of the effects may be a result of suggestion. Patients should speak with their physician if considering Reiki therapy.

Yoga

Yoga is one of several health practices grouped by the NCCAM under the title "Mind-Body Medicine." The yoga philosophy began approxi-

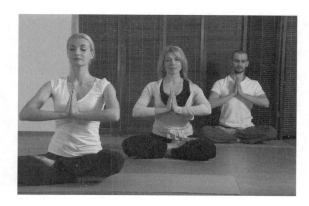

Participants in a yoga class meditating in the lotus position.

mately 5,000 years ago in India. The Indian philosopher and thinker Patanjali is believed to have collated the practice of yoga into the *Yoga Sutra* about 2,000 years ago. The *Sutra* is a collection of 195 statements that serve as the philosophical guidebook for most of the yoga that is practiced today. It also outlines eight limbs of yoga: the *yamas* (restraints or ethical standards), *niyamas* (observances), *asana* (postures), *pranayama* (breathing), *pratyahara* (withdrawal of senses), *dharana* (concentration), *dhyani* (meditation), and *samadhi* (absorption). Exploration of these limbs refines our behavior in the outer world, and then allows us to focus inwardly until we reach *samadhi* (liberation and enlightenment) (Lee, 2004).

Yoga is a philosophy, not a religion. It is, however, sometimes interwoven with Hinduism or Buddhism.

There are six branches of yoga—*hatha, raja, karma, bhakti, jnana,* and *tantra*. Initially, the discipline of hatha yoga—the physical aspect of yoga—was developed as a vehicle for meditation. Hatha yoga prepares the body, and particularly the nervous system, for stillness, creating the necessary physical strength and stamina that allows the mind to remain calm. Hatha is considered the "yoga of activity." It addresses the body and mind and requires discipline and effort. Meditation is the focus of raja, which involves strict adherence to the eight limbs of yoga. Individuals who are introspective and drawn to meditation, especially members of religious orders and spiritual communities, devote themselves to raja. Karma yoga is described as the path of service. The principle of karma yoga is that what we experience today is created by our actions in the past. According to the principle, all of our present efforts become a way to consciously create a future that frees us from being bound by negativity and selfishness. Those practicing karma yoga believe they practice whenever they perform their work and live their lives selflessly. Bhakti yoga describes the path of devotion. Seeing the divine in all of creation, this branch is a positive way to channel emotions. Bhakti yogis express the devotional nature of their path in their every thought and deed. Jnana yoga is the yoga of the mind, of wisdom; it is the path of the sage or scholar. It requires development of the intellect through the study of the scriptures and text of the yoga tradition. Jnana yoga is considered the most difficult and the most direct and will appeal to those more intellectually inclined. Tantra yoga, the sixth branch, is the pathway of ritual that includes consecrated sexuality. In tantric practice, yogis experience the divine in everything they do. It appeals to those who enjoy ceremony (Carrico, 2004a, 2004b).

The practice of yoga has gained in popularity in North America in the past 100 years. Modern yoga proponents feel that infections, injuries, and other problems with a strong physical basis should be handled by conventional medicine. Many advocates believe that sufferers of degenerative disorders and psychosomatic ailments can be helped by the practice of yoga. While traditional yoga philosophy requires that students adhere to its mission constantly through their behavior, diet, and meditation, many people use it simply for flexibility, relaxation, or stress relief. For these purposes, hatha yoga seems most appropriate because it focuses on physical poses and controlled breathing. In the typical hatha yoga class, students focus on 10 to 30 poses. The difficulty of the poses varies greatly. Controlled breathing is an important part of yoga. Enthusiasts believe that if you can control your breathing, you can control your body and gain control of your mind. Various techniques are used to focus your mind on your breathing, and hatha yoga is practiced in several forms.

There are several benefits to yoga, especially relaxation and flexibility. The breathing and relaxation methods used in yoga may be beneficial to sufferers of asthma, carpal tunnel syndrome, osteoarthritis, or memory problems. Yoga can also be helpful when combined with other therapies for heart disease and high blood pressure. It is often used in combination with aerobic exercise, medication, and a vegetarian diet to reduce cardiovascular disease and blood pressure levels (MayoClinic.com, 2004).

Yoga is considered safe if you are generally healthy, although some positions can strain the lower back and joints. Those considering a yoga class should consult a physician if they have high blood pressure, a risk of blood clots, eye conditions such as glaucoma, osteoporosis, or a history of psychotic disorders.

Chiropractic

Chiropractic is a branch of CAM that is based on the concept that a properly functioning nervous system is the key to health. It emphasizes the spine and the nerves extending from the spine to all parts of the body. Chiropractic attempts to address health problems by locating and adjusting a musculoskeletal area of the body, primarily the spine, that is functioning improperly. While chiropractic may emphasize the mind-body relationship in healing and health maintenance, the primary technique applied by chiropractors is spinal manipulation.

The spine is a series of bones called vertebrae that are stacked one on top of the other. Between the vertebrae are disks, made of soft, gel-like material, that absorb shock and keep the vertebrae from contacting one another. The spinal cord, a dense mass of nerves, runs through a channel made by stacked openings in the vertebrae and the disks. Ligaments, muscles, tendons, fascia, and blood vessels are also part of the vertebral

joints. Occasionally, a vertebra or a disk becomes unaligned; this is what chiropractors call a "subluxation." Subluxations may also describe loss of joint mobility in the spine. According to chiropractic, a vast range of health problems is caused by subluxations. In order to treat these problems, chiropractors manipulate the spine to eliminate the subluxation and realign the spine.

Modern chiropractic had its beginnings in the late 1800s when Daniel David Palmer, a self-educated and self-proclaimed healer, performed the first spinal manipulation. Palmer is credited with curing a case of deafness in a janitor who lived in his building by pressing a vertebra that he thought out of position back in place. From this beginning, Palmer leapt to the conclusion that spinal manipulation could cure many illnesses. Later, he delivered a part biological–part theological thesis that held that (1) "Innate Intelligence" or "nerve energy" flows through the nervous system and controls every bodily activity not under voluntary control; (2) even slight spinal misalignments hinder this flow, causing people to become ill; and (3) manual manipulation of the spine is the remedy.

Palmer opened a chiropractic school in 1897 called the Palmer Infirmary and Chiropractic Institute in Davenport, Iowa. It was later renamed the Palmer College of Chiropractic. Palmer's son, Bartlett Joshua, soon took over the daily activities of the school. In 1906, the elder Palmer was arrested along with hundreds of other chiropractors and convicted of practicing medicine without a license.

The "Chart of Effects of Spinal Misalignments" governed the practice of chiropractic almost exclusively for decades. It is claimed that more than 100 health problems, including allergies, amnesia, crossed eyes, hernias, jaundice, and pneumonia, are caused by spinal misalignments. The chart identifies the exact offending area of the spine that is subluxated and in need of manipulation to relieve a specific health problem. Chiropractors who continue to follow the chart to the exclusion of other diagnoses and treatments are referred to as "straights."

Today's chiropractor uses a number of diagnostic techniques. Chiropractors will usually collect a large amount of historical and observational information, such as the patient's description of the pain, the location of the pain, the gait and posture, general range of motion, muscle tone, muscle strength, and balance. Spinal palpation is a process of examining the spine by means of touch. It is the central diagnostic procedure (Strasser, 2004). Chiropractors also make liberal use of x-rays in diagnosing subluxations, including a minority who use full-spine x-rays, that yield little or no diagnostic information but subject the patient's reproductive organs to high levels of radiation (Barrett, Jarvis, Kroger, & London, 2002). Some use dubious methods such as hair analysis, thermography, and various gadgets alleged to detect subluxations.

The primary treatment used in chiropractic is the adjustment of the spine by manipulation. The chiropractor uses his or her hands and body to quickly move the spine to eliminate subluxations. But chiropractic in its present form goes well beyond manual manipulation. The practice now gravitates toward a more holistic approach in treatment of the total person, particularly the relationships among lifestyle, environment, and health. Many chiropractors emphasize nutrition and exercise, as well as lifestyle modification. While they are not allowed to prescribe drugs, many use herbal substances and homeopathic remedies.

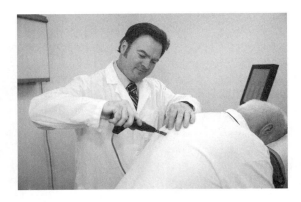

A chiropractor uses a computerized electronic tool to diagnose and adjust a patient.

Although not qualified by training to understand the use of prescription drugs, many chiropractors discourage their use. A few even apply such alternative treatments as reflexology.

Doctors of chiropractic often refer patients to allopathic physicians (MDs) when they feel it is indicated. In some cases, chiropractors, physical therapists, medical doctors, and other health care professionals work together in occupational health, sports medicine, and a variety of other rehabilitation practices. These are practitioners who either do not embrace the "Chart of Effects of Spinal Misalignments" or refer patients to other practitioners for other diagnoses and treatments; they are described as "mixers" as opposed to "straights." While they recognize the importance of germs, hormones, and other factors, many of these practitioners believe that mechanical disturbance to the nervous system is the underlying cause of many, if not most, health problems.

There are currently 16 chiropractic colleges in the United States. More than 14,000 people attend these colleges annually (ChiroFind.com, 2009). The Council on Chiropractic Education, recognized by the U.S. Department of Education as a specialized accrediting agency, has set standards and monitored chiropractic education since 1974.

The practice of chiropractic is licensed and regulated in all 50 states and in more than 30 countries worldwide. State licensing boards regulate, among other elements, the education, experience, and moral character of candidates for licensure. There were about 49,000 practicing chiropractors in 2008; the number is expected to increase by 20 percent by 2018 (U.S. Department of Labor, 2009).

Chiropractic is not without its detractors. William Jarvis, the founder of the National Council Against Health Fraud, studied chiropractic as his doctoral dissertation. He concluded that "chiropractic's uniqueness is not in its manipulation but in its theoretical basis for doing it." He describes chiropractic as "a conglomeration of factions in conflict, bound together only by opposition to outside critics" (Jarvis, 1987). The editors of *Consumer Reports* (1994) warned people to be suspicious of any chiropractor who does any of the following:

- Takes full-spine or repeated x-rays
- Fails to take a comprehensive history and do a clinical examination to determine the cause of your trouble
- Claims that the treatment will improve immune function, benefit organ systems, or cure disease
- Offers to sell you vitamin cures, nutritional remedies, or homeopathic remedies
- Solicits children or other family members
- Advises against the immunization of children
- Wants you to sign a contract for long-term care
- Promises to prevent disease through regular checkups and spinal adjustments

Chiropractic treatment is not effective for conditions such as cancer, fractures, infectious diseases, and neurologic disease processes. Those with conditions that increase vulnerability of the bones or joints may experience harm from chiropractic treatment. Those who have known circulatory problems, especially with a history of thrombosis, should not have spinal manipulation.

The American Medical Association was a frequent critic of chiropractic for decades. However, AMA's Code of Medical Ethics (2008–2009) has stated that it is in the best interests of the patient for physicians and chiropractors to associate professionally. Contrary to previous positions, the AMA now permits member physicians to refer patients to chiropractors.

Acupuncture

Acupuncture has been practiced in China for more than 4,000 years. Chinese medicine practitioners believe in a vital force called *qi* or *chi* that runs throughout the body. Qi is believed to regulate spiritual, emotional, mental, and physical balance and to be influenced by the opposing forces of *yin* and *yang*. Yin represents the feminine, passive, or accepting qualities, and yang the masculine, aggressive, or forceful qualities. According to this notion, when yin and yang are balanced, they work together with the natural flow of qi to help the body achieve and maintain health. Acupuncture, by keeping the normal flow of energy clear and unblocked, is believed to balance yin and yang. Chinese medicine also includes herbs, diet, massage, and meditative physical exercise, all intended to improve the flow of qi.

Acupuncture has been practiced in the United States for more than 200 years. Research on acupuncture began in the United States in 1976. Twenty years later, the Food and Drug Administration approved acupuncture needles as a medical device.

In modern practice in the United States, acupuncture needles are metallic, solid, and very thin. They may be twirled, heated, or even stimulated with weak electrical current, ultrasound, or certain wavelengths of light. Some acupuncturists inject saline water, procaine, morphine, vitamins, or homeopathic solutions through the inserted needles. The exact number of acupuncture points is controversial. Traditional Chinese medicine holds that there are more than 2,000 acupuncture points on the human body, and that these connect with 12 main and eight secondary pathways called meridians. Practitioners believe these meridians conduct the qi throughout the body. Traditional Chinese medicine is not based on modern physiology, biochemistry, nutrition, anatomy, or the known mechanisms of healing. The meridians used in Chinese medicine and the actual position of organs and nerves in the body are not correlated.

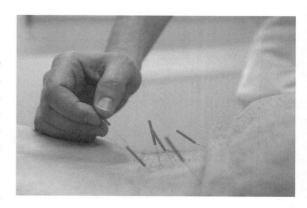

Acupuncture needles being applied to a patient.

Other methodologies also abound both in the United States and in other parts of the world. Acupressure, or manual pressure, is a variation on the use of needles. Auriculotherapy is a method of diagnosis and treatment based on the belief that the ear is the map of the body with certain points on the ear corresponding to parts of the body. Cupping is the process of applying suction by cups containing heated air. Still another method, called moxibustion, involves burning a cone of leaves and herbs at an acupuncture point.

People experience acupuncture differently, but most feel little or no pain. Some people are energized by the treatment, while others feel relaxed (American Academy of Medical Acupuncture, 1996). Soreness or pain during the treatment may be traced to movement of the patient, improper needle placement, or a defective needle (Lao, 1996).

As with many CAM therapies, it is difficult to demonstrate scientifically the powers of acupuncture. Since qi is defined as being undetectable by the methods of empirical science, science can never demonstrate that unblocking qi by acupuncture or any other means is effective against any disease (Skepdic.com, 2003).

Since the practice is used most often in the West for relief of pain, we will concentrate first on acupuncture's alleged analgesic effects. Acupuncture points are thought to stimulate the central nervous system to release chemicals into the muscles, spinal cord, and brain. These chemicals either change the experience of pain or release other chemicals, such as hormones, that influence the body's self-regulating systems. The changes may stimulate the body's natural healing abilities and promote physical and emotional well-being. The National Center for Complementary and Alternative Medicine (2002) identified three main mechanisms purported to explain pain-relieving effects of acupuncture: acupuncture points as conductors of electromagnetic signals; activation of opioids, chemicals in the brain that reduce pain; and changes in brain chemistry, sensation, and involuntary body functions. Still another theory suggests that pain impulses are blocked from reaching the spinal cord and brain at various "gates" to these areas. The National Cancer Institute (2010) described the pain relief mechanisms of acupuncture by stating, "Acupuncture may cause physical responses in nerve cells, the pituitary gland, and parts of the brain. These responses can cause the body to release proteins, hormones, and brain chemicals that control a number of body functions. It is proposed that, by these actions, acupuncture affects blood pressure and body temperature, boosts immune system activity, and causes the body's natural painkillers, such as endorphins, to be released."

As with all therapies, clinical trials should be the basis for judging effectiveness of acupuncture. Studies have been conducted on pain associated with fibromyalgia, carpal tunnel syndrome, migraine, low-back pain, menstrual cramps, osteoarthritis, and postoperative dental pain. The NCCAM (2009) summarized the results of these studies. For the most part, acupuncture was found to be no better than a placebo at relieving pain. For some types of pain, the research results are mixed.

Acupuncture has been studied for conditions other than pain. Studies of cancer patients suggest that acupuncture improves immune system response. Different types of clinical trials using different acupuncture methods have been shown to reduce nausea and vomiting caused by chemotherapy, surgery, and morning sickness.

Some suggest that the effects of acupuncture are due to less than anatomical reasons. The placebo effect, a measurable, observable, or felt improvement not attributable to treatment, may be a reason for some individuals' progress. Most medical conditions fluctuate with no treatment. Failure to recognize this phenomenon and ascribing changes in conditions to some therapy is called the **regression fallacy** (Gilovich, 1993). Other explanations include external suggestion (a form of hypnosis) and cultural conditioning (Barrett, 2004a).

While acupuncture is seen as a primary treatment in China, it is used mainly as a complementary treatment in the United States. For example, physicians may combine acupuncture and drugs to control surgery-related pain. Some have found indicators that using acupuncture lowers the need for conventional pain-killing drugs and reduces the risk of side effects of the drugs (Lewith & Vincent, 1996; Tsibuliak, Alisov, & Shatrova, 1995).

One of the main reasons Americans seek acupuncture is to relieve chronic pain, especially from arthritis and lower back disorders. Some clinical studies show that acupuncture is effective in relieving both chronic and acute or sudden pain, but other research indicates that it provides no relief from chronic pain (Ter Reit, Kleijnen, & Knipschild, 1990). The American College of Rheumatology (2008) stated that relief of pain associated with degenerative arthritis is due to acupuncture's unusually potent placebo effects.

The U.S. Food and Drug Administration approved acupuncture needles for use by licensed practitioners in 1996. The FDA requires manufacturers of acupuncture needles to label them for single use only (U.S. FDA, 1996). This recognition may eventually force insurers to cover acupuncture treatments, although Medicare currently does not.

Millions of Americans spend approximately $500 million a year on acupuncture treatments. They are treated for a range of ailments that include depression, AIDS, allergies, asthma, arthritis, bladder and kidney problems, constipation, diarrhea, colds, flu, bronchitis, dizziness, smoking, fatigue, gynecologic disorders, headaches, migraines, paralysis, high blood pressure, premenstrual syndrome, sciatica, sexual dysfunction, stress, stroke, tendinitis, and vision problems (Skepdic.com, 2003). Acupuncture is being used in drug and alcohol rehabilitation programs.

A person seeking acupuncture treatment may find a practitioner among medical doctors such as anesthesiologists or neurologists, chiropractors, traditional Chinese practitioners, or other CAM practitioners. Regardless of where a patient seeks acupuncture, it is a good idea to apply some simple practices.

- *Check a practitioner's credentials.* A practitioner who is licensed may provide better care than one who is not. Although proper credentials do not ensure competency, they

indicate that the practitioner has met certain standards to treat patients through the use of acupuncture.

- *Check treatment cost and insurance coverage.* A practitioner should inform you about the estimated number of treatments needed and how much it will cost. Check with your insurer to determine if the treatments are covered for your condition.

- *Ask about treatment procedures that will be used and their likelihood of success for your condition or disease.* Be aware that some unscrupulous practitioners may not be honest in their assessments. Make certain that a new set of disposable needles in sealed packaging is used every time. The practitioner should swab the puncture site with alcohol or other disinfectant before inserting the needle.

All states allow acupuncture to be performed, some by laypeople under medical supervision. Most states require a certification or licensure to practice acupuncture. Some states limit it to the practice of physicians or chiropractors or both. Some allow dentists or podiatrists to practice the technique. A few place acupuncture within the scope of practice for naturopaths.

Acupuncture is not without risks. There have been some reports of lung and bladder punctures, broken needles, fainting, local hematoma (bleeding due to a punctured blood vessel), convulsions, and allergic reactions to needles containing substances other than surgical steel. Unsterilized needles may lead to infection such as hepatitis B. Acupuncture may be harmful to a fetus during pregnancy since it may stimulate the production of adrenocorticotropic hormone and oxytocin, which affect labor. The adverse effects of acupuncture are probably related to the practitioner's training. On a global scale, acupuncture is practiced in more than 140 countries and accidents are increasing. Prevention of acupuncture accidents has become a global issue deserving of great attention (Zhang, 2004). Patients can gain some comfort in the fact that two prospective studies (White, Hayboe, Hart, & Ernst, 2001; MacPherson, Thomas, Walters, & Fitter, 2001) reported low complication rates and no serious complications among patients who underwent a total of more than 66,000 treatments.

Reflexology or Zone Therapy

The chart here illustrates the locations or zones of the foot that are connected to other areas of the body, according to practitioners of reflexology. There are similar charts for the other parts of the body, including the top of the foot, the ear, and the hand. Reflexologists believe that the hands and feet are reflections of the body. The effects of reflexology are described in the following quote that appears on several Web sites—e.g., Spirita Health (2010) and DistantHealer.co.uk (2010)—"Pressure applied to the feet generates a signal through the peripheral nervous system. From there it enters the central nervous system where it is processed in various parts of the brain. It is then relayed to the internal organs to allocate the necessary adjustments in fuel and oxygen. Finally a response is fashioned that is sent onto the motor system. This message is fed forward to adjust the body's tone or overall tension level." The colorful description, similar in tone to those of other alternative therapies, offers no real evidence to back claims of therapeutic effects.

According to Barrett (2004b), "Many proponents claim that foot reflexology can cleanse the body of toxins, increase circulation, assist in weight loss, and improve the health of organs throughout the body. Others have reported success in treating earaches, anemia, bedwetting,

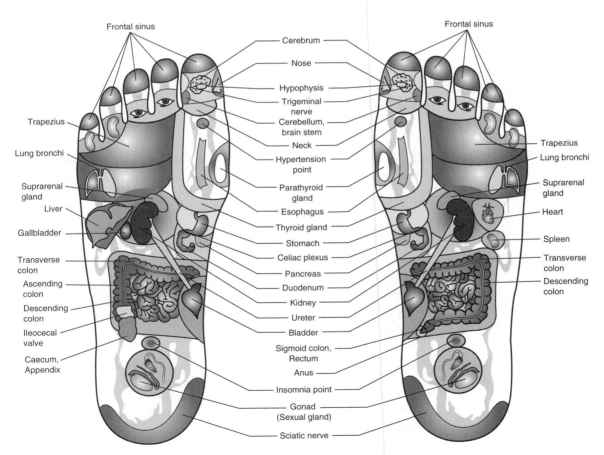

In reflexology, areas of the feet, hands, and ears correspond to parts of the body. By stimulating the areas, reflexologists claim to treat ailments related to the corresponding body parts.

bronchitis, convulsions in an infant, hemorrhoids, hiccups, deafness, hair loss, emphysema, prostate trouble, heart disease, overactive thyroid gland, kidney stones, liver trouble, rectal prolapse, undescended testicles, intestinal paralysis, cataracts, and hydrocephalus."

There seems to be no limit to the list of health problems that reflexologists claim to treat. While a foot massage can feel good and can help a person relax while lessening the stress that may accompany a work day, the research to support claims of therapeutic value is virtually absent.

Religious-Based Practices

Religion and a belief in the capacity of a higher power to heal are as old as humankind. Native Americans believed in the power of nature to heal and used, for example, the pipe ceremony and the purification ceremony as ways to invoke healing powers. Some modern Native Americans still practice these rites. Voodoo, practiced in Haiti and in parts of the southern United States, uses various rituals to release metaphysical healing powers. The merger of religion and healing or maintaining health is both ancient and modern.

Christian Science was discovered or founded in 1866 by Mary Baker Eddy. In 1875, Eddy published the first edition of *Science and Health with Key to the Scriptures,* which has sold more than 10 million copies. Christian Science is more faith than science, relying on a system of spiritual, prayer-based healing. Its practitioners do not accept medical treatment, including vaccinations, in the belief that sickness is an illusion, a "nonreality." Christian Science nurses cannot take a pulse, use a fever thermometer, give an enema, or even administer a backrub. They have no training in recognizing contagious diseases. There are reports that they have been retained to attend sick children and have sat taking notes as the children suffered and died, but have not called for medical care or recommended that parents obtain it.

Christian Science is a form of **faith healing,** but numerous other religious sects have adopted this method and it has been popular throughout history. The notion is that prayer, divine inter-

vention, or the ministrations of an individual healer can cure illness. Miraculous recoveries have been attributed to a myriad of techniques commonly lumped together as faith healing, but documenting a connection between the intervention and the result has been difficult. The fact that the practice relies heavily on faith makes it virtually impossible to validate through science. Some people who visit "healers" may feel better because the experience causes them to relax or because of a placebo effect. However, any benefit of this type should be weighed against the fact that people who are not relieved may conclude that they are "unworthy" and become depressed as a result. Money spent for a fruitless experience with a healer is another negative factor. Many faith healers, most notably Oral Roberts, have amassed great wealth through their practices. Some have been shown to be frauds.

Science-fiction writer L. Ron Hubbard (1911–1986), founded the Church of Scientology in 1953. Hubbard established a philosophy, system of psychotherapy, and quasireligion in the bestseller *Dianetics: The Modern Science of Mental Health,* first published in 1950. The Church of Scientology is often criticized as a cult or a money-making enterprise. It has a devoted following that embraces Hubbard's human division into the mind, body, and spirit. When a person joins the church, he or she goes through an "auditing" process, often using a device called an E-meter. According to Scientologists, auditing discovers destructive elements called engrams and begins a process to eliminate them. The auditing process is quite expensive and generates much income for the organization. Among the "psychosomatic" conditions Dianetics claims to cure or alleviate are asthma, poor eyesight, color blindness, hearing deficiencies, stuttering, allergies, sinusitis, arthritis, high blood pressure, coronary trouble, dermatitis, ulcers, migraine, conjunctivitis, morning sickness, alcoholism, the common cold, and tuberculosis. In total, Hubbard claimed in *Dianetics,* "70% of Man's listed ailments" could be cured through the use of Dianetics.

The Church of Scientology operates a chain of clinics that offer treatments purported to purge drugs and toxins from a person's system through a rigorous regimen of exercise, saunas, and vitamins—a combination intended to dislodge the poisons from fatty tissues and sweat them out. Physicians affiliated with the regimen have touted it as a major breakthrough, and a number of patients who have undergone the treatment say their health improved. Some health authorities dismiss Hubbard's program as a medical fraud that preys upon public fear of toxins. In the mid-1990s, the president of the Church of Scientology International announced plans to eradicate the medical practice of psychiatry.

Herbs and Dietary Supplements

Herbs are popular largely because they are considered natural. Figure 6.7 depicts the popularity of several products, as revealed by the NHIS. This subject will be discussed in more detail in Chapter 7. However, it is worth noting that many of these "natural prod-

ucts" have little or no evidence to support effectiveness for what they are claimed to treat or that they are safe. Since, under federal law, they are not treated as drugs, they can be marketed without testing the veracity of claims of effectiveness of treatment and, until recently, no evaluation of their safety. According to a study published in the *Journal of the American Medical Association,* of 433 complementary and alternative Web sites, most made misleading or unproven health claims about herbal remedies they sold (Morris & Avorn, 2003).

Many FDA medications contain ingredients derived from herbs and other plants. This has led to an assumption that anything that is described as "natural" is safe. Consumers should be careful in using herbal products and dietary supplements. Most have not been demonstrated safe and effective in clinical trials. Many have been shown to be useless, and some have been demonstrated harmful.

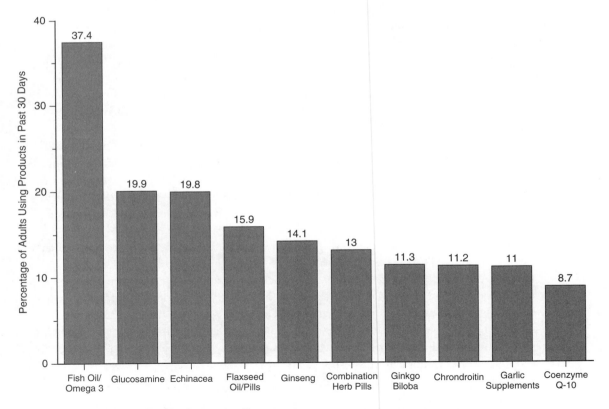

FIGURE 6.7 MOST COMMON "NATURAL" PRODUCTS USED AMONG ADULTS, 2007

Source: Barnes, P. M., Bloom, B., & Nahin, R. (2008). Complementary and alternative health medicine use among adults and children: United States, 2007. CDC National Health Statistics Report no, 12.

OTHER ALTERNATIVE AND COMPLEMENTARY THERAPIES

Aromatherapy: Involves the use of essential oils (extracts or essences) from flowers, herbs, and trees to promote health and well-being.

Biofeedback: The use of high-technology devices that allows the mind to control certain bodily functions.

Dietary supplements: A product (other than tobacco) taken by mouth that contains a "dietary ingredient" intended to supplement the diet. Dietary ingredients may include vitamins, minerals, herbs or other botanicals, amino acids, and substances such as enzymes, organ tissues, and metabolites. Dietary supplements come in many forms, including extracts, concentrates, tablets, capsules, gel caps, liquids, and powders.

Electromagnetic fields (EMFs; also called electric and magnetic fields): Invisible lines of force that surround all electrical devices. The Earth also produces EMFs; electric fields are produced when there is thunderstorm activity, and magnetic fields are believed to be produced by electric currents flowing at the Earth's core.

Esogenic colorpuncture: The practice of applying different-colored light to treat various maladies.

Guided imagery: A therapy based on the body-mind connection that uses directed thoughts and suggestions that guide the imagination toward a relaxed, focused state.

Massage: Manipulation of muscle and connective tissue to enhance function of those tissues and promote relaxation and well-being.

Meditation: A conscious mental process using certain techniques—such as focusing attention or maintaining a specific position—to suspend the stream of thoughts and relax the body and mind.

Qi gong ("chee-GUNG"): A component of traditional Chinese medicine that combines movement, meditation, and regulation of breathing to enhance the flow of *qi* (an ancient term given to what is believed to be vital energy) in the body, improve blood circulation, and enhance immune function.

Shiatsu: An Asian therapy that uses pressure applied with thumbs, fingers, elbows, and palms to the same energy meridians as acupressure and incorporates assisted stretching.

Therapeutic touch: Derived from an ancient technique called laying-on of hands, it is based on the premises that it is the healing force of the therapist that affects the patient's recovery, healing is promoted when the body's energies are in balance, and, by passing their hands over the patient, healers can identify energy imbalances.

Traditional Chinese medicine (TCM): The current name for an ancient system of health care from China. TCM is based on a concept of balanced qi, or vital energy, that is believed to flow throughout the body and which regulates a person's spiritual, emotional, mental, and physical balance and to be influenced by the opposing forces of yin (negative energy) and yang (positive energy). Disease is proposed to result from the flow of qi being disrupted and yin and yang becoming imbalanced. Among the components of TCM are herbal and nutritional therapy, restorative physical exercises, meditation, acupuncture, and remedial massage.

Sources: National Center for Complementary and Alternative Medicine. (2007). *What is CAM?* Retrieved from http://nccam.nih.gov/whatiscam/overview.htm

National Center for Complementary and Alternative Medicine. (2004). *Get the facts: What is complementary and alternative medicine (CAM)?* Retrieved from http://nccam.nih.health/whatiscam

Why Are Alternative and Complementary Treatments So Popular?

Today, many people are apprehensive about modern scientific medicine. Even though medicine as practiced in the United States and other developed nations benefits from many high-technology diagnostic and treatment devices and a wide range of effective medicines, the system is often impersonal and cold. Treatments tend to be invasive and complex in theory and practice. Often, the treatment seems to function completely void of input from the patient. It is no wonder that people often turn to more welcoming environments.

The practitioners of alternative therapies are usually quite personable. They characteristically spend much time with patients and are good listeners. Many of them tell patients exactly what they came to hear. A warm, friendly treatment room with a seemingly caring practitioner is sometimes enough to encourage an individual to give up allopathic medicine.

Many alternative and complementary treatments are effective. It is an undisputed fact that a lot of accepted conventional therapies were once considered "alternative." Some complementary methods are enhanced by conventional treatment and vice versa.

A good many remedies, especially alternative remedies, are without any scientific evidence of their effectiveness. There are a lot of reasons that they are perceived to be effective by their practitioners and/or their recipients. One reason is the placebo effect, accompanied by the power of suggestion. Many of us are so impressed by the surroundings of a treatment setting that we believe strongly in the power of the practitioner to help us. Many diseases, by virtue of the human immune system, dissolve on their own, a process known as natural remission, often leading the patient to believe that some therapy is the cause of his or her good fortune.

Part of the reason that CAM remedies may appear so beneficial relies on basic human nature. After investing time and money in a practitioner, it may be too much of a loss of prestige to admit that we have been duped. It is in our own self-interest to deny the failure of a therapy. It is especially difficult to admit a failed treatment when the patient has a strong commitment to the method, as occurs with the use of prayer and faith healing.

We should not overlook the fact that some CAM remedies make patients feel better. A massage, whether it be through reflexology or some other form of pressure, can relax the patient and produce a feeling of well-being. Some herbs contain small doses of mind-altering chemicals. Some, such as homeopathic remedies, may contain a dose of real medicine or may be adulterated with stimulants or other substances that promote a "feel-good" response (Jarvis, 1997).

Should You Consider an Alternative or Complementary Therapy?

The consumer's best asset is unbiased information. Anyone considering a CAM should discuss the procedure with his or her conventional physician. This is especially true of pregnant or breastfeeding women and adolescents. Make a list of questions and listen carefully to your doctor's responses. Ask about the length of time to give the therapy to show an effect, the scientific record of the method, and the expected cost. Ask if the method is used in conjunction with conventional medicine—i.e., is it complementary? Since many people consider CAM because of the side effects of conventional treatment, ask your physician if there are mainstream methods for dealing with side effects.

Check out the therapy in the scientific literature. Many people feel that, because a therapy may be purchased without a prescription, because the product is touted as being "natural," or because a person delivering the service or product says it is harmless, it is really safe. There are abundant examples of adverse effects. For instance, it is possible to suffer lead poisoning from ayurvedic remedies and nerve damage from spinal manipulation. There may be unexpected interactions with allopathic therapies, causing serious side effects or causing the conventional therapies to be ineffective. For example, oral contraceptives can have negative interactions with the herb St. John's wort. When seeking out information about CAM remedies, ask these questions:

- What claims are being made for the treatment?
- Who is advocating for the treatment? What are the credentials of those supporting the treatment? Will they profit from selling the product or service?
- Have scientific studies backed by clinical trials been done to determine the effectiveness of the method? Were the findings published in scholarly, refereed journals?
- How is the product promoted? Is it promoted only in mass magazines, Internet, infomercials, books, or talk shows rather than in scientific journals?
- Will your insurance cover the treatment? How much will it cost? Include travel costs in that calculation.
- Is it safe? Do scientific studies verify a reasonable margin of safety? Could it interact with your other methods, including medications or supplements?
- Is it widely available for use within the medical community? Is it available only from one practitioner or at one clinic?

Much information about CAM comes from the Internet, the content of which is practically unregulated. A careful consumer looks for information from major medical centers, national professional or nonprofit organizations, universities, and government agencies. If a Web site does not clearly distinguish between scientific evidence and advertising, consider it untrustworthy. Make sure that the information is current. Most Web pages have a date of the last update.

The U.S. Food and Drug Administration (Kurtzweil, 1999) recommends that you watch out for the following claims or practices:

- *Red-flag words or ambiguous language.* "New discovery" is a synonym for untested and unproven. If it were really a cure, it would be widely reported and your doctor would know about it. The words "satisfaction guaranteed" usually mean nothing. Often the people making the guarantee are nowhere to be found when you try to locate them. Do not be fooled by the terms "natural" or "all natural," words that are largely unregulated and are applied to virtually any product. After all, poison ivy is natural, but would you eat it? Promoting a product by saying it will bring relief "in just days" leaves the door open to any number of days, including years.
- *Pseudomedical jargon.* Promoters of sham remedies like to use words like "purify," "detoxify," and "energize" to attract unwary customers. These words are usually used in place of scientific evidence.
- *Cure-alls.* If the manufacturer claims that the product can treat a wide range of symptoms, cure many illnesses, or prevent a number of diseases, the chances are good that it is a sham. No product can treat every condition, and many conditions have no cures, only therapies to manage them. Unfortunately, serious conditions such as AIDS, cancer, and diabetes are favorite targets of these types of practitioners.
- *Quick fixes.* Be cautious of a product that promises a quick cure or quick relief from symptoms, especially if the condition is serious.
- *Anecdotal evidence and testimonials.* Personal testimonies should tip you off to health fraud because they are difficult to prove. Often, they are personal case histories that have been passed on from person to person, made up, or distorted. Some patients' positive experiences with a fraudulent product may be due more to remission in their disease, the placebo effect, or earlier or concurrent use of approved medical treatments rather than the use of the alternative product.
- *False accusations.* The seller accuses the government or the medical establishment of suppressing important information

about the product's benefits. Neither the government nor the medical profession has any reason to withhold information that could help people.

Other tip-offs that the therapy may be risky are claims of no side effects, requirement that you travel to another country, availability from only one person or clinic, and general or vague attacks on the medical or science community.

After all consideration, two important facts remain. First, alternative therapies lack scientific testing for safety and effectiveness. Therefore, their use may carry more and different risks than conventional medicine. Second, many people delay conventional treatment while trying alternative therapies. If the alternative therapy is not successful, the delay can result in the condition becoming more serious, leading to less chance of success with conventional medicine and greater cost of treatment.

SUMMARY

Conventional medicine is the group of diagnostic, treatment, and preventive practices that have been tested and shown to be safe and effective within acceptable standards. Alternative and complementary therapies have not been shown by objective clinical trials to be safe and/or effective. Alternative therapies are used in place of conventional medicine, while complementary therapies are used in conjunction with conventional medicine. This history of alternative therapies has been contaminated by practitioners who used unproven treatments that provided no benefit and often harm to the patient. The establishment of the National Center for Complementary and Alternative Medicine in the National Institutes of Health is an attempt to promote research to determine the safety and effectiveness of CAM remedies.

There are many different CAM remedies. They fall into five domains: alternative "medical" systems, mind-body interventions, biologically based therapies, manipulative and body-based methods, and energy therapies.

CAM remedies are quite popular. Almost two-thirds of the adult U.S. population has used CAM. A sizable proportion of children have experienced CAM treatments or practices. The popularity seems to be growing for a number of reasons, including perceived costs and desperation.

Before deciding to use a CAM therapy, patients should attempt to gather as much information about the treatment as possible. Good sources of information include conventional physicians, government agencies, peer-reviewed journals, and professional organizations.

KEY TERMS

Allopathy: methods of diagnosis, treatment, and prevention that have undergone extensive testing in multiple trials and have been shown to exceed agreed-upon standards of safety and effectiveness; also called conventional medicine

Alternative therapy: a remedy that has not been shown by scientific study to be safe and effective but is used in place of conventional medicine

Anecdotal evidence: evidence based on unscientific observation and accounts of individuals' personal experiences

Complementary therapy: a therapy that has not been accepted as conventional medicine but is used together with conventional medicine

Conventional medicine: methods of diagnosis, treatment, and prevention that have undergone extensive testing in multiple trials and have been shown to exceed agreed-upon standards of safety and effectiveness; also called allopathy or allopathic medicine

Faith healing: a concept that religious belief can bring about healing through prayers, touch, or rituals that evoke a divine power that cures disease or disability

Holistic approach: an approach to treatment that includes the entire person—mind, body, and spirit

Integrative therapy: combining of mainstream medical therapies for which there is some high-quality scientific evidence of safety and effectiveness with alternative or even ancient therapies

Regression fallacy: failure to recognize that health conditions change without treatment and ascribing changes in conditions to some therapy

Vitalism: a doctrine that the processes of life are not explainable by the laws of physics and chemistry alone and that a force courses through the body that affects physical, mental, and spiritual health

STUDY QUESTIONS

1. What are the differences among conventional, complementary, and alternative therapies?
2. Define "integrative therapy" and explain the reasons it is sometimes viewed as a more appropriate term than CAM.
3. Distinguish among the five categories of CAM.
4. What are some of the most commonly used CAMs?
5. How popular is CAM? What are some of the characteristics of people most likely to use CAM therapies?
6. What is anecdotal evidence and how useful is it in evaluating a therapy?
7. What are the foundations and beliefs of homeopathy, chiropractic, acupuncture, and other CAMs?
8. What information would you need to evaluate the benefits and risks of a CAM therapy? From where or whom would you obtain this information?
9. Do you think chiropractic is a valid treatment practice? What about Ayurveda? Why or why not?

REFERENCES

American Academy of Medical Acupuncture. (1996). *Doctor, what's this acupuncture all about? A brief explanation for patients.* Los Angeles, CA: American Academy of Medical Acupuncture.

American Association of Naturopathic Physicians. (2004). *Naturopathic medicine.* Retrieved from http://www.naturopathic.org

American College of Rheumatology. (2008). *Herbal remedies, supplements and acupuncture for arthritis.* Retrieved from http://www.rheumatology.org/practice/clinical/patients/diseases_and_conditions/herbal.asp

American Medical Association. (2008–2009). *Code of medical ethics of the American Medical Association.* Chicago, IL: American Medical Association.

Astin, J. A. (1998). Why patients use alternative medicine: Results of a national study. *JAMA, 279*(19), 1548–1553.

Atwood, K. C. (2004). *Why naturopaths should not be licensed.* Retrieved from http://www.quackwatch.org

Ayurvedic Foundations. (2003). *What is Ayurveda?* Retrieved from www.ayur.com/about.html

Barnes, P. M., Bloom, B., & Nahin, R. L. (2008). Complementary and alternative medicine use among adults and children: United States, 2007. National Health Statistics Report no. 12. Hyattsville, MD: National Center for Health Statistics.

Barrett, S. (2003). *A close look at naturopathy.* Retrieved from http://www.quackwatch.org/01QuackeryRelatedTopics/Naturopathy

Barrett, S. (2004a). *Be wary of acupuncture, qigong, and "Chinese medicine."* Retrieved from http://www.quackwatch.org/01QuackeryRelated Topics/acu.html

Barrett, S. (2004b). *Reflexology: A close look.* Retrieved from http://www.quackwatch.org/01QuackeryRelatedTopics/reflex.html

Barrett, S., Jarvis, W. T., Kroger, M., & London, W. M. (2002). *Consumer health: A guide to intelligent decisions* (7th ed.). New York: McGraw-Hill.

Bullock, M. (1997). Reiki: A comprehensive therapy for life. *American Journal of Hospice and Palliative Care, 14,* 31–33.

California College of Ayurveda. (2004). *Ayurveda for the 21st century.* Retrieved from http://www.ayurvedacollege.com

Carrico, M. (2004a). *A beginner's guide to the history of yoga.* Retrieved from http://www.yogajournal.com/newtoyoga/160.cfm

Carrico, M. (2004b). *The branches of yoga from* Yoga Journal's *yoga basics.* Retrieved from http://www.yogajournal.com/newtoyoga/157_1.cfm

Chan, E. (2008). Quality of efficacy research in complementary and alternative medicine. *JAMA, 299*(22), 2685–2686.

ChiroFind.com. (2009). *Chiropractic licensure and education.* Retrieved from http://www.chiroweb.com/find/licen.html

Chopra, D. (1994). *Growing younger: A practical guide to lifelong youth.* Alexandria, VA: Time Life Video.

Cody, G. (1985). History of naturopathic medicine. In J. E. Pizzorno, Jr., & M. T. Murray (Eds.). *A textbook of natural medicine.* Seattle, WA: John Bastyr College, Palos.

The Council for Homeopathic Certification. (2004). *How certification differs from licensing.* Retrieved from http://www.homeopathicdirectory.com/re_licensing.htm

DistantHealer.co.uk. (2010). *Reflexology—ultimate foot therapy*. Retrieved from http://www.distanthealer.co.uk/reflexology.htm

Editors of *Consumer Reports*. (1994). Chiropractic. *Consumer Reports, 59*, 383–390.

Gilovich, T. (1993). *How we know what isn't so: The fallibility of human reason in everyday life*. New York: Free Press.

Herron, D. (2004a). *Healing through applying universal life force energy (Reiki)*. Retrieved from http://reiki.7gen.com/healing.htm

Herron, D. (2004b). *Using Reiki for healing*. Retrieved from http://reiki.7gen.com/doreiki.htm

Inglis, B., & West, R. (1983). *The alternative health guide*. New York: Alfred A. Knopf.

Jarvis, W. T. (1987). Chiropractic: A skeptical view. *Skeptical Inquirer, 12*(4), 47–55.

Jarvis, W. T. (1997). *Consumer forum: Health fraud leader speaks out on homeopathy*. Retrieved from http://www.fda.gov/fdac/departs/1997/397_form.html

Jarvis, W. T. (1999). *Reiki*. Retrieved from http://www.ncahf.org/articles/o-r/reiki.html

Jiva Institute. (2004). *AyurBasics*. Retrieved from http://www.ayurvedic.org

Kemper, K. J., Vohra, S., & Walls, R. (2008). The use of complementary and alternative medicine in pediatrics. *Pediatrics, 122*(6), 1374–1386.

Kurtzweil, P. (1999). How to spot health fraud. *FDA Consumer Magazine*, November–December 1999. Retrieved from http://www.fda.gov/fdac/features/1999/699_fraud.html

Lao, L. (1996). Safety issues in acupuncture. *Journal of Alternative and Complementary Medicine, 2*(1), 21–29.

Lee, C. (2004). *Yoga teacher and studio owner Cyndi Lee answers your frequently asked questions*. Retrieved from http://www.yogajournal.com/newtoyoga/820.cfm

Lewith, G. T., & Vincent, C. (1996). On the evaluation of the clinical effects of acupuncture: A problem reassessed and a framework for future research. *Journal of Alternative and Complementary Medicine, 2*(1), 79–90.

MacPherson, H., Thomas, K., Walters, S., & Fitter, M. (2001). York acupuncture safety study: Prospective survey of 24,000 treatments by traditional acupuncturists. *British Medical Journal, 322*, 486–487.

MayoClinic.com. (2004). *Yoga: Moving and breathing your way to relaxation*. Retrieved from http://www.mayoclinic.com/invoke.cfm?id=CM00004

MayoClinic.com. (2005). *Complementary and alternative medicine: What is it?* Retrieved from http://www.mayoclinic.com/invoke.cfm?id=PN00001

Morris, C. A., & Avorn, J. (2003). Internet marketing of herbal products. *Journal of the American Medical Association, 290*(11), 1505–1509.

Moukheiber, Z. (1994). Lord of immortality. *Forbes, 153*(8), 132.

Nahin, R. L., Barnes, P. M., Stussman, B. J., & Bloom, B. (2009). Costs of complementary and alternative medicine (CAM) and frequency of visits to CAM practitioners: United States, 2007. National Health Statistics Report no. 18. Hyattsville, MD: National Center for Health Statistics.

National Association of Naturopathic Physicians. (1970). Pp. 734–754 in Social Security Amendments of 1970. Hearings before the Committee on Finance, United States Senate, Ninety First Congress, Second Session, on H.R. 17550. September 14, 15, 16, 17, and 23, 1970. Washington, DC: U.S. Government Printing Office.

National Ayurvedic Medical Association. (2004). *Mission statement*. Retrieved from http://www.ayurveda-nama.org

National Cancer Institute. (2010). *Questions and answers about acupuncture*. Retrieved from http://www.cancer.gov/cancertopics/pdq/cam/acupuncture/patient/53.cdr#Section_53

National Center for Complementary and Alternative Medicine. (2002). *Research report: acupuncture*. NCCAM Publication No. D003. Retrieved from http://nccam.nih.gov/health/acupuncture

National Center for Complementary and Alternative Medicine. (2004). *Get the facts: What is complementary and alternative medicine (CAM)?* Retrieved from http://nccam.nih.gov/health/whatiscam

National Center for Complementary and Alternative Medicine. (2009). *Acupuncture for pain*. Retrieved from http://nccam.nih.gov/health/acupuncture/acupuncture-for-pain.htm

National Council Against Health Fraud. (1994). *NCAHF position paper on homeopathy*. Retrieved from http://www.ncahf.org/pp/homeop.html#cardinal

Pizzorno, J. E., Jr., & Murray, M. T. (Eds.). (1985–1996). *A textbook of natural medicine*. Seattle: John Bastyr College Publications.

Pizzorno, J. E., Jr., & Murray, M. T. (1990). *Encyclopedia of natural medicine*. Rocklin, CA: Prima Publishing & Communications.

Pizzorno, J. E., Jr., & Murray, M. T. (1998). *Encyclopedia of natural medicine* (2nd ed.). Rocklin, CA: Prima Publishing & Communication.

Pizzorno, J. E., Jr., & Murray, M. T. (Eds.). (1999). *A textbook of natural medicine* (2nd ed.). Philadelphia: W. B. Saunders.

Raso, J. (1994). *"Alternative" healthcare: A comprehensive guide*. Amherst, NY: Prometheus Books.

Raso, J. (1998). *Dictionary of metaphysical healthcare*. Self-published.

Relman, A. (2001). *Textbook of natural medicine* (book review). Retrieved from http://www.quackwatch.org/01QuackeryRelatedTopics/Naturopathy/relman.html

Riley, R. W. (2001). Decision of the secretary, Recognition Proceeding, Docket No. 00-06-O.

Sampson, W. (1996). Does homeopathy work? *Healthline, 15*(2), 10–11.

Segen, J. C. (1998). *Dictionary of alternative medicine*. Stamford, CT: Appleton & Lange.

Skepdic.com. (2003). *Acupuncture*. Retrieved from http://skepdic.com/acupunc.html

Skrabanek, P., & McCormick, J. (1990). *Follies and fallacies in medicine*. Amherst, NY: Prometheus Books.

Spirita Health. (2010). *Reflexology*. Retrieved from http://www.spirita.net/reflexology.net

Stehlin, I. (1996). *Homeopathy: Real medicine or empty promises?* Retrieved from http://www.fda.gov/fdac/features/096_home.html

Strasser, A. (2004). *Chiropractic care and back pain: An overview of diagnostic principles and treatment*. Retrieved from http://www.spineuniverse.com

Ter Reit, G., Kleijnen, J., & Knipschild, P. (1990). Acupuncture and chronic pain: A criteria-based meta-analysis. *Clinical Epidemiology, 43,* 1191–1199.

Tsibuliak, V. N., Alisov, A. P., & Shatrova, V. P. (1995). Acupuncture analgesia and analgesic transcutaneous electroneurostimulation in the early postoperative period. *Anesteziologiia I Reanimatologiia, 2*, 93–97.

Turner, R. N. (1990). *Naturopathic medicine: Treating the whole person*. Wellingborough, Northamptonshire, England: Thorsons Publishers.

U.S. Department of Labor. (2009). *Occupational outlook handbook, 2010–11 edition*. Retrieved from http://www.bls.gov/oco/ocos071.htm#outlook

U.S. Food and Drug Administration. (1996). Acupuncture needles no longer investigational. *FDA Consumer Magazine, 30*(5), 2.

White, A., Hayboe, S., Hart, A., & Ernst, E. (2001). Adverse events following acupuncture: Prospective surgery of 32,000 consultations with doctors and physiotherapists. *British Medical Journal, 323*(September 1), 485–486.

Zhang, R. (2004). Accidents in acupuncture treatment: History and current state. *Zhong Xi Yi Jie He Xue Bao, 2*(4), 306–313.

Chapter 7

Dietary Supplements

Chapter Objectives

The student will:

- Define and explain the term "dietary supplements."
- List reasons that people use supplements.
- Discuss the benefits and hazards of supplements.
- Discuss characteristics of people who might benefit from using supplements.
- Explain some of the risks of using herbs as remedies.
- Explain the federal regulation of dietary supplements.

What Are Dietary Supplements?

According to the U.S. Food and Drug Administration (U.S. FDA, 2003a,c), a product is a **dietary supplement** if it meets all of the following conditions:

- It is a product (other than tobacco) that is intended to supplement, or be an addition to, the diet and that contains one or more of the following: vitamins, minerals, herbs or other **botanicals**, amino acids, or any combination of the above ingredients.
- It is intended to be taken in tablet, capsule, powder, softgel, gelcap, or liquid form. (Supplements can be in other forms, such as energy bars and tea bags.)
- It is not represented for use as a conventional food or as a sole item of a meal or the diet.

Dietary supplements are also known as nutritional supplements.

More than 1,000 new supplements are developed each year. In 2009, consumers in the United States spent about $26.7 billion on them ("Dangerous supplements," 2010). These products are often used as alternative or complementary therapies, and some have also become a part of conventional medical therapy. They are marketed in food stores, so-called health food stores, physician and chiropractic offices, and roadside stands, and are available by mail and though the Internet.

There was a time when the only dietary supplements that were commercially marketed were vitamins and minerals. The production of herbs was often a mom-and-pop business, and other types of supplements were largely absent from the marketplace. Today, major drug companies, including pharmaceutical giants Bayer, Novartis, Johnson and Johnson, Pfizer, GlaxoSmithKline, and Boehringer-Ingelheim, produce and market supplements.

Dietary supplements have been touted to cure or prevent almost every condition known to man, including cancer, AIDS, depression, anxiety, syphilis, tuberculosis, diabetes, leprosy, impotence, menopause, prostate problems, fatigue, the common cold, high blood pressure, arthritis, and heart disease. Some marketers of dietary supplements have promised people with cancer that they could cancel their surgery, radiation, or chemotherapy in favor of herbal cures. Most of these claims are backed by little or no evidence beyond the anecdotal. As an example of an all-too-familiar scenario, the Aaron Company of Florida marketed a dietary supplement that allegedly contained suspended particles of silver as an orally taken cure for over 650 diseases (U.S. Federal Trade Commission, 2001). Claims that supplements cure, prevent, or treat diseases should be met with skepticism.

The supplements industry has grown explosively over the past twenty years. Herbal remedies and botanicals have gained in popularity. A botanical is a plant or plant part valued for its medicinal or therapeutic properties. These properties may be manifested in flavor and/or scent. Herbs, non-woody plants or plant parts claimed to have medicinal, therapeutic, or performance-enhancing properties, are a subset of botanicals. Products made from botanicals that are touted to maintain or improve health may be called herbal products, botanical products, or **phytomedicines** (National Institutes of Health, 2007). More recently, hormones, such as melatonin and DHEA, and the amino acids have become popular. Enzymes, organ and glandular tissues, and metabolites are sold as supplements.

People take supplements for a variety of reasons, the most common being for health or a belief that they are good for you (Kaufman, Kelly, Rosenberg, Anderson, & Mitchell, 2002). Some athletes use supplements to increase muscle mass and strength, decrease fat, promote healing, increase endurance, and improve performance. Some use products labeled as dietary supplements that contain hormones or hormone-like substances.

Conventional medical uses of dietary supplements are common. Scientists have found that the vitamin folic acid prevents certain birth defects. A regimen of vitamins and zinc can slow the progression of the age-related eye disease macular degeneration. There are many people who have deficiencies in certain vitamins and minerals and are helped by supplements. Hormone supplements can help some individuals with deficiencies.

In contrast, some supplements are considered complementary or alternative therapy. An example of such a use would be to take 1,500 milligrams of vitamin C per day to prevent or treat a cold; use of vitamin C for this purpose has not been proven to be effective. Another common example is the use of herbal formulas to relieve arthritis pain, an unproven effect.

Reducing Risk When Using Supplements

Of the 54,000 dietary supplement products in the Natural Medicines Comprehensive Database, only about one-third have scientific evidence of some level of safety and effectiveness ("Dangerous supplements," 2010). Before using dietary supplements, the consumer should try to get as much information as possible. The consumer cannot be secure in governmental regulation of these products for safety and effectiveness. Decisions should be made based on evidence derived from scientific testing, rather than from testimonials, word of mouth, or other unscientific information. There are several good sources of information. Consider the following suggestions:

- Ask your health care provider, preferably a physician. Be careful about information from alternative practitioners, especially those who wish to sell the product. Even if your provider does not happen to know about a particular supplement, he or she can access the latest medical guidance about its uses and risks.
- Ask dietitians or pharmacists, who have helpful information.
- Find out if there are any scientific research findings on the supplement in which you are interested. The National Center for Complementary and Alternative Medicine (NCCAM) and other federal agencies have free publications, clearinghouses, and databases with this information.

NCCAM (2007) and the editors of *Consumer Reports* ("Dangerous supplements," 2010) offer several points to keep in mind about safe use of dietary supplements:

- Tell your health care providers about any complementary and alternative practices you use. This includes supplements. Give them a full picture of what you do to manage your health. This will help ensure coordinated and safe care and reduce the likelihood of interactions with medication you may take. It is especially important to talk to your provider if you:
    - Are thinking about replacing your regular medical care with one or more supplements.
    - Are taking any medications (whether prescription or over-the-counter). Some supplements have been found to interact with medications.
    - Have a chronic medical condition.
    - Are planning to have surgery. Certain supplements may increase the risk of bleeding or affect anesthetics and painkillers.
    - Are pregnant or breastfeeding.
    - Are considering giving a child a dietary supplement. Supplements can act like drugs, and many have not been tested in pregnant women, breastfeeding mothers, or children.
- Do not exceed label directions for dosage unless your physician advises you to do so. More is not necessarily better.
- Avoid products claiming "megadoses." It is possible to overdose on supplements, even vitamins and minerals.
- Be especially wary of supplements marketed for weight loss, sexual dysfunction, and bodybuilding. Some products used for these purposes contain hormones, steroids, and other hazardous ingredients. Potentially dangerous side effects include changes in blood pressure, kidney failure, heart attack, stroke, and serious liver injury.
- If you experience any side effects that concern you, stop taking the supplement and contact your health care provider. You can also report your experience to the U.S. Food and Drug Administration's MedWatch program, which tracks consumer safety reports on supplements. The MedWatch telephone number is 1-800-332-1088.
- Look for the "USP Verified" mark indicating that the manufacturer has asked the U.S. Pharmacopeia to verify the quality, purity, and potency of its raw ingredients and final products.
- For current information from the federal government on the safety of particular supplements, check the "Alerts and Advisories" section of the NCCAM Web site or the FDA Web site.

The Internet can be a rich source of information, but it can also contain erroneous or misleading information, especially where dietary supplements are concerned. When searching on the World Wide Web, try using directory sites of respected organizations rather than doing blind searches with a search engine. Follow the recommendations in Chapter 1 for evaluating Web sites. Several good sources of Internet information are listed in the box on page 138 titled "For More Information."

Be savvy. Statements that a product can treat or cure diseases are drug claims and should not be associated with dietary supplements; if you see that kind of claim, avoid the product and report the violation. A corollary to this warning is to avoid products that are claimed to treat a variety of conditions. Supplements that boast that they are totally safe, have no side effects, or are "all natural" should be looked upon with suspicion. Claims of limited availability or money-back guarantees are red flags for trouble. Do not fall for testimonials. Frequently, they are false and are typically delivered by actors. Even if they are true, that is no indication that the supplement will work for all consumers.

The FDA issues warnings and advisories about supplements that pose risks to consumers, including those used in CAM therapies. The FDA issues warnings if it believes the product could damage

FOR MORE INFORMATION

The NCCAM Clearinghouse provides information on CAM and NCCAM, including publications and searches of federal databases of scientific and medical literature. The Clearinghouse does not provide medical advice, treatment recommendations, or referrals to practitioners.

> http://nccam.nih.gov
> E-mail: info@nccam.nih.gov
> Toll-free in the United States: 1-888-644-6226
> TTY (for deaf and hard-of-hearing callers): 1-866-464-3615

The U.S. Food and Drug Administration (FDA) oversees the safety of many products, such as foods (including dietary supplements), medicines, medical devices, and cosmetics.

> http://www.fda.gov
> Web site for alerts and advisories: http://www.fda.gov/food/dietarysupplements
> Toll-free in the United States: 1-888-463-6332

The Center for Food Safety and Applied Nutrition (CFSAN) oversees the safety and labeling of supplements, foods, and cosmetics. Publications include "Tips for the Savvy Supplement User: Making Informed Decisions and Evaluating Information."

> http://www.cfsan.fda.gov
> Toll-free in the United States: 1-888-723-3366

MedWatch, the FDA's safety information and adverse event reporting program, allows consumers and health care providers to file reports on serious problems suspected with dietary supplements.

> http://www.fda.gov/medwatch/report/consumer/consumer.htm
> Toll-free in the United States: 1-888-463-6332

The Federal Trade Commission (FTC) is the federal agency charged with protecting the public against unfair and deceptive business practices. A key area of its work is the regulation of advertising (except for prescription drugs and medical devices).

> http://www.ftc.gov
> Toll-free in the United States: 1-877-382-4357

The Office of Dietary Supplements (ODS), National Institutes of Health (NIH), seeks to strengthen knowledge and understanding of dietary supplements by evaluating scientific information, supporting research, sharing research results, and educating the public. Its resources include publications and the International Bibliographic Information on Dietary Supplements (IBIDS) database.

> http://ods.od.nih.gov
> E-mail: ods@nih.gov

PubMed®, a service of the National Library of Medicine (NLM), contains publication information and (in most cases) brief summaries of articles from scientific and medical journals. CAM on PubMed, developed jointly by NCCAM and NLM, is a subset of the PubMed system and focuses on the topic of CAM.

> http://www.ncbi.nlm.nih.gov/sites/entrez?db=pubmed
> CAM on PubMed: http://nccam.nih.gov/camonpubmed/

The Cochrane Database of Systematic Reviews is a collection of evidence-based reviews produced by the Cochrane Library, an international nonprofit organization. The reviews summarize the results of clinical trials on health care interventions. Summaries are free; full-text reviews are by subscription only.

http://www2.cochrane.org/reviews/

Other Useful Sites

American Dietetic Association, http://www.eatright.org
American Pharmacists Association, http://www.pharmacyandyou.org
Food Marketing Institute, http://www.fmi.org
International Food Information Council Foundation, http://www.foodinsight.org/
AARP, http://www.aarp.org
Consumer Reports Health, http://www.ConsumerReportsHealth.org (subscription required)

health, is contaminated—with other unlabeled substances, pesticides, heavy metals, or prescription drugs—or interacts dangerously with prescription drugs. Portions of a few FDA advisories are contained in the box titled "Excerpts from FDA Advisories."

The following supplements have carried FDA cautions about safety:

- Ephedra
- Kava kava
- Some "dieters' teas"
- L-tryptophan
- GHB (gamma hydroxybutyric acid), GBL (gamma butyrolactone), and BD (1,4-butanediol)
- PC SPES and SPES (herbal combinations for cancer treatment or prostate health)
- Aristolochic acid
- Comfrey
- St. John's wort

EXCERPTS FROM FDA ADVISORIES

The FDA warns consumers not to purchase or consume Actra-Rx (also known as Yilishen), a product promoted as a "dietary supplement" for treating erectile dysfunction and enhancing sexual performance for men. The product is labeled as all natural and sold over the Internet.

The FDA has announced a crackdown on products containing androstenedione, commonly known as "andro." The products are marketed over the counter as dietary supplements that enhance athletic performance. In the body, androstenedione is converted into testosterone and estrogen. While ads claim that andro-containing supplements promote increased muscle mass, research has not shown this to be the case. Studies have shown side effects and potential long-term risks, the same kinds of health risks as anabolic steroids, including shrunken testicles, male-pattern baldness, increased risk of breast cancer in women, and acne in youth.

The FDA warns consumers to avoid ayurvedic products such as spices, herbs, vitamins, proteins, minerals, and metals (e.g., mercury, lead, iron, zinc). Some preparations combine herbs with minerals and metals. These products are commonly sold on the Internet or in stores. "Consumers should know that ayurvedic products are generally not reviewed or approved by the Food and Drug Administration," said Mike Levy of the FDA. Most ayurvedic products are marketed either for drug uses not approved by the FDA or as dietary supplements. As such, consumers should understand that these products have not been approved by the FDA before marketing.

Source: U.S. Food and Drug Administration.

- Certain products, marketed for sexual enhancement and claimed to be natural versions of the drug Viagra®, that were found to contain an unlabeled drug (sildenafil or tadalafil)

Taking a combination of supplements or using these products together with medications, whether prescription or OTC drugs, could, under certain circumstances, produce adverse effects, some of which could be life threatening. A **drug interaction** occurs when the effect of a particular drug is altered when it is taken with another drug or with food. While dietary supplements are not considered to be drugs under the law, they often act like drugs and can cause some serious interactions.

Many athletes fall victim to the desire to excel at all costs. Creatine, which occurs naturally in the body, is touted to enhance muscle mass and strength. Abnormal heart rhythm, loss of kidney function, diarrhea, cramps, and loss of appetite are side effects of creatine supplements. Ephedra, an herbal supplement, has been used by athletes for weight loss and performance enhancement. Hundreds of adverse effects, including death, are associated with use of ephedra. Use of ephedra

increases risk of heart problems, stroke, and psychiatric symptoms.

Just as purveyors of fraudulent products use buzzwords like "natural," so does the dietary supplement industry. What does it mean? The answer is: virtually nothing. It certainly does not mean that a product is safe. Remember, poisonous mushrooms, poison ivy, and animal droppings are all natural, but hardly safe for human consumption.

Research on Dietary Supplements

NCCAM funds numerous studies related to dietary supplements. Some of these studies are designed to determine if the supplements work as claimed. Some go further, asking how they work. Other studies are searching for ways to develop purer and more standardized products. Among substances researchers have studied in recent years are:

- Yeast-fermented rice, to see if it can lower cholesterol levels in the blood
- Ginger and turmeric, to see if they can reduce inflammation associated with arthritis and asthma
- Chromium, to better understand its biological effects and impact on insulin in the body, possibly offering new pathways to treating type 2 diabetes
- Green tea, to find out if it can prevent heart disease
- Glucosamine hydrochloride, to see if it provides relief of knee pain from osteoarthritis
- Black cohosh, to see if it reduces hot flashes and other symptoms of menopause
- Echinacea, to see if it shortens the length or lessens the severity of colds in children
- Omega-3 fatty acids, to see if they affect cognitive performance
- Garlic, to find out if it can lower moderately high cholesterol levels
- Ginkgo biloba, to determine whether it prevents or delays decline in cognitive function in people aged 85 and older

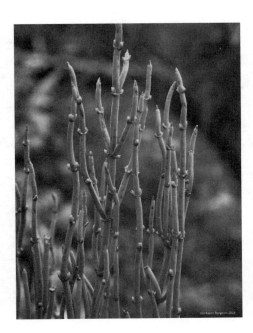

Ephedra plant.

- Chamomile, to see if it has value as a treatment for prostate cancer
- Ginger, to confirm whether it eases nausea and vomiting after cancer chemotherapy

It is important for athletes to note that quality research on herbs, both for health effects and for performance enhancement, is very limited; there is insufficient scientific support for the use of any herb to improve athletic performance (Kundrat, 2005). Scientific evidence is sparse that any of the "muscle builder" supplements, such as amino acids and carbohydrate products, produce noticeable muscle growth beyond that achieved with a sound program of resistance training and good nutrition (Eichner, King, Myhal, Prentice, & Ziegenfuss, 1999). Consuming hormone or hormone-like products for this purpose can be harmful.

Vitamins and Minerals

Vitamins and minerals are basic nutrients that are necessary to sustain life. Vitamins and essential minerals, also called micronutrients, are needed in very small amounts to promote vital biochemical reactions in the body's cells. They are necessary for normal growth and development, digestion, resistance to infection, and enabling the body to use carbohydrates, fats, and proteins for energy. They also act as catalysts, initiating or speeding up chemical reactions.

Vitamins and minerals are widely dispersed in foods. Most nutrition experts believe that most people can acquire all of the vitamins and minerals they need by eating a variety of foods, including fruits, vegetables, legumes, lean meats, and whole grains.

Vitamin and mineral supplements have been widely marketed for many years, some with incredible claims. They are sold in supermarkets, "health food" stores, pharmacies, and virtually every shopping mall in the United States. Many people take single nutrient supplements, and multivitamins are marketed in a dizzying array of formulations. One popular brand markets multivitamins in at least 15 different formulations. Trying to select one over another can be a challenge. Multivitamins are often marketed as a sort of nutritional insurance policy that fills in the gaps created by poor diets. About 37 percent of American adults take a multivitamin supplement each day (Fogle, Anderson, & Wilken, 2007), spending about $4.7 billion in 2008.

The most justifiable reason for taking supplements is to overcome deficiencies. Vitamin deficiencies are not common. Deficiencies result from either inadequate consumption or biological malfunction in which the body cannot absorb or use the vitamin properly. Deficiencies should be diagnosed by a physician to avoid mistakes and overconsumption of these nutrients.

There is very little evidence that taking multivitamins actually improves health in people who do not have nutritional deficiencies. When comparing taking vitamin and mineral supplements, including multivitamins, with not taking a multivitamin, clinical trials have found no lowered risk of disease for those taking the supplements. A study of 35,000 women over 10 years found a significant association between breast cancer and consumption of multivitamins (Larsson, Akesson, Bergkvist, & Wolk, 2010). While the study did not establish a causal relationship, it does provide reason for concern and it adds to the reasons to get nutrients from foods rather than supplements.

Humans need 15 minerals that help regulate cell function and provide structure to cells. Major minerals include calcium, phosphorus, and magnesium. In addition, the body needs smaller amounts of chromium, copper, fluoride, iodine, iron, manganese, molybdenum, selenium, zinc, chloride, potassium, and sodium. Like vitamins, these minerals are readily accessible in foods, and excessive amounts can be toxic. Mineral supplements are sold separately and in multivitamin formulations.

There are some people who should consider taking vitamin or mineral supplements. Examples include:

- ***Persons whose diets are poor.*** If you eat fewer than five total servings of fruits and vegetables daily, you probably are not getting all the vitamins and minerals you need. College students frequently have poor diets and can benefit from taking a multivitamin with minerals.

- **Pregnant women, breastfeeding mothers, or women trying to become pregnant.** Pregnant women and breastfeeding mothers need supplements, especially folic acid, calcium, and iron. Physicians usually recommend a dietary supplement that should be taken before and after becoming pregnant.

- **Young children.** Pediatricians often recommend vitamins for young children until they can eat solid foods. After age two, vitamins are seldom necessary. However, children with poor eating habits or those on weight reduction diets can usually benefit from a multivitamin and mineral supplement. Children should also receive fluoride supplements if the mineral is not in their water supply.

- **Vegetarians.** It is difficult to get sufficient calcium, iron, zinc, and vitamins B_{12} and D from a vegetarian diet, although it is possible with adequate planning.

- **Persons who consume fewer than 1,200 calories a day.** Persons who consume a low number of calories are usually trying to lose weight. Low-calorie diets limit the types and amounts of foods consumed and the amount of nutrients received. These diets are not safe unless monitored by a physician. Some weight loss drugs inhibit absorption of fat-soluble vitamins.

- **Smokers.** Tobacco products decrease the absorption of many vitamins and minerals, so even if you consume them in food, they are not available to the body tissues. Supplements do not make up for the tremendous health risks caused by smoking.

- **Heavy drinkers.** Long-term consumption of large amounts of alcohol can impair the digestion and absorption of several vitamins and minerals, including vitamin B_2, zinc, magnesium, and folic acid. Dietary supplements will not offset the major

health risks caused by excessive alcohol consumption.

- **Postmenopausal women.** To keep bones strong and to reduce bone loss, physicians often recommend that postmenopausal women take calcium and vitamin D, especially if they do not get enough of these nutrients through foods.

- **Elderly persons.** Lack of appetite, loss of taste and smell, and denture problems may contribute to a poor diet. Depression or loneliness may also contribute to lack of interest in eating. After age 65, the body may not be able to absorb vitamins B_6, B_{12}, and D, making supplements beneficial. Older women may need to increase their intake of calcium and vitamin D to reduce the risk of osteoporosis, especially if they do not take estrogen supplements.

- **Women with heavy menstrual bleeding.** Because of depleted iron, women with heavy menstrual flows probably need to take an iron supplement to avoid anemia.

- **People with a medical condition that affects absorption, use, or excretion of nutrients.** Intolerance to certain foods, such as dairy products, or food allergies can result in failure to consume sufficient amounts of certain nutrients. Diseases of the liver, gallbladder, pancreas, or intestines can make it difficult to digest or absorb nutrients. Some surgeries make it difficult to consume, digest, and absorb nutrients properly. Physicians usually recommend dietary supplements in these situations.

How much is enough? The answer depends on your age, health status, and nutritional status. However, the federal government has made several efforts to provide guidance. Initially, the Food and Drug Administration published Minimum Daily Allowances (MDA) for vitamins and minerals. These were amounts deemed necessary to avoid diseases seen with specific deficiencies. In the 1980s, this was revised to Recommended Daily Allowances (RDA). Generally, the requirements were increased above the MDA. RDA considered that low levels might interfere with optimal health even if not severe enough to be considered a deficiency-related disease. More recently, the terminology "Percent Daily Value" (%DV) has been coined. This is the percentage of the daily requirement that a serving of food contains, assuming a 2,000-calorie-a-day diet. Even more recently, Dietary Reference Intake (DRI) has been introduced. DRI is a set of values that serves as the standard for nutrient intake for healthy persons in the United States and Canada of any vitamin or mineral, except on the advice of a physician. It is not advisable to consume more than 100 percent of DRI for any nutrient. Single-nutrient supplements or high-potency vitamin or mineral supplements may be harmful. These megavitamins may contain 10 to over 100 times the DRI and can act like drugs, with potentially serious results (Fogle et al., 2007). Many practitioners and charlatans make large amounts of money selling supplements to people who do not need them, often in amounts that can cause harm.

Many products are marketed as "natural vitamins." Vitamins are chemicals, whether synthetically manufactured or produced in nature. The body treats most natural supplements the same as synthetic vitamins. Products sold as natural supplements are often much more expensive. Vitamin B$_{15}$ (pangamic acid), vitamin B$_{17}$ (laetrile), and vitamin P (bioflavinoids) have been marketed as new vitamins, capable of preventing cancer, improving athletic performance, and promoting overall health. These are not vitamins, and there is no evidence that they are effective. In fact, laetrile contains cyanide, a potent poison.

Some vitamin-mineral supplements are sold as "stress formula," indicating that people under stress need additional nutrients. Emotional stress does not increase nutrient needs, although physiological stress, such as injuries and surgery, does increase nutrient needs and a supplement may be prescribed.

Supplements are often marketed to competitive athletes and others who exercise regularly, suggesting that physical activity increases the need for nutrients. Fogle et al. (2007) responded to this claim by saying, "Athletes and fitness buffs are less likely to need supplements than anyone! When a person eats more calories to meet increased demands, the small amount of extra nutrients are easily supplied" by foods.

Vitamin C and the B complex are water-soluble vitamins. They are not stored in the body and are excreted. However, it is possible to consume enough of the water-soluble vitamins to cause health problems. Vitamins A, D, E, and K are fat soluble. This means that they are stored in body fat and are not excreted. Consuming large amounts of these vitamins can cause serious health problems. Table 7.1 depicts the major food sources, positive physiological effects in the body, and effects of overconsumption of fat-soluble vitamins.

Table 7.2 contains a list of food sources of water-soluble vitamins, positive function of those vitamins in the body, and effects of overconsumption. Overconsumption is much less likely with water-soluble vitamins, but it does occur, almost always as a result of overuse of supplements.

Minerals are necessary nutrients. They may also be consumed in excessive amounts, usually in supplements, resulting in health problems. Table 7.3 presents information about minerals.

According to the American Dietetic Association, the National Academy of Sciences, the National Research Council, and other major medical societies, healthy people can and should obtain all the vitamins and minerals they need from eating a variety of foods (Doctors Corner Internet Group, 2004). Supplements are no guarantee against disease. Taking self-prescribed single-nutrient supplements can be dangerous and should be done only after consulting a physician or registered dietician. Taking a multiple vitamin-mineral supplement with dose levels no higher than 100 percent DRI is probably not harmful but, given the cost, is unnecessary for most healthy individuals.

Persons who choose to use vitamin and mineral supplements should observe the following:

- ***Look for "USP" on the label.*** This ensures that the supplement meets the standards for strength, purity, disintegration,

TABLE 7.1 FACTS ABOUT FAT-SOLUBLE VITAMINS

Vitamin	Sources	Physiological Functions	Effects of Overconsumption
A (retinol) (provitamin A, such as beta carotene)	Liver, vitamin A fortified milk and dairy products, cheese, egg yolk. Provitamin A: carrots, leafy green vegetables, sweet potatoes, pumpkins, apricots, cantaloupe.	Helps form skin and mucous membranes and keeps them healthy, thus increasing resistance to infections; essential for night vision; promotes bone and tooth development. Beta carotene is an antioxidant and may protect against cancer.	Mild: nausea; fatigue; irritability; blurred vision; dry, itchy skin; diarrhea. Severe: irregular periods, growth retardation, rashes, enlargement of liver and spleen, hair loss, bone pain, increased pressure in skull.
D	Vitamin D–fortified dairy products, fortified margarine, fish oils, egg yolk; sunlight enables the body to make vitamin D.	Helps build and maintain teeth and bones; increases absorption of calcium.	Mild: nausea, weight loss, irritability. Severe: calcium deposits in organs, fragile bones, kidney and cardiovascular damage, mental and physical growth retardation.
E	Corn, soybean, and cottonseed oils; butter; brown rice; nuts; wheat germ; green and leafy vegetables; liver; whole-grain products.	Helps form red blood cells, muscles, and other tissues; protects vitamins A and C and fatty acids; prevents damage to cell membranes.	Nontoxic under normal conditions. Severe: nausea, blood clots, digestive tract disorders; tumors in the breast.
K	Dark-green leafy vegetables, liver; also made by bacteria in the intestine.	Helps blood to clot.	Jaundice in infants.

TABLE 7.2 FACTS ABOUT WATER-SOLUBLE VITAMINS

Vitamin	Sources	Physiological Functions	Effects of Overconsumption
C (Ascorbic acid)	Citrus fruits, broccoli, strawberries, green pepper, tomatoes, dark green vegetables, potatoes.	Helps bind cells together and strengthens blood vessel walls; assists in wound healing; helps maintain gums, teeth, and bones; aids in absorption of iron, calcium, and folacin; contributes to production of brain hormones.	Rebound scurvy when high doses are discontinued; diarrhea; bloating; cramps; increased incidence of kidney stones.
B_1 (Thiamin)	Pork, liver, whole grains, sunflower seeds, dried beans, peas.	Necessary for carbohydrate metabolism; helps release energy from foods; promotes proper nerve function and muscle coordination; promotes normal appetite.	Unknown, although excess of one B vitamin may cause deficiency of others.

TABLE 7.2 (CONTINUED)

Vitamin	Sources	Physiological Functions	Effects of Overconsumption
B_2 (Riboflavin)	Liver, milk, dark-green vegetables, whole- and enriched-grain products, eggs, mushrooms.	Necessary for metabolism of all foods; helps release energy from foods to cells; promotes good vision and healthy skin; necessary for the functioning of vitamin B_6 and niacin.	Unknown, although excess of one B vitamin may cause deficiency of others.
B_3 (Niacin)	Liver, fish, poultry, meat, mushrooms, peanuts, whole- and enriched-grain products.	Energy production from foods; aids digestion; promotes normal appetite; promotes healthy nerves and skin.	Hot flashes; cramps; nausea; irritability; ulcers; liver disorders; high blood sugar and uric acid; cardiac arrhythmias.
B_6 (Pyridoxine)	Meats, bananas, whole grains and cereals, legumes, green leafy vegetables.	Necessary for protein metabolism and absorption and carbohydrate and fat metabolism; helps form red blood cells; promotes nerve and brain function.	Nerve damage.
Folic Acid (Folacin)	Green leafy vegetables, orange juice, organ meats, sprouts, fish, whole and fortified grains and cereals, citrus fruits.	Promotes red blood cell formation; aids in protein metabolism; prevents birth defects of spine and brain; lowers hemosystein levels and coronary heart disease risk; essential for production of genetic material.	Convulsion in persons with seizure disorders; may mask pernicious anemia (vitamin B_{12} deficiency).
B_{12}	Animal products.	Builds genetic material; helps form red blood cells.	Unknown, although excess of one B vitamin may cause deficiency of others.
B_5 (Pantothenic Acid)	Animal products, whole-grain cereals, legumes, egg yolks.	Helps in formation of hormones and chemicals that regulate nerve function; necessary for protein metabolism and absorption.	Unknown, although excess of one B vitamin may cause deficiency of others.
Biotin	Liver, kidney, egg yolk, fresh vegetables, cheese, cauliflower, peanut butter.	Needed for metabolism of glucose and formation of certain fatty acids.	Unknown, although excess of one B vitamin may cause deficiency of others.

and dissolution established by the U.S. Pharmacopeia, a testing organization.

- *Check the label for contents.* Product labels carry information identifying the active ingredient or ingredients, the serving size, and the amount of the nutrients in each serving.

- *Reject supplements that provide "megadoses."* Megadoses of water-soluble vitamins are wasted because they are flushed

TABLE 7.3 FACTS ABOUT MINERALS

Mineral	Sources	Physiological Functions	Effects of Overconsumption
Calcium	Dairy products, yogurt, sardines, leafy vegetables.	Builds bones and teeth; promotes nerve and muscle function; promotes blood clotting; helps convert food to energy.	Kidney stones, constipation, calcium deposits in body tissues; hinders absorption of other minerals.
Iron	Liver, lean meats, kidney beans, enriched breads, raisins, dried fruit, egg yolk.	Necessary to make hemoglobin.	Toxic buildup in liver and heart.
Phosphorus	Chicken breast, milk, egg yolks, nuts, cheese, legumes.	Helps build bones and teeth; promotes metabolism and nerve and muscle function.	Interferes with absorption of calcium.
Magnesium	Dark leafy greens, broccoli, tofu, popcorn, nuts, cashews, wheat bran, legumes, milk.	Helps release energy in the body; necessary for genetic material and bone and tooth growth; promotes bowel function.	Nervous system disorders, nausea, low blood pressure, fatal to people with kidney disease.
Zinc	Crab, shrimp, oysters, beef, turkey, peanuts, beans, whole grains, eggs.	An essential element in many enzymes that are necessary to digestion and metabolism; aids sexual maturation; promotes wound healing; increases immunity.	Vomiting, diarrhea, abdominal pain, gastric bleeding.
Potassium	Broccoli, sunflower seeds, beans, peanuts, bananas, orange juice, green beans, mushrooms, dark leafy vegetables.	Maintains regular fluid balance; necessary for nerve and muscle function.	Rare: irregular heartbeat.
Selenium	Seafood, kidney, liver, grains.	Interacts with vitamin E to prevent breakdown of fats and body chemicals; constituent of red blood cell enzymes.	Hair loss; fingernail changes.
Molybdenum	Milk, beans, bread and cereals.	Necessary component of enzymes that promote metabolism; regulates iron storage.	Goutlike pain.
Copper	Liver and other organ meats, seafoods, nuts, seeds, legumes.	Component of several enzymes that make skin and hair; stimulates iron absorption; helps to make red blood cells, connective tissue, and nerve fibers.	Liver disease, vomiting, diarrhea.

from the body. Large doses of fat-soluble vitamins and minerals may be harmful.

- *Beware of label and advertising claims.* Proclaiming a vitamin to be "doctor-tested," "organic," or "natural" is an attempt to convince the buyer that it is superior to synthetics, which it is not. Touting added herbs, amino acids, or other substances may increase cost and produce harmful interactions, but seldom provides any benefit.
- *Observe expiration dates.* Supplements lose potency over time. Discard supplements when they expire.
- *Store supplements wisely.* The bathroom is the worst room in the house for storing supplements and drugs. Heat and humidity contribute to rapid breakdown and chemical changes. Store supplements away from children's reach. Even water-soluble vitamins may be toxic to a small child. Storing in a locked cabinet is preferable.
- *Take supplements carefully.* As any parent knows, young children imitate adults. Do not take supplements in front of children. Take them as directed at a regular time each day.

Amino Acids

Proteins are necessary nutrients, providing energy and contributing to the construction and maintenance of the body's tissues. Amino acids are the constituent parts of proteins. Amino acids that the body cannot manufacture, **essential amino acids**, must be consumed. Consumption of foods containing intact proteins ordinarily provides sufficient amounts of the essential amino acids required for growth and development in children and for health maintenance of adults.

When marketed as dietary supplements, amino acids are sold in different forms: single compounds, in combinations of two or more amino acids, as components of protein powders, and as chelated single compounds or in chelated mixtures. The term "**chelator**" refers to a substance consisting of molecules that bind tightly to metal atoms, thus forcing the metal atoms to go

wherever the chelator goes. The bound pair—chelator plus metal atom—is called a **chelate**. Amino acids can act as chelators when they react with positively charged metal atoms, forming a strong chemical bond. The metal atoms of interest here are those that serve as dietary minerals, including zinc, iron, chromium, copper, and magnesium (Hashimoto, 2003). Too little published research exists to provide evidence of the safety and effectiveness of chelated amino acids.

The Federation of American Societies for Experimental Biology warned that consuming amino acids in dietary supplement form posed potential risks for several subgroups of the general population, including women of childbearing age (especially if pregnant or breastfeeding), infants, children, adolescents, the elderly, individuals with inherited disorders of amino acid metabolism, and individuals with certain diseases (Center for Food Safety and Applied Nutrition, 1993).

At least two of the amino acids consumed in dietary supplements have been associated with serious injuries in healthy adults. In 1989, the supplement l-tryptophan was associated with an epidemic of an immune system disorder called eosinophilia-myalgia syndrome (EMS). At least 38 patients are known to have died, although the true incidence of l-tryptophan-related EMS is thought to be much higher. Phenylalanine supplementation has been associated with EMS, scleroderma, and scleroderma-like illnesses occurring in children with poorly controlled blood phenylalanine levels, as well as in those with phenylketonuria, a genetic disorder characterized by the inability to metabolize phenylalanine.

Ironically, years later, consumers have even fewer safeguards for dietary supplements than when these tragedies began occurring. The following statement, under the title "Current policy on the marketing of dietary supplements containing l-tryptophan and related compounds," explains the legal impotence of the U.S. Food and Drug Administration (Center for Food Safety and Applied Nutrition, 2001) to protect the public from questionable dietary supplements:

Although FDA continues to enunciate its concern about the safety of dietary supplements containing L-tryptophan and related compounds such as L-5-hydroxytryptophan, this does not mean that FDA prohibits the marketing of dietary supplements that contain L-tryptophan. Under the Federal Food, Drug and Cosmetic Act (the Act), as amended by the Dietary Supplement Health and Education Act of 1994 (DSHEA), the manufacturer is responsible for ensuring that its products are safe. A firm is not required to obtain premarket review or approval from the FDA of its products before marketing them as dietary supplements. Moreover, a firm is not required to submit scientific evidence to FDA of the safety of its products or ingredients. While we are unaware of conclusive scientific data that would establish that a dietary supplement L-tryptophan would be safe, if a firm has information that it believes establishes that a product containing L-tryptophan is safe within the meaning of the Act, it could market such a product as a dietary supplement. The burden and responsibility for assuring that such a product is not adulterated under the Act is with the firm and not FDA.

We shall examine the DSHEA later in this chapter.

What About Herbs?

Herbs are naturally occurring substances taken from parts of plants and are a subset of botanicals; the two terms are often used synonymously. There is a history in native and ancient cultures of using herbs for medicinal purposes dating back hundreds of years. No doubt, many herbal remedies are effective. In fact, many modern FDA-approved medications are derived from herbs. Dietary supplements that contain herbs may contain one or more ingredients derived from herbs.

Herbal supplements may act in the same way as drugs. Therefore, they can cause medical problems even if used in accordance with label directions. Taking herbs in large amounts is very risky. Women who are pregnant should be especially cautious. This caution applies to treating children with herbal supplements.

The active ingredients in many herbs and herbal supplements are not known. There may be dozens, even hundreds, of compounds in an herbal

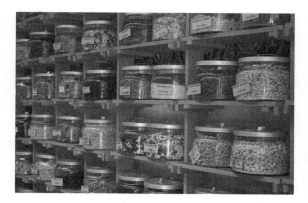

Rows of herbs labeled for sale.

supplement. Identifying the active ingredients in herbs and understanding how herbs affect the body are important research areas (NCCAM, 2006), but for now, it is "buyer beware."

Herbs may interact with prescription medications, over-the-counter drugs, vitamins, and minerals in unpredictable ways. For example, ginkgo taken with aspirin may lead to spontaneous and/or excessive bleeding (Blumenthal, Goldberg, & Brinckmann, 2000). For this reason, patients should make their health care providers aware of all herbs they are taking. If any unusual side effects occur, they should be reported immediately to a physician.

People with compromised immune systems such as the elderly or those with HIV should avoid herbs except on the advice of a physician. Those with liver disease or kidney disease or anyone undergoing surgery should not take herbal preparations. Pregnant or lactating women are advised to avoid herbs. Herbal products are also not recommended for children under age six. Few herbal supplements have been tested on children, and safe doses for children have not been established (MayoClinic.com, 2010).

Herbal supplements do not always contain the ingredient(s) listed on the label, and for those that do, the amounts of the ingredient(s) listed on the label are not always accurate. Furthermore, some herbal supplements have been found to be contaminated with metals, unlabeled prescription drugs, microorganisms, or other substances (DecisionNewsMedia, 2003; Lallanilla, 2005).

Information from friends or from salespersons may not be accurate or based on scientific inquiry. If you choose to use herbal supplements, you should do so under the guidance of a professional who has been properly trained in herbal therapy. If this person is not a conventional practitioner— i.e., an MD or DO— you should consult with a conventional practitioner for a second opinion and monitoring for adverse effects.

Research on the health benefits is lacking, especially with well-controlled studies. While NCCAM has sponsored some studies on this issue, our understanding is largely anecdotal. All of the short-term and long-term benefits associated with herbs are not known (Anderson, 2007). Marcus (2010), writing in a publication of the American College of Rheumatology, goes even further, stating, "There are no herbal medicines whose health claims are supported by sound scientific evidence."

Table 7.4 summarizes claims about commonly used herbs and the documented side effects. It also provides information about the results of research on the herbal product.

As with many other products, herbs are often labeled with the term "natural," leading many people to believe that herbs are healthier or gentler than conventional medicines. Consumers should be aware of three important points about the use and abuse of the term. First, so-called natural products are often synthetic. This is not illegal given the state of regulation of dietary supplements and the lack of an FDA-approved legal definition of the term "natural." Second, ingredients carrying this moniker may be extracted with powerful solvents that may leave contaminant residue, or even created by genetically engineered bacteria. Third, even if the product meets the consumer's definition of "natural," that does not equate with "safe" or "effective." Many plants occurring in nature are toxic, some to the point of being fatal if ingested. For example, wild almonds, cashews, and mushrooms contain lethal poisons. Germander, comfrey, and chapparal can cause severe liver damage. Plants grown beside a busy highway or near an industrial plant or waste disposal area could easily absorb heavy metals such as lead, mercury, and arsenic.

In 1993, Varro E. Tyler, former dean of Purdue University and a leading authority on the science of medicines from natural sources, observed (Tyler, 1993):

> The literature promoting herbs includes pamphlets, magazine articles, and books ranging in quality from cheaply printed flyers to elaborately produced studies in fine bindings with attractive illustrations. Practically all of these writings recommend large numbers of herbs for treatment based on hearsay, folklore, and tradition. The only criterion that seems to be avoided in these publications is scientific evidence. Some writings are so comprehensive and indiscriminate that they seem to recommend everything for anything. Even deadly poisonous herbs are sometimes touted as remedies, based on some outdated report or a misunderstanding of the facts. Particularly insidious is the myth that there is something almost magical about herbal drugs that prevents them, in their natural state, from harming people.

All of the precautions mentioned above are necessary to make intelligent, informed decisions, especially in light of the federal government's reluctance to protect consumers (see the next section). However, it is also important to point out that many herbs do provide medicinal benefit. In fact, many of our most important medicines originate from plants, including herbs.

Regulation of Dietary Supplements

The U.S. Federal Trade Commission has primary responsibility for regulating the advertisement and labeling of dietary supplements within strict limitations. When the FTC finds evidence that false and unsubstantiated claims have been made, the agency can take a variety of actions to terminate the advertisement. Between 2008 and 2010, the FTC filed or settled 30 cases against supplement marketers, charging them with making illegal claims. In one case, the FTC reached a $7.5 million settlement with the QVC home-shopping channel. The U.S. Postal Inspection

Table 7.4 Commonly Used Herbs

Common Name	Primary Uses and Apparent Efficacy	Probable Side Effects	Comments
Echinacea	Prevents colds*; reduces duration of colds**; boosts immune system†; heals wounds†.	Minor gastrointestinal symptoms; chills; short-term fever reaction; nausea and vomiting; allergic reactions, including anaphylaxis, increased asthma, rashes.	Side effects are less common when taken by mouth.
Asian Ginseng	Improving health of people recovering from illness**; increases stamina**; improved mental and physical performance**; treating hepatitis C**; erectile dysfunction**; reducing symptoms of menopause**; lowering blood glucose**, controlling blood pressure**.	Headaches; sleep problems; gastrointestinal problems; allergic reactions.	When taken by mouth, usually well tolerated producing few side effects. Can increase the stimulant effects of caffeine (as in coffee, tea, and colas). It can also lower blood sugar levels, creating the possibility of problems like low blood pressure when used with diabetes drugs.
Garlic	Prevent heart disease†; lowered blood cholesterol**; lowered blood pressure**; improving clotting disorders†; cancer prevention**; antibacterial, antiviral**.	Breath and body odor; heartburn; upset stomach; allergic reactions.	Serious side effects are rare. Since garlic can thin the blood, it may be a problem during or after surgery. Garlic has been found to interfere with Saquinavir, a drug used to treat HIV infection.
Saw Palmetto	Reducing benign prostatic hyperplasia**; improve overall prostate health*; enhance sexual vigor*.	Gastrointestinal disturbances; headaches; diarrhea in large amounts.	
St. John's Wort	Reducing depression**; reducing premenstrual depression**; treating seasonal affective disorder**.	Photosensitivity; allergic reactions; anxiety and dizziness; dry mouth; gastrointestinal symptoms; fatigue; headache; sexual dysfunction.	It is not a proven therapy for depression and, when combined with certain antidepressants, may increase side effects. Using it for treatment of depression without consulting a physician can be hazardous. St. John's wort interacts with several medications, such as warfarin, an anticoagulant. It can interfere with drugs used to treat HIV infection, to treat cancer, for birth control, or to prevent the body from rejecting transplanted organs; it can increase the effects of anti-depression drugs.

TABLE 7.4 (CONTINUED)

Common Name	Primary Uses and Apparent Efficacy	Probable Side Effects	Comments
Kava Kava	Reducing anxiety†, tension**, restlessness**; enhanced sleep**; treatment of asthma**; reducing menopausal symptoms**.	Hepatitis, cirrhosis and liver failure; abnormal muscle spasms; scaly, yellow skin (long-term use); drowsiness.	Kava kava may interact with many drugs. NCCAM-funded studies were suspended after an FDA warning linking product to liver damage.
Ginkgo Biloba	Improved memory in Alzheimer's patients**; improved blood flow**; treatment of sexual dysfunction**.	Can cause seizures in people with epilepsy; allergic skin reactions; headaches; gastrointestinal upset.	Do not take with blood-thinning drugs or high doses of garlic or vitamin E. Studies have shown promise in treating Alzheimer's symptoms, but larger studies are needed.
Black Cohosh	Treating rheumatism**; reducing menopausal symptoms**; menstrual irregularities**.	Headaches; stomach discomfort.	Black cohosh does not appear to interact with most prescription drugs, although it may make chemotherapy drugs less effective. It is not clear if it is safe for women who have had breast cancer or for pregnant women. It should not be confused with blue cohosh, a different herb with different effects.
Evening Primrose Oil	Reduced menopausal symptoms*; treatment of allergic skin rash (eczema)**; treating rheumatoid arthritis; cancer treatment**; diabetes treatment**.	Headaches; gastrointestinal distress at high doses.	It is well tolerated by most people and appears to be safe for use during pregnancy, although data are limited.
Ginger	Improving motion sickness**; reducing pregnancy-related nausea**; digestive aid**; treatment of rheumatoid arthritis**.		People with gallstones should not use without consulting a doctor. Many digestive, antinausea, and cold and flu dietary supplements contain ginger extract.

*Research shows the product to be ineffective and/or unsafe.

**Clinical evidence is inconclusive.

†Research supports the efficacy and safety of this product when used appropriately.

   Note: Research on herbs is continuous and information is frequently changing. Herbs are not generally recommended for people suffering from autoimmune disorders or liver disease, people undergoing surgery or other invasive medical procedures, pregnant or lactating women, or infants and small children. Use herbs only for minor conditions and only for the short term. Discontinue if you experience any adverse side effects (Anderson, 2007). Consult a physician before taking herbal supplements.

Service regulates advertising and promotional material received in the mail under different laws.

The U.S. Food and Drug Administration regulates dietary supplements, aside from advertising. This regulation is somewhat hollow because these products are regulated more as foods than drugs. The Federal Food, Drug, and Cosmetic Act defines a drug as any article, excluding devices, "intended for use in diagnosis, cure, mitigation, treatment, or prevention of disease." Knowing that drugs of abuse may have no medical use, we define the term move broadly as "a nonfood substance that, when taken into the body or applied to its surface, affects the structure or function of the body." Since supplements are intended to alter the structure or function of the body, they fit the common definition of a drug, yet by law, they are treated as foods. Outright claims that a supplement prevents, treats, or cures a disease are not allowed, as these are drug claims. Promoters of supplements are usually careful to imply or allude to their products' use for diagnosis, cure, and prevention rather than making outright claims, a practice that often misleads the uninformed consumer.

Laws about putting foods on the market and keeping them there are less strict than the laws for drugs. Since supplements are considered foods under the law, the less-strict standards apply to them. Specifically, research studies in people to demonstrate a supplement's safety are not required before the supplement is marketed, unlike for drugs. The manufacturer does not have to prove that the supplement is effective—i.e., that it does what it is intended to do—unlike for drugs.

The FDA does not analyze the content of supplements. Except in the case of a "new dietary ingredient," one not sold in the United States in a dietary supplement before October 15, 1994, the manufacturer does not have to provide the FDA with evidence to substantiate safety or effectiveness of the ingredient before or after marketing the product. Since there is no authoritative list of dietary ingredients that were marketed before 1994, manufacturers and distributors are responsible for determining if a dietary ingredient is "new."

FDA regulations require that dietary supplement labels contain a descriptive name of the product stating that it is a supplement; the name and place of business of the manufacturer, packer, or distributor; a complete list of ingredients; and net contents of the product. Each supplement, except for some small-volume products or those produced by eligible small businesses, must have nutrition labeling in the form of a "Supplement Facts" panel that identifies ingredients. Ingredients not listed in the "Supplement Facts" panel must be listed in the "other ingredients" statement beneath the panel. Examples of "other ingredients" would be water, sugar, coloring, preservatives, and processing aids such as gelatin. Serving size, or dosage, is determined entirely by the manufacturer.

The issue of ingredient lists is, in some cases, moot, since actual ingredients may not match those listed on the label or, in the case of botanicals, the correct plant species. Gilroy, Steiner, Byers, Shapiro, and Georgian (2003) analyzed 59 preparations of echinacea and found that about half did not contain the species listed on the label. Biochemists at the Stanford Research Institute International analyzed 10 different samples of the widely marketed human sex hormone DHEA. Three samples contained no identifiable DHEA, three more had at least 25 percent less than claimed on the label, and one sample provided a 50 percent overdose (Parasrampuria, Schwartz, & Petesch, 1998). Supplement products may contain higher or lower amounts of the active ingredient that is claimed on the label. An NCCAM-funded study (Harkey, Henderson, Gershwin, Stern, & Hackman, 2001) found that most of the ginseng products studied contained less than half the amount of ginseng listed on the labels. Supplement products may also be contaminated (NCCAM, 2007). Supplements and their ingredients are often imported, many from China. Although several Chinese products have been found to be contaminated and China is a main supplier of supplement ingredients, the FDA has not inspected even one factory there.

There is no practical way for the FDA to make sure that ingredients listed on labels are actually in the products. It cannot ensure that the amounts of ingredients are accurate. In many cases, contents and amounts have been discovered to be erroneous, but only after the product has been sold. FDA Commissioner Jane E. Henney (1999) testified before a congressional committee: "Products that contain substances similar to those found in prescription drugs are marketed for children as dietary supplements. Likewise, products with ingredients that simulate illicit street drugs are marketed as dietary supplements to adolescents via the Internet and shops specializing in drug paraphernalia."

There is no standard dosage or serving size for dietary supplements. There are no rules that limit a serving size or the amount of an ingredient in supplements. Dosage decisions are made by the manufacturer and do not require FDA approval.

The Dietary Supplement Health and Education Act of 1994 (DSHEA) is the federal law governing the regulation of dietary supplements. Rather than establishing consumer protections, the DSHEA severely limits the FDA's ability to regulate these products.

The history of the passage of the DSHEA is interesting and infamous. In the early 1990s, the U.S. Congress considered two bills designed to strengthen the ability of federal agencies to fight health fraud. Lobbyists for the "health-food" industry rallied consumers to complain to the Congress that the two bills would damage consumers' freedom to choose dietary supplements and might even take away their right to purchase vitamins. While both assertions were false, as a result of vigorous lobbying and pressure from ill-informed consumers, the DSHEA was passed.

The DSHEA defined dietary supplements as a separate regulatory category (i.e., not drugs) and liberalized the information that could be distributed by their sellers. By defining supplements so they are not considered drugs, although many of them are, the FDA was hindered from conducting the regulatory actions that it was originally intended to do.

The DSHEA protects ingredients that are useless but harmless. Even more serious, the act prohibits the FDA from banning suspicious

ingredients. In the backward world of DSHEA, the FDA must demonstrate the product to be unsafe before it can ban it. Rather than the burden of proof being placed on the company marketing the product and making claims about it, the burden is on the FDA. In the words of former FDA commissioner David Kessler (2000), "Congress has put the FDA in the position of being able to act only after the fact and after substantial harm has already occurred." Here are a few examples of herbal supplements that have a questionable past:

- A Chinese herbal product that contained aristologic acid, a known carcinogen, found in an herb called *Aristolochia fangi*.
- Germander, associated with acute hepatitis.
- Comfrey, associated with hepatic veno-occlusive disease, blockage of veins in the liver.
- Ephedra, associated with death from cardiovascular problems. It was highlighted in the news because it was linked to the death of professional baseball player Steve Bechler. Ephedra was officially banned only after the publicity surrounding Bechler's death.
- Yohimbe, associated with seizures and renal failure.

The FDA has authority to stop the marketing and sale of products with unsubstantiated "drug claims"—cure, treatment, or prevention. Supplement manufacturers have still managed to evade regulation of health claims by promoting such claims in books, magazines, newsletters, pamphlets, and on the Internet. They support lectures and radio and television broadcasts, some of them infomercials that make claims that appear to be "medicinal." Retailers often make oral preventive and therapeutic claims to customers without meaningful oversight.

To further confuse consumers, dietary supplements may legally bear "statements of support." These statements may claim a benefit related to classical nutrient deficiency disease, describe how ingredients affect the structure or function of the body (compare this with the classical definition of "drug"), characterize the documented mechanism by which ingredients act to maintain structure or function, and describe intended benefits of using the product. A "nutritional support statement" must not be a "drug claim," although the distinction between a drug claim and a health or nutrient claim is very thin. This means the statement cannot suggest that the product or ingredient is intended for prevention or treatment of disease. Nevertheless, an iron supplement label may say that "iron is essential to make hemoglobin," a calcium supplement label may say "calcium builds strong bones and helps prevent osteoporosis," and a vitamin supplement label may say "folic acid may reduce the risk of neural tube defect–affected pregnancies." In order to make statements such as these, there must be evidence to support them. Sometimes evidence of the health claim is strong, but the linkage to the actual product is weak. Under the DSHEA, when a manufacturer makes claims on a label that describe the role of a nutrient or dietary ingredient intended to affect the structure or function of the body, the label must contain the statement: "This statement has not been evaluated by the FDA. This product is not intended to diagnose, treat, cure, or prevent any disease." While the presence of the statement may serve as a warning to astute consumers, it is really a disclaimer that provides legal protection to supplement manufacturers if they are sued because of a claim found to be false.

Morris and Avorn (2003) demonstrated the lack of enforcement related to health claims made on the Internet. The researchers analyzed the health content of all Web sites listed on the five most commonly used search engines when entering the names of the eight most widely used herbal supplements. Among 443 Web sites evaluated, 338 were retail sites either selling a product or directly linked to a vendor. A total of 273 of the retail Web sites made one or more health claims; of these, 149 claimed to treat, prevent, diagnose, or cure specific diseases. More than half of the sites with a health claim omitted the standard federal disclaimer.

In 2000, the FDA (U.S. FDA, 2000) published a revised rule on health claims for dietary supplements. The rule prohibited express disease claims, such as saying that the product "prevents high blood pressure," and implied disease claims, such as the product "prevents fragile bones in postmenopausal women," including claims made through a product's name or through pictures or symbols. The rule allowed health-maintenance claims, such as "maintains a healthy circulatory system," other non-disease claims, such as "helps you relax," and claims for common, minor symptoms associated with pregnancy, menopause, or other life changes, such as "for hot flashes." These changes still allow a great deal of misunderstanding and misinformation.

The FDA's 2003 Consumer Health Information for Better Nutrition Initiative provided for the use of qualified health claims when there is emerging evidence for a relationship between a food, food component, or dietary supplement and reduced risk of a disease or health-related condition. In this case, evidence is emerging but not well enough established to meet significant scientific agreement standard required for the FDA to issue an authorizing regulation (U.S. FDA, 2003a). This represents a low standard for making such a claim.

Congress mandated in 1994 that the FDA issue a rule governing the manufacturing practices of dietary supplements. The FDA did not finalize the rule, the Dietary Supplement Current Good Manufacturing Practices (cGMPs) and Interim Final Rule (U.S. FDA, 2007), until 2007. As of 2011, the standards were not fully implemented. In the meantime, because of the absence of good manufacturing practice regulations, dozens of supplements have been purposely and illegally laced with prescription drugs in an attempt to produce an effect. The final rule is relevant only to dietary supplements, and not to dietary ingredients, a fine but significant difference. It applies to individuals or companies that manufacture, package, or hold dietary supplement products but not to dietary ingredient manufacturers, suppliers, or retailers. The rule is relevant to all dietary supplements sold or offered for sale in the United States, including those manufactured by foreign companies.

Under the final rule, manufacturers are required to evaluate the identity, purity, strength, and composition of their dietary supplements. Every dietary ingredient used in a dietary supplement will be required to meet "100 percent identity testing," such that manufacturers will be required to "conduct at least one appropriate test or examination to verify the identity of any component that is a dietary ingredient." Manufacturers will also be required to "confirm the identity of other components." If dietary supplements contain contaminants or do not contain the dietary ingredient they are represented to contain, the FDA would consider the products to be adulterated or misbranded. The consumer should note that it is the manufacturer, not the FDA or any enforcement agency, that conducts the testing.

The FDA must "exercise enforcement discretion" with regard to products made by practitioners, such as acupuncturists and herbalists, who are "adequately trained in their profession," and who use the products that they make in a "one-on-one consultation." This means that there is no specific requirement that these practitioners be monitored to determine if they follow cGMPs when using or producing supplements.

Manufacturers may request exemption to the cGMP requirement for 100 percent identity testing. They must provide sufficient documentation that the reduced frequency of testing would still ensure the identity of the dietary ingredient.

Most manufacturers probably attempt to maintain high standards. Since the DSHEA eliminated FDA authority to require pre-market testing for safety and efficacy (Wolfe, 2007), and the new cGMP rule relies on the integrity of the manufacturer to be accountable and meet expectations for purity, safety, and proper labeling, consumers should not be complacent.

The DSHEA has facilitated the dispersal of misinformation to customers by expanding the types of products that can be marketed as supplements, including hormones, herbs, amino acids, vitamins, and minerals. The range of products includes concentrates, metabolites, extracts, constituents, or a combination of any such ingredients. Often, these substances are marketed as preventive or therapeutic, but the DSHEA limits the FDA in regulating them.

All of these problems are a result of the lobbying power and the ability to arouse consumers to pressure members of Congress. Kessler (2000) summed up the political problems with regulating nutritional supplements by saying, "Congress has shown little interest in protecting consumers from the hazards of dietary supplements, let alone from the fraudulent claims that are made, since its members apparently believe that few of these products place people in real danger. Nor does the public understand how potentially dangerous these products can be."

Since the DSHEA allows manufacturers of supplements to place products on the market without submitting safety information, the FDA must rely on adverse event reports, product sampling, information from scientific literature, and other sources of evidence. This usually requires personal harm to have already taken place.

For years after passage of the DSHEA, manufacturers were not required to inform the FDA if they received reports of serious adverse events. In 2006, Congress passed the Dietary Supplement and Nonprescription Drug Consumer Protection Act. This legislation came in response to concern about the difficulty to ban ephedra, highlighted by the death of Steve Bechler and the press coverage it generated. This law requires manufacturers of dietary supplements and nonprescription drugs to notify the FDA about serious adverse events related to their products, including deaths, life-threatening experiences, inpatient hospitalizations, persistent or significant disability or incapacity, birth defects, or the need for medical intervention to prevent any such problems. The agency does not routinely publish adverse effects reports to the public, so it is difficult for consumers to be informed. Manufacturers must place a telephone number or address on product labels to facilitate consumer reports. After the loophole was closed, the FDA said it received 1,359 reports of serious adverse effects from manufacturers and 602 from consumers and health professionals in 2008 and 2009. One can only wonder how many serious events went unreported before 2008. Without

---

REQUIREMENTS UNDER THE cGMP RULE

Manufacturers are required to:

- Employ qualified employees and supervisors
- Design and construct their physical plant in a manner to protect dietary ingredients and dietary supplements from becoming adulterated during manufacturing, packaging, labeling, and holding
- Use equipment and utensils that are of appropriate design, construction, and workmanship for the intended use
- Establish and use master manufacturing and batch production records
- Establish procedures for quality control operations
- Hold and distribute dietary supplements and materials used to manufacture dietary supplements under appropriate conditions of temperature, humidity, light, and sanitation so that the quality of the dietary supplement is not affected
- Keep a written record of each product related to cGMPs
- Retain records for one year past the shelf-life date, if shelf-life dating is used, or two years beyond the date of distribution of the last batch of dietary supplements associated with those records

Source: U.S. Food and Drug Administration. (2009). *Dietary supplement current good manufacturing practices (CGMPs) and interim final rule (IFR) facts*. Retrieved from http://www.fda.gov/Food/DietarySupplements/GuidanceCompliance RegulatoryInformation/RegulationsLaws/ucm110858.htm

---

systematic safety and efficacy testing, there is a lack of scientific information to provide warning flags to consumers and a lack of information about what clues to look for when problems arise. In the relatively few cases that result in reports, the FDA is not adequately staffed and funded to pursue them. The system lacks adequate safeguards to protect the consumer from harmful or ineffective supplements. As Moore (1999) stated, "Never have so many people consumed so many medical products about which we know so little."

SUMMARY

The dietary supplement industry provides access to a variety of nutritional products. Most Americans have little need for supplements, but the business remains robust.

Certain people need some supplements. For example, pregnant women, the elderly, and those on low-calorie diets should take certain supplements based on their individual needs. Those needs can best be assessed by a physician.

Some supplements have no demonstrated health benefits. Most can result in health problems if taken in excess, and many can interact with drugs, foods, and other supplements to cause interactions that can be harmful. Therefore, consumers should become informed before using supplements. There are a number of good sources of information, but most patients should begin with a conversation with their family doctor.

The Federal Trade Commission regulates the advertising of dietary supplements, and the Food and Drug Administration regulates the production and labeling of the products and investigates complaints about supplements. The Dietary Supplement Health and Education Act of 1994 reduced the power of the FDA to exercise regulatory authority over supplements. Rather than treating supplements as drugs, they are regulated more like foods. The onus to demonstrate lack of safety or effectiveness is on the FDA, and product testing is not required before marketing.

KEY TERMS

Botanical: a plant or plant part valued for its medicinal or therapeutic properties

Chelate: chelator plus metal atom bound together

Chelator: a substance consisting of molecules that bind tightly to metal atoms, thus forcing the metal atoms to go wherever the chelator goes

Dietary supplement: a product (other than tobacco) that is intended to supplement, or be an addition to, the diet and is not represented for use as a conventional food or as a sole item of a meal or the diet and that contains one or more of the following: vitamins, minerals, herbs or other botanicals, amino acids, or any combination of the above ingredients

Drug interaction: when the effect of a particular drug is altered when it is taken with another drug, a supplement, or with food

Essential amino acids: those that cannot be manufactured by the body and must be consumed

Phytomedicines: products made from botanicals that are touted to maintain or improve health; also called herbal products or botanical products

STUDY QUESTIONS

1. Explain what dietary supplements are.
2. What are the reasons for using dietary supplements?
3. What are some of the benefits of taking vitamin, mineral, and amino acid supplements?
4. What are some of the risks of taking vitamin, mineral, and amino acid supplements?
5. Who would benefit from consuming dietary supplements?
6. Is it safe to use herbal remedies?
7. What are the main elements of the Dietary Supplement Health and Education Act of 1994?
8. What kinds of claims about supplements are allowed by law? What claims are not allowed?
9. How would you strengthen consumer protection with regard to dietary supplements?

REFERENCES

Anderson, J. (2007). *Herbals for health?* Retrieved from http://www.ext.colostate.edu/pubs/foodnut/09370.html

Blumenthal, M., Goldberg, A., & Brinckmann, J. (Eds.). (2000). *Expanded Commission E monographs.* Austin, TX: American Botanical Council.

Center for Food Safety and Applied Nutrition, U.S. Food and Drug Administration. (1993). *Illnesses and injuries associated with the use of selected dietary supplements.* Retrieved from http://vm.cvsan.fda.gov/~dms/ds-ill.html

Center for Food Safety and Applied Nutrition, U.S. Food and Drug Administration. (2001). *Information paper on l-tryptophan and 5-hydroxy-l-tryptophan.* Retrieved from http://cfsan.fda.gov/~dms/ds-tryp-1.html

Dangerous supplements. (2010). *Consumer Reports,* September, 16–20.

DecisionNewsMedia. (2003). *Herbal contamination continues to damage industry.* Retrieved from http://www.nutraingredients.com/news/ng.asp?ID=38615-herbal-contamination-continues

Doctors Corner Internet Group. (2004). *Vitamin and mineral supplements: Sorting fact from fiction.* Retrieved from http://your-doctor.com/patient_info/nutrition_supplements/vitamins.html

Eichner, E. R., King, D., Myhal, M., Prentice, B., & Ziegenfuss, T. N. (1999). *"Muscle builder" supplements.* SSE Roundtable #37. Retrieved from http://www.gssiweb.com/Article_Detail.aspx?articleid=76

Fogle, C., Anderson, J., & Wilken, K. (2007). *Foods vs. pills.* Retrieved from http://www.ext.colostate.edu/pubs/foodnut/09338.html

Gilroy, C. M., Steiner, J. F., Byers, T., Shapiro, H., & Georgian, W. (2003). Echinacea and truth in labeling. *Archives of Internal Medicine, 163*(6), 699–704.

Harkey, M. R., Henderson, G. L., Gershwin, M. E., Stern, J. S., & Hackman, R. M. (2001). Variability in commercial ginseng products: An analysis of 25 preparations. *American Journal of Clinical Nutrition, 73*(6), 1101–1106.

Hashimoto, A. (2003). *The Delano report.* Retrieved from http://www.delano.com/articles/Mineral-forms-compared.html

Henney, J. E. (1999, March 25). Statement by Jane E. Henney, M.S., Commissioner, Food and Drug Administration, Department of Health and Human

Services, Before the Committee on Government Before U.S. House of Representatives.

Kaufman, D. W., Kelly, J. P., Rosenberg, L., Anderson, T. E., & Mitchell, A. A. (2002). Recent patterns of medication use in the ambulatory adult population of the United States: The Sloan survey. *Journal of the American Medical Association, 287*(3), 337–344.

Kessler, D. (2000). Cancer and herbs. *New England Journal of Medicine, 342,* 1742–1743.

Kundrat, S. (2005). Herbs and athletes. *Sports Sciences Exchange 96, 18*(1). Retrieved from http://www.gssiweb.com/Article_Detail.aspx?articleid=704

Lallanilla, M. (2005). *How safe are herbal supplements?* Retrieved from http://abcnews.go.com/Health/story?id=403037

Larsson, S. C., Akesson, A., Berkgvist, L., & Wolk, A. (2010). Multivitamin use and breast cancer incidence in a prospective cohort of Swedish women. *American Journal of Clinical Nutrition, 91*(5), 1268–1272.

Marcus, D. M. (2010). *Herbal remedies, supplements and acupuncture for arthritis.* Retrieved from http://www.rheumatology.org/practice/clinical/patients/diseases_and_conditions/herbal.asp

MayoClinic.com. (2010). *Herbal supplements: What to know before you buy.* Retrieved from http://www.mayoclinic.com/health/herbal-supplements/SA00044/

Moore, T. J. (1999). *A booming industry.* Retrieved from http://www.thomasjmoore.com/pages/dietary_part2.html

Morris, C. A., & Avorn, J. (2003). Internet marketing of herbal products. *Journal of the American Medical Association, 290*(11), 1505–1509.

National Center for Complementary and Alternative Medicine. (2006). *Herbal supplements: Consider safety, too.* Retrieved from http://nccam.nih.gov/health/supplement-safety/

National Center for Complementary and Alternative Medicine. (2007). *What's in the bottle? An introduction to dietary supplements.* Retrieved from http://nccam.nih.gov/health/bottle

National Institutes of Health, Office of Dietary Supplements. (2007). *Botanical dietary supplements: Background information.* Retrieved from http://ods.od.nih.gov/factsheets/BotanicalBackground.asp

Parasrampuria, J., Schwartz, K., & Petesch, R. (1998). Quality control of dehydroepiandrosterone dietary supplement products. *Journal of the American Medical Association, 280*(18), 1565.

Tyler, V. E. (1993). The overselling of herbs. In S. Barrett & T. Jarvis (eds.). *The health robbers: A close look at quackery in America.* Amherst, NY: Prometheus Books.

U.S. Federal Trade Commission. (2001). *"Operation cure.all" wages new battle in ongoing war against internet health fraud.* Retrieved from http://www.ftc.gov/opa/2001/06/cureall.shtm

U.S. Food and Drug Administration. (2000). *FDA finalizes rules for claims on dietary supplements.* FDA Talk Paper T00-1. January 5. Retrieved from http://vm.cfsan.fda.gov/~lrd/tpdsclm.html

U.S. Food and Drug Administration, Center for Food Safety and Applied Nutrition. (2003a). *Claims that can be made for conventional foods and dietary supplements.* Retrieved from http://www.cfsan.fda.gov/~dms/hclaims.html

U.S. Food and Drug Administration. (2003b). *Dietary Supplement Health and Education Act of 1994.* Retrieved from http://fda.gov/opacom/laws/dshea.html

U.S. Food and Drug Administration, Center for Food Safety and Applied Nutrition. (2003c). *Dietary supplements: overview.* Retrieved from http://cfsan.fda.gov/~dms/supplmnt.html

U.S. Food and Drug Administration, Center for Food Safety and Applied Nutrition. (2007). *Dietary Supplement Current Good Manufacturing Practices (cGMPs) and Interim Final Rule (IFR) facts.* Retrieved from http://www.cfsan.fda.gov/~dms/dscGMPs6.html

Wolfe, S. (2007). *June 22—FDA rule still won't ensure safety and efficacy of dietary supplements.* Retrieved from http://www.citizen.org/hot_issues/print_issue.cfm?ID=1646

Chapter 8

Weight Management

Chapter Objectives

The student will:

- Describe the epidemic of overweight and obesity in the United States.
- Describe the human and financial costs of obesity.
- Explain the body mass index.
- Explain the standard recommendations for weight control.
- Explain the role of physical activity in weight management.
- Compare and contrast some commercial diets.
- State the nature, design, and effects of restricted carbohydrate diets.
- List several over-the-counter weight reduction products and their ingredients.
- Explain how prescription weight loss medications work.
- Discuss fad diets.
- Explain the types of bariatric surgery.

America's Weight Problem

Overweight and obesity are at epidemic proportions in the United States and much of the industrialized world. They are directly related to cardiovascular disease, type 2 diabetes, hypertension, liver and gallbladder disease, sleep apnea, and some forms of cancer. According to 2007–2008 data from the National Health and Nutrition Examination Survey (NHANES) (Flegal, Carroll, Ogden, & Curtin, 2010), about one-third of U.S. adults are obese. About two-thirds of adults are either overweight or obese. The body mass index (BMI) is used to determine overweight and obesity and is considered a reliable measure of fatness. BMI is calculated by dividing a person's weight in pounds by height in inches squared, then multiplying by 703.

Applying gender-specific 2000 Centers for Disease Control and Prevention (CDC) weight-for-recumbent-length growth charts, about 10 percent of infants and toddlers carried excess weight in the 2007–2008 NHANES. Children and adolescents aged 2 through 19 years of age who are at or above the 95th percentile of BMI for age are usually described as overweight. About 17 percent of those between 2 and 19 years were at or above the 95th percentile, and about 12 percent were above the 97th percentile of the BMI-for-age growth charts (Ogden, Carroll, Curtin, Lamb, & Flegal, 2010). The percentage of children and adolescents who are overweight has more than quadrupled since the early 1970s (National Center for Health Statistics, 2006). The majority of overweight children between ages 5 and 10 years have at least one risk factor for cardiovascular disease.

Obesity is not evenly distributed in the population. While widespread geographically, it is

TABLE 8.1 BODY MASS INDEX TABLE

Body Weight (pounds)

Height (inches)	Normal						Overweight					Obese										Extreme Obesity														
BMI	19	20	21	22	23	24	25	26	27	28	29	30	31	32	33	34	35	36	37	38	39	40	41	42	43	44	45	46	47	48	49	50	51	52	53	54
58	91	96	100	105	110	115	119	124	129	134	138	143	148	153	158	162	167	172	177	181	186	191	196	201	205	210	215	220	224	229	234	239	244	248	253	258
59	94	99	104	109	114	119	124	128	133	138	143	148	153	158	163	168	173	178	183	188	193	198	203	208	212	217	222	227	232	237	242	247	252	257	262	267
60	97	102	107	112	118	123	128	133	138	143	148	153	158	163	168	174	179	184	189	194	199	204	209	215	220	225	230	235	240	245	250	255	261	266	271	276
61	100	106	111	116	122	127	132	137	143	148	153	158	164	169	174	180	185	190	195	201	206	211	217	222	227	232	238	243	248	254	259	264	269	275	280	285
62	104	109	115	120	126	131	136	142	147	153	158	164	169	175	180	186	191	196	202	207	213	218	224	229	235	240	246	251	256	262	267	273	278	284	289	295
63	107	113	118	124	130	135	141	146	152	158	163	169	175	180	186	191	197	203	208	214	220	225	231	237	242	248	254	259	265	270	278	282	287	293	299	304
64	110	116	122	128	134	140	145	151	157	163	169	174	180	186	192	197	204	209	215	221	227	232	238	244	250	256	262	267	273	279	285	291	296	302	308	314
65	114	120	126	132	138	144	150	156	162	168	174	180	186	192	198	204	210	216	222	228	234	240	246	252	258	264	270	276	282	288	294	300	306	312	318	324
66	118	124	130	136	142	148	155	161	167	173	179	186	192	198	204	210	216	223	229	235	241	247	253	260	266	272	278	284	291	297	303	309	315	322	328	334
67	121	127	134	140	146	153	159	166	172	178	185	191	198	204	211	217	223	230	236	242	249	255	261	268	274	280	287	293	299	306	312	319	325	331	338	344
68	125	131	138	144	151	158	164	171	177	184	190	197	203	210	216	223	230	236	243	249	256	262	269	276	282	289	295	302	308	315	322	328	335	341	348	354
69	128	135	142	149	155	162	169	176	182	189	196	203	209	216	223	230	236	243	250	257	263	270	277	284	291	297	304	311	318	324	331	338	345	351	358	365
70	132	139	146	153	160	167	174	181	188	195	202	209	216	222	229	236	243	250	257	264	271	278	285	292	299	306	313	320	327	334	341	348	355	362	369	376
71	136	143	150	157	165	172	179	186	193	200	208	215	222	229	236	243	250	257	265	272	279	286	293	301	308	315	322	329	338	343	351	358	365	372	379	386
72	140	147	154	162	169	177	184	191	199	206	213	221	228	235	242	250	258	265	272	279	287	294	302	309	316	324	331	338	346	353	361	368	375	383	390	397
73	144	151	159	166	174	182	189	197	204	212	219	227	235	242	250	257	265	272	280	288	295	302	310	318	325	333	340	348	355	363	371	378	386	393	401	408
74	148	155	163	171	179	186	194	202	210	218	225	233	241	249	256	264	272	280	287	295	303	311	319	326	334	342	350	358	365	373	381	389	396	404	412	420
75	152	160	168	176	184	192	200	208	216	224	232	240	248	256	264	272	279	287	295	303	311	319	327	335	343	351	359	367	375	383	391	399	407	415	423	431
76	156	164	172	180	189	197	205	213	221	230	238	246	254	263	271	279	287	295	304	312	320	328	336	344	353	361	369	377	385	394	402	410	418	426	435	443

Source: Adapted from *Clinical Guidelines on the Identification, Evaluation, and Treatment of Overweight and Obesity in Adults: The Evidence Report.*

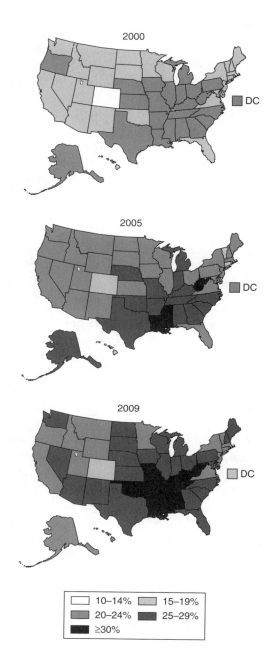

2000

2005

2009

10–14%	15–19%
20–24%	25–29%
≥30%	

FIGURE 8.1 OBESITY TRENDS BY STATE. SELF-REPORTED PREVALENCE OF OBESITY* AMONG ADULTS—BEHAVIORAL RISK FACTOR SURVEILLANCE SYSTEM, UNITED STATES, 2000, 2005, AND 2009

*Body mass index (BMI) ≥30.0

Source: U.S. Centers for Disease Control and Prevention. (2010). Vital signs: State-specific obesity prevalence among adults—United States, 2009. *MMWR, 59* (early release), 1–5.

more concentrated in the South (see Figure 8.1). African Americans have 51 percent higher obesity prevalence and Hispanics have 21 percent higher obesity prevalence compared with whites (CDC, 2010).

Genetics play a role in body type and weight, including obesity. Genes can directly cause obesity in disorders such as Bardet-Biedl syndrome and Prader-Willi syndrome. Genes and behavior may both be needed for a person to be overweight or obese. In most cases, multiple genes may increase one's susceptibility for obesity and outside factors, such as abundant food supply, social reinforcement for consuming high-calorie foods, or little physical activity, are also required. This is made obvious by the fact that overweight and obesity have increased in developed countries much faster than changes in genetic makeup take place in populations.

The cost of the obesity and overweight epidemic to the health care system, including government treasuries, was $78.5 billion in 1998 (Finkelstein, Trogdon, Cohen, & Dietz, 2009). Annual cost of treating adult non-institutionalized obesity has swollen to over $168 billion, or 16.5 percent of national medical care spending (Cawley & Meyerhoefer, 2010).

Americans spend between $55 billion and $60 billion each year on weight control products, many of which seem to have no lasting effect on weight loss. The overweight and obese often become desperate, and there is no shortage of people, from qualified physicians to greedy hucksters, who offer help. Cable television is replete with **infomercials** touting weight loss products. Newspapers carry full-page ads on programs and services, many of which have no basis in science. Magazine articles and books hype worthless lose-weight-fast programs.

A recent example of extremely questionable publishing is the book titled *The Weight Loss Secret They Don't Want You to Know About* by convicted felon Kevin Trudeau, who is not recognized by health or nutrition authorities as having expertise in the field. The book rocketed to the top of most best-seller lists. It claims that a cure for obesity was discovered almost 50 years ago but was

TABLE 8.2 STEPS TO HELP PREVENT AND DECREASE OVERWEIGHT AND OBESITY

Home	Reduce time spent watching television and in other sedentary behaviors.
	Build physical activity into regular routines.
School	Ensure that the school breakfast and lunch programs meet nutrition standards.
	Provide food options that are low in fat, calories, and added sugars.
	Provide all children, from pre-kindergarten through grade 12, with quality daily physical education.
Work	Create more opportunities for physical activity at work sites.
Community	Promote healthier choices, including at least five servings of fruits and vegetables a day, and reasonable portion sizes.
	Encourage the food industry to provide reasonable food and beverage portion sizes.
	Encourage food outlets to increase the availability of low-calorie, nutritious food items.
	Create opportunities for physical activity in communities.

Source: U.S. Department of Health and Human Services. (2001). *The Surgeon General's Call to Action to Prevent and Decrease Overweight and Obesity 2001*. Rockville, MD: U.S. Public Health Service.

suppressed by the American Medical Association and the U.S. Food and Drug Administration. The Federal Trade Commission recently filed suit against Trudeau for allegedly violating a court order by misrepresenting the contents of his book. (See "An Infomercial Star Falls and Rises" in Chapter 9.) Nevertheless, the book was a best seller for many weeks, demonstrating the desperation and gullibility of many consumers.

The keys to health and weight management are healthy eating and physical activity. A joint working group of the National Heart, Lung, and Blood Institute and the North American Association for the Study of Obesity (2000) issued a guide reinforcing this fact and a treatment model in which diet, exercise, and behavior therapy are the cornerstones of weight management. Prevention of overweight and obesity is more prudent than dealing with the problems after they develop. *The Surgeon General's Call to Action to Prevent and Decrease Overweight and Obesity 2001* identified action steps for several locations that may help prevent and decrease obesity and overweight. Table 8.2 provides examples of these steps.

Many people in industrialized nations, such as the United States and Canada, who are dealing with overweight and obesity try other methods of varying quality. This has led to the introduction of many commercial and proprietary weight loss programs. Unfortunately, little published information is available to guide practitioners or consumers in the selection of a commercial weight loss program (Tsai & Wadden, 2005).

Dieting alone is almost certain to lead to long-term failure. As many as 95 percent of people who try to lose weight by only dieting gain the weight back in five years or less. Controlling weight is an overall lifestyle choice, including increasing physical activity and balancing caloric intake and expenditure. We need to consume, on average, about 15 calories per pound of body weight per day. A large percentage of Americans consume much more without the expenditure of energy necessary to burn those calories.

Standard Recommendations for Weight Control

For decades the standard recommendations for weight control have emphasized caloric balance. Each pound of fat contains about 3,500 calories. In order to lose one pound, an individual would have to reduce the number of calories consumed and/or increase the number of calories burned by a total of 3,500. The beauty of this advice is that it incorporates physical activity that has a multitude of benefits on its own.

A person who consumes 3,000 calories per day could reduce that amount by 500. At the end of a week, he or she would have reduced by 3,500 calories, or one pound. Another option would be to reduce calories by 300 per day and burn 200 per day with extra activity. Again, at the end of seven days, 3,500 calories would be eliminated. Health experts advise losing no more than two pounds per week. Gradual weight loss is more likely to be sustained and is much healthier than sudden large shifts in weight.

A person who is following the standard recommendation for weight control should make sure that he or she is obtaining the proper nutrients while reducing calories. Because many obese and overweight individuals have health problems that may restrict their physical activity, these individuals should consult a physician before beginning any weight reduction regimen.

Most diets work, at least for a while, because of their novelty. Their longer-term success depends on the ability of the dieter to continue to adhere to the plan for a long time. For this reason, weight management should be a lifetime commitment to healthy behaviors, including nutritious food consumption and physical activity, in order to achieve long-term success.

The Role of Physical Activity in Controlling Weight

It is difficult to exaggerate the role of physical activity in controlling weight and reducing obesity and overweight. Activity burns calories. In addition, regular physical activity increases resting metabolism that, in turn, burns more calories even when at rest.

This relationship between sedentary lifestyle and overweight has been understood for decades. This result is particularly distressing in youth, where overweight is often rooted and where behavioral patterns are established. Dietz and Gortmaker (1985) showed that among 12- to 17-year-olds, the prevalence of obesity is related to the number of hours spent watching television. The same authors (1993) stated that "29% of the cases of obesity could be prevented by reducing television viewing to 0 to 1 hours per day." Gortmaker et al. (1996) concluded, "Estimates of attributable risk [of overweight] indicate that more [than] 60% of overweight incidence in [children ages 10 to 15] can be linked to excess television viewing time." Similar links between television viewing and overweight, obesity, body fat, and/or high BMI were reported in several studies (Anderson, Crespo, Bartlett, Cheskin, & Pratt, 1998; Crespo et al., 2001; Lowry, Wechsler, Galuska, Fulton, & Kann, 2002; Proctor et al., 2003). These studies have been supplemented by others (Epstein et al., 1995; Klesges, Shelton, & Klesges, 1993) that expanded sedentary activity to include watching videos and playing video games and computer games; these activities were also related to incidence of obesity and overweight in youth.

Reducing children's time spent in front of screen media has potential for reducing body weight (Robinson, 1999; Epstein et al., 1995). However, it does not necessarily hold that reducing screen time increases physical activity among youth. It is important that parents encourage and

GUIDELINES FOR WEIGHT LOSS AND MAINTENANCE
- Select a program with which you are comfortable. If you need support, take that into consideration. If you are uncomfortable with group weigh-ins, avoid programs that require them.
- Use a program that is based on real, healthy foods. This allows you to learn how to prepare foods and govern portion sizes. If this is already done for you with prepackaged food, you are unlikely to learn necessary skills when you grow tired of purchasing packaged meals.
- Consume a wide variety of foods. Try new foods, especially fruits and vegetables.

(continues)

- Include regular physical activity. The exercise routine is nearly as important as dietary habits. Regular activity increases the **basal metabolic rate**, the rate at which we burn calories when at rest.
- Avoid diet pills unless you are obese and the use of the pills is monitored by a physician. Pills are not something you can or should use for a lifetime.
- Avoid fad diets.
- Seek out a flexible program, one that accommodates travel and socializing.
- Set realistic, attainable goals. Remain positive toward those goals even when setbacks occur.
- Develop a healthy lifestyle; look at weight management as a lifelong commitment. Stress management, physical activity, and healthy social relationships are also important parts of overall health.
- Eat more slowly. It takes 20 minutes for your brain to send the signal that you have had enough to eat. During that 20 minutes you may eat a lot of food and consume more calories that you do not need.

provide opportunity for activity and for schools to include daily physical activity in their plans.

The Mediterranean Diet

Several years ago, it was observed that individuals in the region of the Mediterranean Sea had lower rates of heart disease and death rates than people in other developed countries, including the United States. These advantages were present even though the diets derived a large percentage of their calories from fat. Speculation centered around the so-called Mediterranean diet. Nineteen countries border the Mediterranean, and diets vary among these countries and even within regions of individual countries. Although there is no single Mediterranean diet, the commonalities among the Mediterranean diets are healthy nutrition, natural products, and inclusion of almost any type of food except artificial ones, such as hydrogenated fats. The common elements of the various diets in the region are consumption of:

- Fruits, vegetables, bread and other cereals, potatoes, beans, nuts, and seeds
- Olive oil, a source of monounsaturated fat
- Dairy products, fish, and poultry in small to moderate amounts, and small portions of red meat

- Eggs no more than four times a week
- Wine in low to moderate amounts

It was the presence of wine that first attracted many scientists to the Mediterranean diet.

As the popularity of the Mediterranean diet increased, it was studied and promoted as a way to lose weight. The diet has been touted for weight control and incorporated into other programs. Whether or not it is an effective long-term weight management tool, the principles behind the Mediterranean diet are solid when considering improving overall health.

Very-Low-Calorie and Low-Calorie Diets

Very-low-calorie diets (VLCDs) are defined as diets providing fewer than 800 calories per day. VLCDs are not for the average person who wants to lose a few pounds. They are generally recommended only for the obese, people whose BMI exceeds 30, and people with weight-related morbidity. **Low-calorie diets** (LCDs) provide 800 to 1,500 calories per day.

VLCDs are generally used as part of a comprehensive intervention that includes medical monitoring and a program of lifestyle modification (Tsai & Wadden, 2006). The care is frequently provided by a team that includes a physician, psychologist, dietitian, and exercise physiologist. The program usually includes 12 weeks of weight loss followed by 12 to 14 weeks of reintroduction of conventional foods and weight stabilization. Physician attention is important because during the initial weeks, patients are at increased risk of gallstones, cold intolerance, hair loss, headache, fatigue, dizziness, muscle cramps, and constipation (Mustajoki & Pekkarinen, 2001; National Task Force on the Prevention and Treatment of Obesity, 1993; Wadden, Stunkard, & Brownell, 1983). VLCDs can lead to dramatic shifts in fluid and electrolyte balance and can lead to loss of lean body mass. Serious complications, even death, have been reported in obese persons who consumed very-low-calorie diets without medical supervision (Wadden, Stunkard, & Brownell, 1983; Wadden, Van Itallie, & Blackburn, 1990).

A large analysis of several studies (Tsai & Wadden, 2006) found that VLCDs induced significantly greater short-term weight loss than LCDs but greater weight regain in the long term. Generally, the research indicates that VLCDs are not as effective as LCDs for long-term weight loss. Any long-term success with VLCDs seems to be associated with one to two years of participation in an integrated weight maintenance program that includes lifestyle interventions including dietary change, nutrition education, behavior therapy, and increased physical activity. Still, the quick weight loss associated with VLCDs often produces improvement in patients with obesity-related conditions such as diabetes, high cholesterol, joint problems, sleep apnea, and hypertension.

VLCDs often result in a loss of lean body mass, or muscle. This can be mitigated somewhat by engaging in regular exercise. Constipation is also a common side effect, one that can be helped by increased intake of fiber. Perhaps the greatest problem with VLCDs is that most people regain the weight they lost. Given the complications associated with VLCDs, the costs, and the relative effectiveness, the expert panel of the National Heart, Lung, and Blood Institute (1998) concluded that VLCDs should not be recommended over LCDs composed of conventional foods.

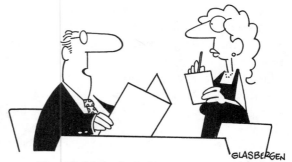

"I can't drink alcohol on my low-carb diet. I'll just have a couple shots of gravy with a twist of bacon."

Source: © Randy Glasbergen, used with permission from www.glasbergen.com.

LCDs in which women consume 1,000 to 1,200 calories per day and men consume 1,200 to 1,600 calories per day will help most people lose weight safely. The upper range of calories per day may also benefit women who weigh more than 165 pounds. For overweight children or teens, it is important to slow the rate of weight gain. Reduced-calorie diets are not advised without consultation with a health care provider. The overall success is dependent on consuming a healthy selection of foods and comes with the caveat that physical activity is an important part of a weight loss program.

Commercial Weight Loss Programs

A number of commercial weight loss programs are available. Many of them are major national and international chains. Persons considering the use of commercial weight loss programs should realize that these programs have not been carefully studied, especially in the long term, and that they vary greatly in cost (Tsai & Wadden, 2005). Most of them market themselves with before-and-after pictures and testimonials instead of solid research. Some of the most recognizable names are Weight Watchers, eDiets.com, Health Management Resources, OPTIFAST, Jenny Craig, and Nutrisystem. Many of these companies offer a variety of programs.

Federal monitoring of these programs is by the Federal Trade Commission. Thus, the oversight of these programs is largely related to their advertising rather than safety and efficacy, for which they are not required to submit any data. The FTC occasionally intervenes when it suspects that companies are making false or misleading claims.

A coalition of weight loss programs (Partnership for Healthy Weight Management, 1999) developed the *Voluntary Guidelines for Providers of Weight Loss Products or Services*. The guidelines include provision of information concerning the staff qualifications and central components of the program, the risks of overweight and obesity, risks associated with the provider's product or program or components of the program, and total and periodic costs. Since the guidelines are voluntary, it is not known how many programs actually follow them or the accuracy of the information that is provided.

Those considering a commercial weight loss program should ask about the qualifications of the staff and whether counseling is available. They should also investigate whether scheduling of meetings, consultations, and counseling sessions are flexible enough to meet their needs.

We shall explore some of the better-known commercial programs. This is not meant to be an exhaustive listing and description of the programs because there are many in number, they sometimes change their program components, and some are short-lived.

Weight Watchers

Weight Watchers is one of the oldest and largest commercial weight loss programs. In 2009, consumers spent over $4 billion on Weight Watchers–branded products and services. Each week approximately 1.3 million members attend almost 50,000 Weight Watchers meetings (WeightWatchers.com, 2010). This figure does not include the customers who use Weight Watchers Online.

There have been several versions of Weight Watchers programs, but the focus has always been on long-term weight management. The program claims to provide "an integrated approach emphasizing good eating choices, healthy habits, a supportive environment and exercise" (WeightWatchers.com, 2010). It also proclaims that it allows you to eat what you like, with an emphasis on nutrition and advice on staying satiated.

Much of the satisfaction that clients report with Weight Watchers is undoubtedly based on the support component of the program. Members pay a fee and attend regular group meetings where they are weighed confidentially. The weekly meetings are conducted by a Weight Watchers leader. The leaders are satisfied customers, called

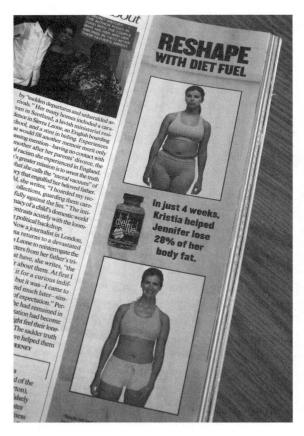

Before-and-after photos are typical advertising ploys used to promote weight loss programs and products. They usually do not reflect typical results, nor do they indicate the "after that," the way the person looks a year or two after the diet.

Lifetime Members, who have undergone extensive training. Group support and access to information via the company's Web site and message boards are important keys.

The program is based on the Weight Watchers *POINTS®* Food System, which is designed to allow the consumer to eat any food as long as he or she keeps track and controls how much is consumed. Every food has a *POINTS* value, a number based on the calories, grams of total fat, and grams of dietary fiber of a specific portion of the food. Clients consume a self-selected diet of conventional foods rather than products sold by the company. The program attempts to control calories by focusing eating on a core list made up of foods from all the food groups: fruits and vegetables; grains and starches; lean meats, fish, and poultry; eggs; and dairy products.

It is to the program's credit that physical activity is emphasized through a "Get Moving" booklet and DVDs. In the beginning, clients are encouraged to reduce sedentary habits. Later, a formula is used, based on body weight, the amount of time the activity is done, and the level of intensity to plan regular physical activity. The objective is to enable the client to do any exercise or activity that is enjoyable and fits within his or her lifestyle.

Weight Watchers is considered one of the best commercial weight loss programs. It generally gives good nutritional advice. The system of counting points is not something most people will carry out all of their lives, but if the process leads to forming good eating habits, it is beneficial. As with any approach, the discipline and commitment of the client is the most important element. It appears that the persistence rate is good for Weight Watchers clients in comparison with those of other commercial programs.

Weight Watchers charges a membership fee of $29 to $35 and weekly, pay-as-you-go fees that are around $10 to $15 per meeting. Fees vary by region and are subject to change. The estimated cost of a three-month program in 2004 was about $170 (Tsai & Wadden, 2005). Weight Watchers' online program costs $29.95 to sign up, then a monthly fee of $16.95 per month, with a discount for signing up for a three-month package. Weight Watchers frequently offers reduced membership fees and coupons.

Jenny Craig

The Jenny Craig method (WebMD.com, 2010a) is a three-level plan to help people lose weight and keep it off. The first level of the program teaches clients how to eat the foods they want in sensible, frequent portions and how to plan healthy menus. The second level teaches how to increase energy levels through physical activity; this includes strategies to avoid everyday barriers to activity. Level three teaches clients how to build more balance into their lives in order to maintain weight loss and healthy diet. This includes maintaining motivations and building a supportive environment.

The Jenny Craig program does not exclude any foods, but calorie counts are important. Counselors train clients to develop menus that are based on individual goals, height, and weight.

As opposed to the group sessions of Weight Watchers, Jenny Craig provides individual counseling at one of over 650 centers in the United States, Canada, Puerto Rico, New Zealand, and Australia as well as telephone counseling 24 hours a day, seven days a week. It can be a problem that clients do not get the same counselors on each call. Jenny Craig facilitates online chats with other clients and counselors. The program includes weekly weighing.

Jenny Craig requires clients to purchase the company's prepackaged meals, which can be expensive. The meals reflect the 2005 federal nutritional guidelines and the U.S. Department of Agriculture's food pyramid. The nutrition in the meals may be sound, but the cost of the food may be prohibitive for many people. In addition, the use of prepackaged meals does not encourage clients to learn to cook for themselves or make healthful decisions on foods. The ultimate goal is to wean clients from the prepackaged meals while continuing the same eating habits.

This program has been around since the mid-1980s, so it must be either satisfying many customers, marketed extremely well, or both. Still, there is not a lot of research, especially long-term studies, to evaluate its effectiveness. A notable exception (Rock, Pakiz, Flatt, & Quintana, 2007) found that Jenny Craig facilitated weight loss that was maintained at one year. In one study touted on the Jenny Craig Web site, less than 7 percent of males who entered the Platinum Program were retained for a year. However, those who stayed in the program showed substantial weight loss after a year (Finley et al., 2007).

There is an initial membership fee and a charge for a weight loss manual. The prepackaged food costs around $85 to $140 per week, depending on choices, plus shipping and handling charges. There are frequent special offers, but some of them are conditioned on eventual weight loss.

OPTIFAST

OPTIFAST is considered a medically based program; clients begin with a medical evaluation. Following the evaluation, the program offers a three-phase meal replacement and lifestyle modification program. The program consists of 12 to 18 weeks of rapid weight loss, a transition phase of three to eight weeks, and long-term maintenance. OPTIFAST recommends a very-low-calorie diet of fewer than 800 calories per day. Clients are seen by physicians regularly and undergo laboratory tests, support and counseling, and lifestyle modification education.

OPTIFAST is based on the use of meal replacements during the active weight loss phase of the program. Participants purchase the OPTIFAST brand of prepackaged liquid meals and nutrition bars. The program boasts of high-quality, pre-portioned products providing complete nutrition and freedom from having to make a food choice (OPTIFAST, 2010). This latter quality seems at odds with the concept of teaching people to choose healthy foods for a lifetime.

The program includes one-on-one counseling with a nutritionist or physician and small group discussions with a counselor. There are also activity plans customized for the individual's needs and time constraints.

People lose weight during the initial phase of the program. However, the very-low-calorie diet can put many people at risk, which explains the physician monitoring. Few people would stay on a VLCD or a liquid diet for very long, so the long-term benefits are in question. The program is expensive. WebMD.com (2010b) estimated the cost of a three-month OPTIFAST program to be $1,700 to $2,000.

Medifast

Like OPTIFAST, Medifast offers a medically based low-calorie replacement program. Medifast also offers a nonmedical do-it-yourself option. A majority of clients buy Medifast products directly from the company and do not participate in the medically supervised portion. Both options are considered a soy-based liquid supplement modified fasting program. A relatively new product, Momentum by Medifast, is said to burn extra calories, boost metabolism, and decrease appetite. It contains caffeine and an antioxidant found in green tea.

Medifast does not require an initial membership fee or medical evaluation. Fees are based on the meal plan. Physician visits are recommended and subject to an additional fee. Estimated cost of a three-month program is about $840 (WebMD.com, 2010b); costs may increase with the medical plan. Medifast offers both low-calorie-diets and very-low-calorie diets, the latter requiring medical monitoring. However, the company does not require written documentation of such monitoring for clients to purchase its meal replacements. The National Task Force on the Prevention and Treatment of Obesity (1993) suggested that consumer safety when using a VLCD is dependent on physician monitoring.

Medifast may be a good program for those who need to lose a substantial amount of weight, as long as the client is monitored by a physician, since diets with fewer than 1,200 calories per day can pose health risks. The program is easy to use, although there is quite an adjustment from solid food to liquid and back to solid.

Nutrisystem

Since its inception in 1972, Nutrisystem has undergone many changes, but one feature has been consistent—convenience. It markets its own line of meals. The company operates mainly through the Internet and direct mail with some television sales. Counseling and behavior modification services are available at no charge, but the counseling is not face-to-face. Counselors may be dietitians, health educators, nurses, or others. There are exercise DVDs for the Nutrisystem Advanced participants.

The 12-week plan includes three meals a day plus snacks. The underpinning of the Nutrisystem plan is eating high-fiber, low-fat foods with optimal amounts of lean protein to curb cravings and satisfy hunger on fewer calories.

The plan is based on the **glycemic index**, a method of ranking foods based on a "good carbs—bad carbs" scale and the effects of carbohydrates on blood sugar. The principle behind the glycemic index is to avoid foods that cause a quick rise in blood sugar. While the science behind the index is sound, the problem is that we eat foods in combinations, making it difficult to predict the blood-sugar response.

Women on Nutrisystem usually consume 1,200 calories, and men consume 1,500 per day. The client supplements the packaged foods by purchasing fruit, milk, and vegetables; six servings of fruits and vegetables per day are recommended. All products are solid foods, not liquid products. There is no need to record calories, count points, or deal with recipes, a factor that adds to the convenience of the program. Meals can usually be prepared in less than five minutes. The cost of monthly shipments of food ranges from about $290 to $330, including shipping charges. Nutrisystem also sells vitamin and protein supplements.

Recently, Nutrisystem has attempted to attract specific audiences with vegetarian, diabetic, and men's plans. The program is not what one would call long term, although there is online guidance over time and the Mindset guide that addresses a wide range of long-term issues.

While Nutrisystem offers a sound dietary program, a common criticism is that dieters do not learn to plan meals, gauge portion size, or cook for themselves after they have lost the desired amount of weight on the program. In addition, experts' opinions are mixed on the glycemic approach to weight loss. Some think it's just another gimmick—but say that if it helps people eat in a more healthy way, the gimmick can be successful (Zelman, 2010).

It is difficult to gauge the long-term effects of the program. Nutrisystem does not appear to have been used in clinical trials reported in the medical literature, possibly because of its heavy commercial emphasis as well as the number of different subprograms it markets. The average customer stays on the plan for about nine weeks and loses an average of 20 pounds; about a third of customers will return to the plan within a year. Most, however, regain the lost weight (Diet.com, 2010).

Volumetrics Diet

This diet, developed by nutritionist Barbara Rolls (Rolls & Barnett, 2000), focuses on foods that have fewer calories per serving, so that people can eat more and feel satisfied, but consume fewer calories. Rolls uses the term "low energy density" to mean few calories per serving. Some examples of low-energy-density foods are nonstarchy vegetables, fruits, soup broth, whole grains, and nonfat milk products.

The central tenet of the diet is to consume foods that create a feeling of fullness. Rolls believes that water is the key to creating fullness and that foods high in water are critical to limiting calories and still feeling full. For example, the diet would advocate getting 100 calories from 1 2/3 cups of grapes (high water content) to 100 calories from ¼ cup of raisins (low water content). To this end, she has created 125 recipes that are contained in her second book (Rolls, 2005). A benefit of this approach is the opportunity to learn how to prepare healthy foods, something missing from prepackaged diet food.

The overall plan of the Volumetrics diet includes physical activity, keeping a journal of exercise and what is consumed, and learning to calculate energy density foods. It also includes water and fiber consumption. To her credit, Rolls advocates loss of only one or two pounds per week.

There seem to be few risks with the plan, but Smith (2005) cautions that the Volumetrics diet has the potential for muscle loss rather than fat loss. Some people may grow hungry quickly, once the water is absorbed from the stomach.

While the basic idea of Volumetrics is based on years of research, there is a shortage of controlled studies that actually demonstrate its value. It is generally accepted by registered dietitians and nutritionists as a sensible, effective, and nutritionally balanced eating plan. In 2004, the Tufts University Health and Nutrition Letter named *The Volumetrics Eating Plan* one of the three best diet books on the market. In addition, the American Dietetic Association includes the book on its 2007 Good Nutrition Reading List.

Online Commercial Weight Loss Programs

The most recent development in commercial weight loss programs is Internet-based interventions. Examples include Nutrisystem.com, Weight Watchers Online, Dietwatch.com, Caloriescount .com, and eDiets.com. There are indications that they can be useful tools if they include personalized feedback, especially a therapist-led intervention (Gold, Burke, Pintauro, Buzzell, & Harvey-Berino, 2007).

The most studied of these programs is eDiets .com. The program supports with peer groups and expert registered dietitians and over a dozen different approaches to dieting along with individualized eating plans, including a version of the Mediterranean diet. eDiets provides home-delivered meals as well as counseling and information at low cost, about $3 per week. The program appears to result in average to below average weight loss when compared with other programs.

While there are some data on the short-term results of online weight loss programs, there is a stark lack of published research on the long-term effectiveness and safety of these programs. There is not enough evidence to recommend commercial Internet-based programs.

Organized Self-Help Programs

The two largest organized self-help programs are Take Off Pounds Sensibly (TOPS) and Overeaters Anonymous (OA), both of which are nonprofit and are organized and led by volunteers. Costs of self-help programs are generally very low or free. Self-help programs are based on the belief that people who have the same condition can provide empathy and support to one another.

TOPS recommends a low-calorie exchange diet and provides a curriculum on diet, physical activity, and behavior modification (Take Off Pounds Sensibly, 2007). Members meet weekly in over 10,000 local chapters in the United States and Canada. The program offers a system of competition, awards, and recognition for success, effort, and support.

OA supporters believe that obesity results from compulsive eating that is considered the consequence of sadness, loneliness, and other troublesome emotions. Participants frequently feel that they are addicted to food. The philosophy and 12-step approach are similar to those of Alcoholics Anonymous, including a strong spiritual component (Overeaters Anonymous, 2007).

Carbohydrate-Restricted Diets

Diets based on restricting carbohydrates are not new. Low-carbohydrate and very-low-carbohydrate diets have become extremely popular, primarily because of the publicity the approach has received, clever marketing, and the proliferation of low-carb products, even in fast food chains. The commercial part of these enterprises comes from selling literature and packaged foods. The popularity has at least partly been driven by the success that many people have experienced and many studies that have demonstrated the ability of restricted-carb diets to produce weight loss in the short term.

Low-carb is big business, and companies that are not ostensibly part of the weight loss industry have gotten involved. The American Italian Pasta Company launched a low-carb pasta. Purveyors of protein are getting into the trend. Sales of carb-free macadamia nut oil, made from Australian macadamia nuts, have skyrocketed. The stock of Cal-Maine Foods, the leading U.S. fresh egg producer, was up over 800 percent in 2003. Sales by pork and beef processors rose dramatically as low-carb diets gained popularity. Even low-carb beers have hit the market. Companies like Atkins Nutritionals, Carbolite, CarbSense, and Keto Foods introduced low-carb packaged foods at a rate of almost two products a day in 2003. There are over 250 low-carb specialty stores.

Malik and Hu (2007) pointed out that low-carbohydrate diets are attractive because they promise rapid weight loss without having to count calories. By contrast, traditional dietary recommendations for weight loss endorse a fat-restricted and calorie-restricted diet high in complex carbohydrates. Evidence appears to indicate that low-carb diets can be effective in terms of short-term weight loss relative to traditional low-fat diets (Gardner et al., 2007). In comparison with the prescription drug orlistat combined with a low-fat diet, a low-carbohydrate **ketogenic diet** produced similar results (Yancy et al., 2010). Foster et al. (2010), in one of the most lengthy studies, compared low-carbohydrate and low-fat diets over a two-year period and concluded that successful weight loss can be achieved with either diet coupled with behavioral treatment. Beyond this study, little is known about the long-term utility and safety of low-carb, high-protein diets.

The Atkins Diet

One of the most popular and best publicized low-carbohydrate diets is the Atkins Diet, developed and promoted by the late Dr. Robert Atkins. Atkins gained a huge following through his diet empire, which includes books, journals, multimedia programs, and its own line of nutritional products. Because of its popularity and controversy, we will discuss this diet more thoroughly than others.

The Atkins Nutritional Principles form the core of the Atkins Nutritional Approach. Perhaps the most important of the four principles are that the individual will achieve good health and will lay the permanent groundwork for disease prevention, especially weight-related conditions.

The Atkins Diet allows unlimited consumption of protein and fat but drastically limits carbohydrates. Unlike conventional diets, it does not limit calories or require weigh-ins or keeping food records.

The body burns both carbohydrates and fats for energy. Atkins contends that his approach shocks the metabolism into a new gear, in which the body generates energy by burning its stored fat rather than burning glucose derived from carbohydrates. Once this "metabolic advantage" is turned on, a dieter can stop worrying about calories.

The Atkins Nutritional Approach (Atkins Nutritionals, 2010) is a four-phase eating plan. Phase 1, Induction, restricts carbohydrate consumption to 20 grams each day, primarily from salads and other nonstarchy vegetables. Bread, pasta, potatoes, rice, grains, most fruit, nuts, and sugar are discouraged. Dieters can eat all the fish, fowl, and meat they want, although they should restrict bacon, ham, and organ meat. Dieters are encouraged to eat butter and not skimp on fat. Losing up to 15 pounds in two weeks is mentioned as a kick start. In Phase 2, Ongoing Weight Loss, the user increases carbohydrates as weight loss slows. Individuals are supposed to discover their ideal carbohydrate intake for weight maintenance. During the second phase, carbohydrates come from fiber-rich, nutrient-dense foods. By Phase 3, Pre-Maintenance, the dieter is within 10 pounds of target weight. This phase makes the transition from weight loss to weight maintenance by increasing daily carbohydrate intake as long as very gradual weight loss is maintained. In Phase 4, Lifetime Maintenance, the user stabilizes the target weight and continues to count carbohydrates for the rest of his or her life with minor accommodations for life changes. The dieter selects a wide variety of foods while controlling carbohydrate intake. The individual's ideal amount of daily carb intake is discovered in the previous phases and maintained. This is supposed to ensure weight maintenance and a sense of well-being.

The Atkins program recommends an array of nutritional supplements produced and sold by Atkins Nutritionals. The program encourages exercise and dietary fiber.

The burning question around the Atkins Diet as well as other low-carbohydrate diets is: Does it work? It does appear that, at least in the short term, Atkins is effective at weight reduction (Acheson, 2004; Agnew, 2004; Foster et al., 2003).

The Atkins Diet boasts effects other than weight loss. Some studies (Agnew, 2004; Acheson, 2004) have shown that low-carbohydrate dieters posted significant improvement in cardiovascular biomarkers such as triglycerides; low-density lipoprotein (LDL), the "bad" cholesterol that accumulates on artery walls and increases risk of heart disease; and high-density lipoprotein (HDL), the "good" cholesterol that helps sweep LDL away. Johnston, Tjonn, and Swann (2004) reported reduced total cholesterol, insulin, and uric acid concentration in the blood and found that those on high-protein diets experience more satisfaction and less hunger than those on low-fat diets. Sharman, Gomez, Kraemer, and Volek (2004), in a short-term study of overweight men, found that a very-low-carb, low-calorie diet significantly improved biomarkers associated with metabolic syndrome, including triglycerides and LDL particle size. High levels of triglycerides and LDL are associated with elevated risk of heart disease, while HDL is associated with reduced risk of heart disease. Foster et al. (2010)

found that during the first six months, the low-carbohydrate diet group had greater reductions in diastolic blood pressure, triglyceride levels, and very-low-density-lipoprotein cholesterol levels, but lesser reductions in LDL cholesterol and more adverse symptoms than the low-fat diet group. They also found that the low-carbohydrate group had greater increases in HDL levels at two years. Yancy et al. (2010), in comparing the low-carb ketogenic diet with a combination of prescription orlistat and a low-fat diet, found similar results in measures of serum lipids and glycemic parameters and greater effect for lowering blood pressure with the low-carb diet. Three other recent studies (Foster et al., 2003; Samaha, Iqbal, & Seshadri, 2003; Westman, Yancy, & Edman, 2002) suggested that the Atkins Diet is superior to a low-fat diet with respect to short-term changes in weight, triglycerides, and HDL.

The vast majority of the studies on the Atkins Diet have been done in the short term and most recommended longer-range studies. Some comparison studies (Dansinger, Gleason, Griffith, Selker, & Schaefer, 2005; Morgan et al., 2009) found Atkins to not be superior to other diets for weight loss over months to a year. There is a great need for study of the effects of the diet three, five, or more years later.

Many medical experts question the health safety of the Atkins Diet over the long term. There are concerns about the effects of large amounts of protein on kidney function and the impact of saturated fats on cholesterol and heart disease. It has been known for a long time that a diet low in complex carbohydrates, antioxidants, certain vitamins and minerals, and fiber is associated with some forms of cancer. Calcium depletion, dehydration, and electrolyte loss may occur. Cardiovascular medications, diuretics, and diabetes medications, including insulin, when combined with this diet, may produce dangerous effects. Other medications may change the effects of the diet.

Two caveats are important in considering this diet. First, the long-term effects have not been adequately studied, so it is premature to state that any short-term benefits are likely to be sustained or whether the diet affects cardiovascular health.

However, there is little evidence supporting any advantage of the low-carb/high-protein formula over traditional diets that restrict fats and calories over the long term. Second, it is critical to discuss the choice with a physician before beginning the diet.

The South Beach Diet

The South Beach Diet is championed by Dr. Arthur Agatston in his book *The South Beach Diet* (2003). While Agatston claims this is not a low-carb or a low-fat diet, instead focusing on the "right" carbs and fats, it has similarities to the low-carbohydrate Atkins Diet. The diet also promises large loss of weight in a short period of time, a serious red flag to those who want to lose weight in a slower, healthy fashion.

The diet is divided into three phases. Phase 1, which lasts two weeks, is designed to eliminate cravings for sugar and refined starches, by stabilizing blood sugar. This phase is characterized by consumption of lean protein, high-fiber vegetables, reduced-fat cheeses, low-fat dairy, and extra-virgin olive oil and canola oil. During this phase, large weight losses, 8 to 13 pounds, are promised and may leave the client feeling weak and wobbly (Bellow, 2007). Vitamins and minerals may be sacrificed because of restriction of fruits.

Phase 2 is the long-term weight loss phase. In addition to the foods encouraged in Phase 1, whole-grain bread, brown rice, whole-wheat pasta, fruits, and more vegetables are added. Snacks and desserts with emphasis on dark chocolate are encouraged.

Phase 3 begins once the individual has reached a healthy weight. The principles from the first two phases are continued, but almost every kind of food, some in the form of occasional indulgences, is allowed. This is a maintenance phase in which the client hopes to maintain ideal weight throughout the life span.

The South Beach Diet differs from the Atkins Diet in several ways. First, the Atkins Diet advocates unlimited amounts of foods high in saturated fats; the South Beach Diet does not.

Second, Atkins is stricter on carbohydrate limitation, even limiting fruits and vegetables. South Beach encourages a diet that includes fruits and vegetables after Phase 1. After that phase, South Beach meets several of the criteria for a healthy diet advocated by nutritionists and government officials (Better Health USA, 2007; WebMD.com, 2004). However, there is a distinct lack of controlled studies on the South Beach Diet.

Possible Negative Effects of Restricted Carbohydrate Diets

Skeptics suspect that there may be serious negative side effects to the restricted-carbohydrate diets. Much of this suspicion is based on the fact that these diets are high in fats and proteins. Headaches, muscle weakness, and either diarrhea or constipation are reported more often by Atkins dieters than those on conventional diets (Astrup, Larsen, & Harper, 2004). Westman, Yancy, and Edman (2002) found that 70 percent of patients on an Atkins Diet for six months were constipated, 65 percent had halitosis, 54 percent reported headaches, and 10 percent had hair loss. Johnston, Tjonn, and Swann (2004) stated that low-carbohydrate, high-protein, high-fat diets such as Atkins have been associated with adverse changes in blood and renal biomarkers. Fleming (2000) also found that high-protein diets diminished blood flow to the heart and produced increased inflammatory markers that predict heart attacks.

The rapid weight loss in the early stages of restricted carb diets can throw off the electrolyte balance. This is because much of the weight loss is from reduction in water weight, not fat.

Cardiovascular medications, diuretics, and diabetes medications, including insulin, when combined with restricted carbohydrate diets, may produce dangerous effects. Other medications may change the effects of the diet on metabolism.

High protein intake, a hallmark of some low-carb diets, may accelerate renal decline in women (Knight et al., 2003). In a randomized control trial, ketogenic diets such as the Atkins Diet impaired cognitive performance and higher-order mental processing after only one week (Wing, Vazquez, & Ryan, 1995).

There is evidence that the Atkins Diet may increase postprandial lipemia, an increase of fats in the blood a few hours after ingestion of fatty foods, and increase free fatty acids that may have harmful effects on platelet aggregation, and it may also promote ventricular arrythmias (Oliver & Yates, 1972; Peyreigne et al., 1999).

Low-carbohydrate dieters, because they consume so much meat and little fruit or vegetables, may suffer from a dietary shortage of fiber. Complex carbohydrates and whole foods are rich in phytochemicals, bioflavonoids, carotenoids, retinols, sulforaphanes, isoflavones, polyphenols, and other substances that may reduce the risk of many chronic diseases. These foods are low in cholesterol, saturated fat, oxidants, and other disease-promoting substances. Diets low in complex carbohydrates, antioxidants, certain vitamins and minerals, and fiber are associated with some forms of cancer. In addition, fiber from whole grains, but not refined grains, was inversely associated with all-cause mortality in 11,040 postmenopausal women followed for 11 years (Jacobs, Pereira, Meyer, & Kushi, 2000).

Diets that contain high levels of fat, especially saturated fats, have the potential to elevate cholesterol, especially LDL, and triglycerides. Should this occur, it can result in cardiovascular disease.

Burning fat produces ketones that might set off ketoacidosis, a particular danger to people with diabetes. Diabetics should be especially cautious about trying low-carb diets unless they are under the supervision of a physician. Drastically reducing carbohydrate intake without adjusting insulin or other diabetes medicines can quickly raise insulin levels and bring on low blood glucose, or hypoglycemia, that could cause coma or death.

Long-term carbohydrate restriction could conceivably cause kidney damage, bone mineral loss, urinary blockage, high cholesterol, and even damage to the brain and nervous system, which are fueled primarily by glucose derived from carbohydrates.

The American Heart Association (2007a) expressed concerns that a diet high in protein and fat and low in nutrient-rich fruits and vegetables can contribute to osteoporosis, heart disease, stroke, kidney stones, liver problems, cancer, and diabetes.

Amid all this skepticism, Agnew (2004) reported that, according to a flurry of respected medical journals, the Atkins Diet seems to work at least as well as other weight loss programs, there are signs it may even work better, and it does not seem to do any serious harm to people who follow it. The South Beach Diet has shown some comparable results. Acheson (2004) stated that while evidence is accumulating in favor of Atkins-type diets, the safety and efficacy of low-carbohydrate, high-protein diets require further long-term verification. Before attempting restricted carbohydrate diets, consumers should consider that there is insufficient research following people on these diets for adequate periods of time to determine the long-term effects.

Diet Pills and Drinks

Over the years, many pills, drinks, and potions have been marketed as diet aids. The record of these products is discouraging, especially those available without a prescription. The ingredients in these preparations were usually stimulants. Products appear in "health food stores," on the Internet, on television, or in stores that specialize in herbs. These products often claim some mysterious value based on originating in Asia, Europe, or South America—as if that would indicate any superiority to American products. They are described as appetite suppressants, sometimes herbal, or fat burners. Usually, they come with extravagant claims. Sensible consumers consult a physician before using these products.

Many experts claim that liquid diets causing rapid weight loss tend to overuse lean muscle and slow the metabolism, making it more difficult to maintain weight loss. People who are only mildly obese lose too much lean body mass, which increases their chance of cardiac dysfunction. The intensity of protein in the liquid diets can cause an electrolyte imbalance and irregular heartbeat.

About 25 percent of the people on liquid diets develop gallstones (Hemphill, 2010).

Most experts advise against using pills or drinks to lose weight except under the direction of a physician. Using pills does not establish healthy lifestyle habits. Although some initial weight loss may occur, in the long term, most individuals gain back the weight they lost.

Available Without a Prescription

Alli

Alli is the only over-the-counter weight loss aid for adults that has been approved by the FDA. The active ingredient in Alli is orlistat, which is also the ingredient in the prescription drug Xenical but in lower dosage. Alli is meant to be used with a reduced-calorie, low-fat diet accompanied by regular exercise. Orlistat works by reducing the absorption of fats, fat calories, and fat-soluble vitamins. Studies show that most people taking Alli lose five to 10 pounds over six months.

Ephedra and Ephedrine

Ephedra, also known as ma huang, a Chinese herb, was once legally marketed in the United States as a weight loss product. Its active ingredient is ephedrine, a chemical that stimulates the heart and nervous system. Ephedra was banned as a weight loss ingredient by the FDA in 2004 because the agency found that there is an unreasonable risk of illness or injury from the use of the drug (U.S. FDA, 2004). The agency concluded that "the totality of the available data showed little evidence of ephedra's effectiveness except for modest, short-term weight loss without any clear health benefit." Pills containing ephedrine or ephedra still appear, especially on the World Wide Web.

Ephedrine made in laboratories is used in drugs to treat asthma and other respiratory conditions. Ephedrine has also been found to suppress appetite, boost metabolism, enhance sports performance, and increase energy. As a result, until recently, ephedra was often found in many so-called natural diet pills and supplements designed for athletes. While many manufacturers removed ephedra from their products in response to the FDA ban, it is still possible to buy products on the Internet that contain or claim to contain ephedra.

Ephedra and ephedrine have been linked to psychiatric problems, depression, nervousness, insomnia, and rapid heart rate. They have also been found to raise blood pressure and put additional stress on the circulatory system, leading to heart attacks and strokes.

It may be true that a person will lose weight while taking diet pills that contain ephedrine, but once the individual is off of these pills, he or she will likely regain the weight. Given the health risks, it is best to avoid ephedra and ephedrine.

Ephedrine is sometimes combined with caffeine and aspirin and marketed as a weight loss product that boosts metabolism. Any product that contains ephedrine, even in combination with other ingredients, carries the same or worse risks as ephedrine alone. In particular, the combination of ephedrine and caffeine or aspirin is potentially lethal for anyone with a heart condition or high blood pressure because the drugs all act as stimulants.

A number of variations on the formula have emerged following the ban on ephedra. Similar products have sprung up in their place using bitter orange extract or *Sida cordifolia,* a plant native to India that contains ephedrine, instead of ephedra. Guarana or kola nut extract are often used to supply a source of caffeine.

Caffeine

Caffeine is frequently used as an ingredient in diet pills. A stimulant of the central nervous system, it may appear in combination with ephedrine or another stimulant. The caffeine in these pills is often from plant extracts such as guarana, yerba mate, green tea, and kola nuts. As a result, these products are often described as being "herbal" or "natural" in an attempt to convince the consumer that they are completely safe.

High-caffeine products can produce anxiety, increased heart rate, raised blood pressure, nausea, diarrhea, restlessness, shaking, irritability, and insomnia. Caffeine can cause dependency. While high doses of caffeine, such as those that may appear in diet aids, are not recommended for anyone, they can be especially dangerous in people with high blood pressure, thyroid disease, diabetes, or heart problems.

Slim-Fast

The Slim-Fast plan calls for a Slim-Fast diet shake at breakfast and lunch, and then a sensible dinner, although the sensible dinner may be substituted for the noon meal. Dieters are also allowed two additional pieces of fruit and a Slim-Fast nutrition bar as needed during the day. The Slim-Fast diet, which averages about 1,200 calories a day, will cause weight loss for most people, as it is at least 500 calories less than the average female consumes and at least 1,000 calories less than the average male consumes. There are healthful aspects to the Slim-Fast meal plan, as the shakes contain the vitamins and minerals that humans need. The Slim-Fast program also encourages exercise and the consumption of several cups of water daily.

One pitfall of Slim-Fast is the fact that it is very difficult to get all of the vitamins, minerals, and other nutrients that are necessary for good health in a calorie-restricted diet. It is important to concentrate on consuming wholesome and nutritious foods during the sensible meal. The shakes contain only added vitamins and minerals. A key problem is the unlikelihood of continuing the program for years. Drinking two shakes each day is not something that most people will do for the rest of their lives. So while Slim-Fast may be a fairly healthy way to lose weight in the short term, maintenance over the long term is improbable.

Phenylpropanolamine

Phenylpropanolamine (PPA) was once a popular ingredient in OTC diet pills. On May 11, 2000, the FDA received results of a study conducted by scientists at Yale University School of Medicine that showed an increased risk of hemorrhagic stroke (bleeding of the brain) in people who were taking PPA (Horwitz, Brass, Kernan, & Viscoli, 2000). The FDA advisory panel confirmed the results of the Yale study. In 2005, the FDA advised that PPA is not generally recognized as safe and effective for over-the-counter use. As a result, this product has been removed from over-the-counter diet pills. It may still appear in imported products or those that have escaped FDA scrutiny.

Other Nonprescription Products

Chromium picolinate, a combination of the element chromium and picolinic acid, is often sold as a dietary supplement that can melt fat, drastically reduce appetite, and increase metabolism. Some claim it will increase muscle mass and tone. Scientific research has not supported the claims regarding weight loss and muscle mass. It is a common ingredient in many herbal weight loss concoctions available for over-the-counter sale at drugstores or on the Internet. Because it is marketed as an herbal dietary supplement, the FDA has little regulatory control over the products that contain it.

Diuretics, so-called water pills, promote the removal of fluids from the body through urination. Most OTC diuretics are derivatives of caffeine. Laxatives promote bowel movements, often producing watery stools. Herbal diuretics and herbal laxatives are often marketed for weight loss. Any weight loss from these products is water weight, not fat. Therefore, they are not effective for weight control. They can also lower the body's potassium levels, which may cause heart and muscle problems. They may also interact with medications.

Hoodia gordonii (hoodia) is a succulent South African plant. Hoodia is widely sold over the World Wide Web and in health food and discount stores, in the form of capsules or tablets. It is also available in milk chocolate chews. Advocates say that hoodia tricks the brain into thinking you are full. While there have been some studies on hoodia, they generally use small sample sizes and questionable research design; they are seldom published in peer-reviewed journals. To complicate the issue, a lot of fake hoodia is being sold.

Prescription Weight Loss Products

Obesity is a chronic condition and may require long-term treatment beyond lifestyle change. However, most weight loss drugs approved by the FDA are for short-term use, meaning a few weeks or months. Patients generally lose 5 to 22 pounds. Most of the weight loss occurs in the first six months, and evidence is lacking on the long-term effectiveness of prescription weight loss products. There are two types of prescription weight loss drugs—those that block or reduce absorption of fats and those that suppress appetite.

Xenical (orlistat) reduces the absorption of fats and fat calories by preventing the body from breaking down and absorbing fat eaten with meals. The unabsorbed fat is eliminated in bowel movements. Side effects include oily and loose stools or diarrhea. People taking orlistat should take multivitamin supplements due to possible loss of some vitamins.

Meridia is a commonly prescribed appetite suppressant. It affects appetite by increasing serotonin or catecholamine, brain chemicals that affect mood and appetite. Side effects include constipation, increased heart rate and blood pressure, stuffy nose, and insomnia.

These drugs are not intended for long-term use. Therefore, patients should make lifestyle changes such as regular physical activity and eating habits.

Fad Diets

A **fad diet** is a diet that has little or no nutritional value or scientific credibility and that usually has short-term popularity. It is unfortunate that many people desperately search for a quick and easy answer to their weight control problems. These people are vulnerable to hucksters and scam artists who develop a plan to make money while providing little of value to clients. Marketers of these plans often promise quick weight loss, sometimes while eating anything you want, usually with no physical activity, and frequently with money-back guarantees that they have no intention of honoring.

A few examples of fad diets include the Negative Calorie Diet, the Master Cleanse or Lemonade Diet, the Cabbage Soup Diet, the Hollywood 48-Hour Miracle Diet, the Bread and Butter Diet, the Russian Airforce Diet, the Chocolate Diet, the Grapefruit Diet, the Apple Cider Vinegar Diet, and the Chicken Soup Diet. It is instructive to note that many of these diets concentrate on

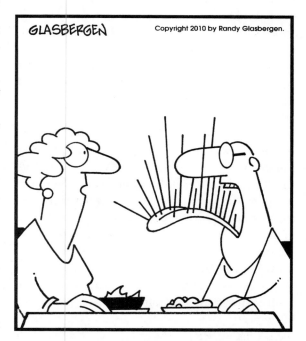

"Tell me more about the Acupuncture Diet. Does it really work?"

Source: © Randy Glasbergen, used with permission from www.glasbergen.com.

one food, something that no serious nutritionist would advocate. The American Heart Association (2007b) summed up the nature of these plans by saying, "Quick-weight loss diets usually overemphasize one particular food or type of food. They violate the first principle of good nutrition: Eat a balanced diet that includes a variety of foods. . . ." The AHA also said that "these diets also violate a second important principle of good nutrition: Eating should be enjoyable. These diets are so monotonous and boring that it's almost impossible to stay on them for long periods."

It could be argued, however, that the lack of ability to stay on these diets for long is really an asset.

Do Diet Programs Work?

Tsai and Wadden (2005) reviewed several studies of commercial weight loss programs. They concluded that with the exception of one trial of Weight Watchers, the evidence to support the use of major commercial and self-help programs is insufficient to recommend them.

The Consumers Union (2007) rated several weight loss programs based on results of clinical published studies. The overall scale score was based on nutritional analysis and the critiques of a panel of diet experts. Specific components of the rating included short-term weight loss and dropout rate, one year weight loss and dropout rate, and nutrition analysis. The highest rated plan was Volumetrics, followed closely by Weight Watchers and Jenny Craig. Even the highest rated diets generally produced less than a 10 percent weight loss after a year and had dropout rates of more than one in five participants. There is a need for research on the long-term results of these and other diets.

Although the marketers of many weight loss programs claim to have clinical proof or scientific studies that their programs work, there are not many peer-reviewed published studies to back up the claims we see in ads. In fact, the claims often have nothing but testimonials, before-and-after photos, and case studies to support them.

In one of the most thorough studies (Shai et al., 2008) to date, moderately obese subjects were randomly assigned to one of three diets: low-fat, restricted-calorie; Mediterranean, restricted-calorie; or low-carbohydrate, non-restricted-calorie. Subjects received approximately the same amount of physical activity. Mean weight loss among the three diets varied by less than four pounds. While none of the diets led to a great amount of weight loss for an obese person, the relative effectiveness of the low-carbohydrate diet was a surprise to many. Although the participants followed their diets for two years, a long time for a study of weight loss, questions about the long-term effects are still unanswered.

Bariatric Surgery

Surgery for weight loss, or **bariatric surgery**, is usually reserved for men who are at least 100 pounds over their desired weight and women who are at least 80 pounds over their desired weight, or those who have a body mass index of 40 or higher. Surgery always carries risks, especially in individuals who have other medical conditions, as obese people often do. Surgical procedures for weight loss carry risks of gallstones, nutritional deficiencies, nausea, increased gas, and vomiting. The good consumer will discuss this option with more than one physician and become educated about the various options and the risks involved.

Restrictive Procedures

When you feel full, you are more likely to have reduced feelings of hunger and will no longer feel deprived. The result is that you are likely to eat less. Restrictive weight loss surgery works by reducing the amount of food consumed at one time. It does not, however, interfere with the normal absorption or digestion of food. In a restrictive weight loss procedure, the surgeon creates a small upper stomach pouch. The pouch may be created by placing a bracelet-like band around the top of the stomach. The pouch, with a capacity of approximately ½ to 1 ounce, connects to the rest of the stomach through an outlet known as a stoma.

In the Roux-en-Y gastric bypass procedure, food intake is restricted and absorption of food is decreased. Food intake is limited by constructing a small pouch. In addition, absorption of food in the digestive tract is reduced by excluding most of the stomach, duodenum, and upper intestine from contact with food by routing food directly from the pouch into the small intestine. Roux-en-Y gastric bypass is generally considered the most effective weight loss surgery and is the most common procedure performed in the United States (MayoClinic.com, 2007).

Another restrictive procedure is removing a portion of the stomach. In either case, the capacity of the stomach is reduced and the individual feels full after consuming small amounts of food. In a cooperative and compliant patient, the reduced stomach capacity, along with behavioral changes, can result in consistently lower caloric intake and consistent weight loss.

Malabsorptive Procedures

These types of procedures alter digestion. Most digestion and absorption take place in the small intestine. Surgery to this area shortens the length of the small intestine and/or changes where it connects to the stomach, limiting the amount of food that is completely digested or absorbed, causing malabsorption. These surgeries are often used in conjunction with restrictive procedures. Some of these techniques involve a bypass of the small intestine, thus limiting the absorption of calories. The risk of complications and side effects generally increases with the lengthening of the small intestine bypass (Ethicon Endo-Surgery, 2008).

Other bypass methods divert the bile and pancreatic juices so they join the ingested food nearer the middle or the end of the small intestine.

SUMMARY

Numerous products and programs are available for weight loss. Many of these provide short-term results; few have been demonstrated to have lasting benefits. There are several commercial programs available to consumers who wish to lose weight. They vary in quality and cost. Counseling, group support, prepackaged foods, and weigh-ins are some of the features of these programs. Some commercial programs have an online component. Totally online options are also available.

Restricted carbohydrate programs have been hyped in the media and advertising. While these programs often produce short-term results, the long-term benefits are not well documented. Health problems may also follow use of these programs.

Many products are available for weight loss, including over-the-counter and prescription drugs and herbal products. FDA-approved drugs offer science-based claims of weight loss for several months. OTC and herbal products, with the exception of Alli, have little research to back their claims.

In order to prevent weight gain and to lose weight, standard medical advice is to reduce caloric intake moderately and increase physical activity. The resulting reduction in calories retained should allow for weight reduction. There are some diets that can assist with the process of reducing calories while meeting the body's nutritional needs.

KEY TERMS

Bariatric surgery: surgery performed on obese people for the purpose of helping them lose weight

Basal metabolic rate: the rate at which we burn calories when at rest

Fad diet: a diet that has little or no nutritional value or scientific credibility and that usually has short-term popularity

Glycemic index: a system that ranks carbohydrates in individual foods on a gram-for-gram basis in regard to their effect on blood glucose levels in the first two hours after a meal

Infomercial: a broadcast advertisement filling an entire program slot

Ketogenic diet: a high-fat, high-protein diet that includes very few carbohydrates

Low-calorie diet: a diet providing between 800 and 1,500 calories per day

Very-low-calorie diet: a diet providing fewer than 800 calories per day

STUDY QUESTIONS

1. What is the extent of the overweight and obesity problem in the United States? What are its costs?
2. What is body mass index?
3. What are the standard recommendations for weight management? What are some guidelines for weight loss and management?
4. How does physical activity enhance weight management?
5. What are the foundations of some commercial weight loss programs? What are the strengths and weaknesses of some of these programs?
6. What are the principles behind prominent restricted-carbohydrate diets? What do we know about their ability to promote weight loss? What about health effects?
7. What are the pros and cons of over-the-counter weight loss products?
8. How do Xenical and Meridia work? Are they safe and effective?
9. What are fad diets? Why should consumers avoid them?
10. What is bariatric surgery? What are the different forms of it?

REFERENCES

Acheson, K. J. (2004). Carbohydrate and weight control: Where do we stand? *Current Opinion in Clinical Nutrition and Metabolic Care, 7*(4), 485–492.

Agatston, A. (2003). *The South Beach Diet: The delicious, doctor-designed, foolproof plan for fast and healthy weight loss.* New York: Rodale Press.

Agnew, B. (2004). Rethinking Atkins. *Diabetes Forecast, 57*(4), 64–66, 68–70.

American Heart Association. (2007a). *High protein diets.* Retrieved from http://216.185.112.5/presenter.jhtml?identifier=11234

American Heart Association. (2007b). *Quick-weight loss or fad diets.* Retrieved from http://www.americanheart.org/presenter.jhtml?identifier=4584

Anderson, R., Crespo, C., Bartlett, S., Cheskin, L., & Pratt, M. (1998). Relationship of physical activity and television watching with body weight and level of fatness among children. *Journal of the American Medical Association, 279*(12), 938–942.

Astrup, A., Larsen, T. M., & Harper, A. (2004). Atkins and other low-carbohydrate diets: Hoax or an effective tool? *The Lancet, 364*(9437), 897–899. doi:10.101615014-6736(04)16986-9

Atkins Nutritionals. (2010). *The program.* Retrieved from http://www.atkins.com/Program/ProgramOverview.aspx

Bellow, J. (2007). *South Beach under the spotlight.* Retrieved from http://www.weightlossresources.co.uk/diet/south_beach_review.htm

Better Health, USA. (2007). *Rating the South Beach Diet: Advantages and disadvantages.* Retrieved from http://www.betterhealthusa.com/public/251.cfm

Cawley, J., & Meyerhoefer, C. (2010). *The medical care costs of obesity: An instrumental variables approach.* NBER Working Paper no. 16467. Cambridge, MA: National Bureau of Economic Research.

Centers for Disease Control and Prevention. (2010). *US obesity trends.* Retrieved from http://www.cdc.gov/obesity/data/trends.html#Race

Consumers Union. (2007, June). *Top diets reviewed.* Retrieved from http://www.consumerreports.org/cro/food/diet-nutrition/diets-6-07/overview/0607_diets_ov.htm

Crespo, C., Smit, E., Troiano, R., Bartlett, S., Macera, C., & Anderson, R. (2001). Television watching, energy intake, and obesity in U.S. children. *Archives of Pediatrics and Adolescent Medicine, 155*(3), 360–365.

Dansinger, M. L., Gleason, J. A., Griffith, J. L., Selker, H. P., & Schaefer, E. J. (2005). Comparison of the Atkins, Ornish, Weight Watchers, and Zone diets for weight loss and heart disease risk reduction. *Journal of the American Medical Association, 293*(1), 43–53.

Diet.com. (2010). *Nutrisystem.* Retrieved from http://new.diet.com/encyclopedia-of-diets/nutrisystem

Dietz, W., & Gortmaker, S. (1985). Do we fatten our children at the TV set? Obesity and television viewing in children and adolescents. *Pediatrics, 75*(5), 807–812.

Dietz, W., & Gortmaker, S. (1993). TV or not TV: Fat is the question. *Pediatrics, 91*(2), 499–500.

Epstein, L., Voloski, A., Vara, L., McCurley, J., Wisniewski, L., Kalarchian, M. A., Klein, K. R., & Shrager, L. R. (1995). Effects of decreasing sedentary behavior and increasing activity on weight change in obese children. *Health Psychology, 14*(2), 109–115.

Ethicon Endo-Surgery. (2008). *How surgery loses weight.* Retrieved from http://www.weightlosssurgeryinfo.com/dtcf/pages/HowSurgeryReducesWeight.htm

Finkelstein, E., Trogdon, J., Cohen, J., & Dietz, W. (2009). Annual medical spending attributable to obesity: Payer- and service-specific estimates. *Health Affairs, 28*(5), w822–831. doi:10.1377/hlthaff.28.5.w822

Finley, C., Barlow, C. D., Green Way, F. L., Rock, C. L., Rolls, B. J., & Blair, S. N. (2007, June). Retention rates and weight loss in a commercial weight management program. *International Journal of Obesity, 6,* 292–298. doi:10.1038/sj.ijo.0803395

Flegal, K. M., Carroll, M. D., Ogden, C. L., & Curtin, L. R. (2010). Prevalence and trends in obesity among US adults, 1999–2008. *Journal of the American Medical*

Association, *303*(3), 235–241. doi:10.1001/jama.2009.2104

Fleming, R. M. (2000). The effect of high-protein diets on coronary blood flow. *Angiology, 51*(10), 817–826.

Foster, G. D., Wyatt, H. R., Hill, J. O., Makris, A. P., Rosenbaum, D. L., Brill, C., . . . Klein, S. (2010). Weight and metabolic outcomes after 2 years on a low-carbohydrate versus low-fat diet: A randomized trial. *Annals of Internal Medicine, 153*(3), 147–157.

Foster, G. D., Wyatt, H. R., Hill, J. O., McGuckin, B. G., Brill, C., Mohammed, B. S., . . . Klein, S. (2003). A randomized trial, of a low-carbohydrate diet for obesity. *New England Journal of Medicine, 348*(21), 2082–2090.

Gardner, C. D., Kiazand, A., Alhassan, S., Kim, S., Stafford, R. S., Balise, R. R., . . . King, A. C. (2007). Comparison of the Atkins, Zone, Ornish, and LEARN diets for change in weight and related risk factors among overweight premenopausal women: The A to Z Loss Study: A randomized trial. *Journal of the American Medical Association, 297*(9), 969–977.

Gold, B. C., Burke, S., Pintauro, S., Buzzell, P., & Harvey-Berino, J. (2007). Weight loss on the Web: A pilot study comparing a structured behavioral intervention to a commercial program. *Obesity, 15*(1), 155–164. doi:10.1038/oby.2007.520

Gortmaker, S., Must, A., Sobol, A., Peterson, K., Colditz, S., & Dietz, W. (1996). Television viewing as a cause of increasing obesity among children in the United States, 1986–1990. *Archives of Pediatrics and Adolescent Medicine, 150*(4), 356–362.

Hemphill, E. (2010). *Liquid diets: Safe and effective?* Retrieved from http://www.vanderbilt.edu/AnS/psychology/health_psychology/LiquidDiets.htm

Horwitz, R. I., Brass, L. M., Kernan, W. N., & Viscoli, C. M. (2000). Phenylpropanolamine and risk of hemorrhagic stroke: Final report of the Hemorrhagic Stroke Project. New Haven, CT: Yale University.

Jacobs, D. R., Pereira, M. A., Meyer, K. A., & Kushi, L. H. (2000). Fiber from whole grains, but not refined grains, is inversely associated with all-cause mortality in older women: The Iowa Women's Health Study. *Journal of the American College of Nutrition, 19*(Suppl. 3), 326S–330S.

Johnston, C. S., Tjonn, S. L., & Swann, P. D. (2004). High-protein, low-fat diets are effective for weight loss and favorably alter biomarkers in healthy adults. *Journal of Nutrition, 134*(3):586–591.

Klesges, R., Shelton, M., & Klesges, L. (1993). Effects of television on metabolic rate: Potential implications for childhood obesity. *Pediatrics, 91*(2), 281–286.

Knight, E. L., Stampfer, M. J., Hankinson, S. E., Hankinson, S. E., Spiegelman, D., & Curhan, G. C. (2003). The impact of protein intake on renal function decline in women with normal renal function or mild renal insufficiency. *Annals of Internal Medicine, 138*(6), 460–467.

Lowry, R., Wechsler, H., Galuska, D., Fulton, J., & Kann, L. (2002). Television viewing and its association with overweight, sedentary lifestyle, and insufficient consumption of fruits and vegetables among US high school students: Differences in race, ethnicity and gender. *American Journal of School Health, 72*(10), 413–421.

Malik, V. S., & Hu, F. B. (2007). Popular weight loss diets: From evidence to practice. *National Clinical Practice of Cardiovascular Medicine, 4*(1), 34–41.

MayoClinic.com. (2007). *Gastric bypass surgery for weight loss.* Retrieved from http://www.mayoclinic.com/health/gastric-bypass/MM00703

Morgan, L. M., Griffin, B. A., Millward, D. J., DeLooy, A., Fox, K. R., Baic, S., . . . Truby, H. (2009). Comparison of the effects of four commercially available weight loss programmes on lipid-based cardiovascular risk factors. *Public Health Nutrition, 12*(6), 799–807.

Mustajoki, P., & Pekkarinen, T. (2001). Very low energy diets in the treatment of obesity. *Obesity Review, 2*(1), 61–72.

National Center for Health Statistics. (2006). *Health, United States, 2006.* Hyattsville, MD: U.S. Department of Health and Human Services.

National Heart, Lung, and Blood Institute. (1998). *Clinical guidelines on the identification, evaluation, and treatment of overweight and obesity in adults: The evidence report.* Bethesda, MD: National Institutes of Health/National Heart, Lung, and Blood Institute.

National Heart, Lung, and Blood Institute & North American Association for the Study of Obesity. (2000). *Practical guide to the identification, evaluation, and treatment of overweight and obesity in adults.* Bethesda, MD: National Institutes of Health.

National Task Force on the Prevention and Treatment of Obesity, National Institutes of Health. (1993). Very low-calorie diets. *Journal of the American Medical Association, 270*(8), 967–974.

Ogden, C. L., Carroll, M. D., Curtin, L. R., Lamb, M. M., & Flegal, K. M. (2010). Prevalence of high body mass index in US children and adolescents, 2007–2008. *Journal of the American Medical Association, 303*(3), 242–249. doi:10.1001/jama.2009.2012

Oliver, M. F., & Yates, P. A. (1972). Induction of ventricular arrhythmias by elevation of arterial free fatty acids in experimental myocardial infarction. *Cardiology, 56*(3), 359–364.

OPTIFAST. (2010). *Weight loss and you.* Retrieved from http://www.optifast.com

Overeaters Anonymous. (2007). *OA program of recovery.* Retrieved from http://www.oa.org/index.htm

Partnership for Healthy Weight Management. (1999). *Voluntary guidelines for providers of weight loss products or services.* Washington, DC: Federal Trade Commission.

Peyreigne, C., Bouix, D., Aissa Benhaddad, A., Raynaud, E., Pérez-Martin, A., Mercier, J., & Brun, J. F. (1999). Hemorheologic effects of a short-term ketogenic diet. *Clinical Hemorheologic Microcirculation, 21*(1), 147–153.

Proctor, M., Moore, L., Gao, D., Cupples, L., Bradlee, M., Hood, M., & Ellison, R. (2003). Television viewing and change in body fat from preschool to early adolescence: The Framingham Children's Study. *International Journal of Obesity, 27*, 827–833. doi:10.1038/sj.ijo.0802294

Robinson, T. (1999). Reducing children's television to prevent obesity: A randomized control trial. *Journal of the American Medical Association, 282*(16), 1561–1567.

Rock, C. L., Pakiz, B., Flatt, S. W., & Quintana, E. L. (2007). Randomized trial of a multifaceted commercial weight loss program. *Obesity, 15*(4), 939–949. doi:10.1038/oby.2007.111

Rolls, B. (2005). *The Volumetrics eating plan.* New York: HarperCollins.

Rolls, B., & Barnett, R. A. (2000). *The Volumetrics weight-control plan.* New York: HarperCollins.

Samaha, F. F., Iqbal, N., & Seshadri, P. (2003). A low-carbohydrate diet as compared with a low-fat diet in severe obesity. *New England Journal of Medicine, 348*(21), 2074–2081.

Shai, R. D., Schwarzfuchs, D., Henkin, Y., Shahar, D. R., Witkow, S., Greenberg, I., . . . Stampfer, M. J. (2008). Weight loss with low-carbohydrate, Mediterranean, or low-fat diet. *New England Journal of Medicine, 359*(3), 229–241. doi:10.1056/NEJMoa0708681

Sharman, M. J., Gomez, A. L., Kraemer, W. J., & Volek, J. S. (2004). Very low-carbohydrate and low-fat diets affect fasting lipids and postprandial lipemia differently in overweight men. *Journal of Nutrition, 134*(4), 880–885.

Smith, M. (2005). *Volumetrics adverse events—two potential outcomes.* Retrieved from http://ezinearticles.com/?Volumetrics-Adverse-Events—Two-Potential-Outcomes&id=20582

Take Off Pounds Sensibly, Inc. (2007). *Take off pounds sensibly with TOPS.* Retrieved from http://www.tops.org

Tsai, A. G., & Wadden, T. A. (2005). Systematic review: An evaluation of major commercial weight loss programs in the United States. *Annals of Internal Medicine, 142*(1), 56–66.

Tsai, A. G., & Wadden, T. A. (2006). The evolution of very-low-calorie diets: An update and meta-analysis. *Obesity, 14*(8), 1283–1293. doi:10.1038/oby.2006.146

Tufts University Health and Nutrition Letter. (2004). *Weighing in on the South Beach Diet.* Retrieved from http://www.healthletter.tufts.edu/issues/2004-05/southbeach.html

U.S. Department of Health and Human Services. (2001). *The Surgeon General's call to action to prevent and decrease overweight and obesity 2001.* Rockville, MD: U.S. Public Health Service.

U.S. Food and Drug Administration. (2004). *FDA issues regulation prohibiting sale of dietary supplements containing ephedrine alkaloids and reiterates its advice that consumers stop using these products.* Retrieved from http://www.cfsan.fda.gov/~ldr/fpephed6.html

Wadden, T. A., Stunkard, A. J., & Brownell, K. D. (1983). Very low calorie diets—their efficacy, safety, and future. *Annals of Internal Medicine, 99*(5), 675–684.

Wadden, T. A., Van Itallie, T. B., & Blackburn, G. I. (1990). Responsible and irresponsible use of very-low-calorie diets in the treatment of obesity. *Journal of the American Medical Association, 263*(1), 83–85.

WebMD.com. (2004). *The South Beach Diet: What it is.* Retrieved from http://www.webmd.com/diet/south-beach-diet-what-it-is

WebMD.com. (2010a). *Jenny Craig weight loss program.* Retrieved from http://www.webmd.com/diet/jenny-craig-what-it-is

WebMD.com. (2010b). *Key components of a popular weight loss program.* Retrieved from http://www.webmed.com/diet/weight-loss-programs-chart

WeightWatchers.com. (2010). *WeightWatchers.* Retrieved from http://www.WeightWatchers.com

Westman, E. C., Yancy, W. S., & Edman, J. S. (2002). Effect of a 6-month adherence to a very-low-carbohydrate diet program. *American Journal of Medicine, 113*(1), 3–36.

Wing, R. R., Vazquez, J. A., & Ryan, C. M. (1995). Cognitive effects of ketogenic weight-reducing diets. *International Journal of Obesity Related Metabolic Disorders, 19*(11), 811–816.

Yancy, W. S., Westman, E. C., McDuffie, J. R., Grambow, S. C., Jeffreys, A. S., Bolton, J., . . . Oddone, E. Z. (2010). A randomized trial of a low-carbohydrate diet vs Orlistat plus a low-fat diet for weight loss. *Archives of Internal Medicine, 170*(2), 136–145.

Zelman, K. M. (2010). *The Nutrisystem diet.* Retrieved from http://www.webmd.com/diet/features/the-nutrisystem-diet

Chapter 9

Advertising

Chapter Objectives

The student will:

- Describe the different types of advertising.
- Explain various advertising techniques.
- Discuss the pros and cons of direct-to-consumer prescription drug advertising
- Describe the regulation of direct-to-consumer drug advertisements.
- Explain how marketers target specific groups of people.
- List ways that parents can protect children from inappropriate advertising.
- Define and explain "unmeasured media."
- Explain the problems associated with infomercials.
- Describe ways to reduce the chances of being cheated when purchasing on the Internet.

Advertising has infiltrated virtually all aspects of our lives—home, recreation, entertainment, work, school, travel. It is difficult to think of a location or situation that is not laden with advertising. Flat-panel screens with videos plugging everything from abdominals machines to zucchini greet you at the grocery store, coffee shop, bank, and gas pump. Pop-up ads pester us on the Internet. Ads even appear in restrooms, mounted on hand dryers and placed above urinals. Cinemas carry advertisements before the movie. Television programming time seems to continually shrink as ads take more and more. It seems as if some of the cable news channels are only a series of commercials interrupted by occasional bits of news. Arenas, theaters, university buildings, parks, and museums sell naming rights to corporations so that the companies' names and logos dominate the facades of public buildings. The Russian space agency launched a rocket that carried a 30-foot-long Pizza Hut logo. The photos demonstrate the extremes to which advertisers will go to market their products.

Advertising has multiple objectives. One of the primary objectives is to create a need or the perception of need. As an example, humans need

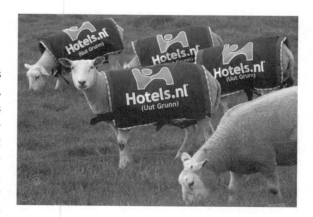

There seems to be no limit to the creativity of advertisers.

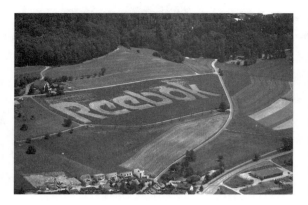

While expensive and massive, relatively few people can actually see this advertisement.

to eat, but we do not need processed meats, sugary cereals, sodas, or fast food. Advertising has influenced people to believe that they need these items; many of us would be unhappy without them. Another objective of advertising is to create or reinforce discontent. There is no inherent need to cover up the natural smells of the body with artificial fragrances, but the unpleasantness we feel with body odor is reinforced by advertising for deodorants. Advertising slogans and images are effective symbols. The McDonald's slogan "You deserve a break today" is linked in the minds of consumers with the Golden Arches as an idyllic place that is a far cry from the hectic life that people are forced to endure. Burger King's longtime slogan "Have it your way"

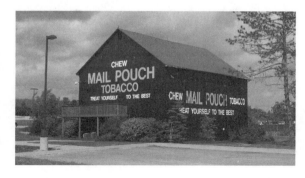

Advertising on the sides and roofs of barns, especially advertising for tobacco products, was common during the twentieth century. This example, photographed in Pennsylvania in 2009, is a rare example of contemporary use of barns for this purpose.

reminds us that in a world of bosses and family responsibilities, this restaurant is one place where the consumer calls the shots. Do burger stores cause discontent or do they exploit it? Maybe it's both. Some ads have the objective of increasing consumer awareness, such as those that tell us specific information about a truck. Regardless of the objectives of any single advertisement, the ultimate goal is to sell a product or service. Consumers of health-related products or services should keep this in mind.

Types of Advertising

There are several ways to classify advertisements and many different forms of advertising. Most fall within three groups: informative, misleading or deceptive, and puffery. Some ads are hybrids of these.

Informative advertising provides the potential buyer with useful information about the product. For example, advertisements for automobiles may state technical information about the specifications of the vehicle, and ads for prescription drugs may state the purpose of use and side effects. Classified ads in newspapers and magazines are among the purest of informative advertisements.

Misleading or **deceptive advertising** intentionally deceives or confuses consumers. Examples include:

- The makers of a therapeutic device claiming effects for which there is no documented evidence
- Claims that studies show the superiority of a product when no such studies exist or those that do exist are flawed or biased

Others use **testimonials**, anecdotes from users or people who are paid to say they are users. These statements are frequently deceptive. It is best to place value in a testimonial or endorsement only if the endorser is truly an expert in an area in which he or she is speaking. It is often difficult to determine the actual qualifications of an "expert" since anyone can put on a lab coat or pretend to be a doctor in an advertisement.

Deceptive advertising can take many forms. Some that are commonly used, often in violation of state laws, include "palming off," misrepresentation, product disparagement, and bait-and-switch advertising. **"Palming off"** occurs when an advertiser creates the impression that its products or services are those that are furnished by a competitor. For example, a manufacturer may market a sunscreen product with a similar name and packaging to another that actually provides superior protection. **Misrepresentation** occurs when an advertiser makes false or misleading claims about its products or services. For example, Listerine was once advertised as being effective at preventing colds; the Federal Trade Commission ruled that it is not. Use of flawed and insignificant research is a form of misrepresentation. Under the Lanham Act of 1946, this means "representations found to be unsupported by accepted authority or research or which are contradicted by prevailing authority or research." An example is claims made by Ralston Purina about its pet food products that were based on statistically insignificant test results. The company was forced to issue a corrective release. **Product disparagement** occurs when an advertiser intentionally makes false or misleading negative remarks about a competitor's goods or services, causing the competitor to lose sales. An example would be an organic food producer stating in advertisements that its competitors sell food that is dangerous, unless the organic food producer could provide evidence of the claim. **Bait-and-switch** occurs when the goods or services are advertised at a low price—the bait. When the customer tries to purchase the product, he or she is told it either is sold out or is an inferior product. The salesperson then tries to convince the customer to purchase a more expensive substitute—the switch. We see this in sales of goods such as computers or appliances, when the advertised product is suddenly not available.

Puffery uses exaggeration, hyperbole, or imagery to market products. It seldom provides useful information unless combined with informative techniques. Terms like "the best" or "the greatest" are frequently used. Idyllic scenes and inflated depictions of sexual attractiveness, vitality, strength, or fun are examples of puffery. This type of advertising is often used when objective data cannot be obtained.

Puffery creates hype and draws attention to the product. Often, puffery is seen as a defense against claims of misleading or deceptive advertising. The Federal Trade Commission has defined puffery as claims that (1) reasonable people do not believe to be true product qualities and (2) are incapable of being proved either true or false (University of Texas, 2000).

Examples of puffery abound. Here are a few examples:

- A restaurant that advertises that its food has the finest taste in town
- The Energizer Bunny that keeps going and going and going . . .
- A tampon that purports to produce the freshest feeling ever
- Tony the Tiger describing Kellogg's Frosted Flakes by saying, "They're GREAT!"
- "Advil just works better"
- "The antidote for civilization" (ClubMed)
- "Bayer works wonders"

The line between puffery and misleading ads is not always clear. As Hoffman (2004) wrote in summarizing several court decisions on puffery, "The line between statements of fact which, if false or misleading can be actionable, and mere puffery is vague and uncertain and have [sic] to be determined on a case by case basis."

Advertising Techniques and Tricks

Advertisers and marketers have an impressive arsenal of techniques at their disposal. Frequently, they combine techniques and use them in informative ads, puffery, or even misleading ads.

Word-of-Mouth Marketing

Word-of-Mouth Marketing can take any form of peer-to-peer communication, such as a chat with a relative, Web log (blog), a social networking Web site, or the comments of a stranger on a bus.

Blogs are easy targets for word-of-mouth marketing. Users frequently comment on products they have used. It is easy for marketing companies to flood blogs with positive statements about their products. It is equally simple to produce negative statements about competitors' products.

A marketing campaign for a Sony Ericsson mobile digital camera and mobile phone drew attention and complaints. The "Fake Tourist" initiative involved placing 60 actors posing as tourists at attractions in New York and Seattle to demonstrate the camera phone. The actors asked passersby to take their photo, which demonstrated the camera phone's capabilities. In another example, Tremor, a marketing division of Procter & Gamble, assembled a volunteer force of 250,000 teenagers to promote the company's products to friends and relatives. The Federal Trade Commission issued a staff opinion noting that such marketing could be deceptive if consumers were more likely to trust the product's endorser "based on their assumed independence from the marketer" (Shin, 2006).

Although word-of-mouth marketing can be misused, people will always communicate with one another. The consumer should be alert to information that can be useful, such as a friend's experience at a restaurant, the taste of pizza sauce, or the length of time spent in a physician's waiting room.

Testimonials and Endorsements

Testimonials and **endorsements** are favorites of advertisers. They are depicted as representing the opinions of experts, including individuals and organizations, or users of the products.

The Federal Trade Commission treats endorsements and testimonials identically. Endorsement means: "Any advertising message (including verbal statements, demonstrations, or depictions of the name, signature, likeness or other identifying personal characteristics of an individual or the name or seal of an organization) which message consumers are likely to believe reflects the opinions, beliefs, findings, or experience of a party other than the sponsoring advertiser" (15 U.S.C. 55, 45 FR 3872, January 18, 1980).

In order to be legal, endorsements must reflect the honest opinions, findings, beliefs, or experience of the endorser. They must not contain any representations that would be deceptive. If the advertisement represents that the endorser uses or used the endorsed product, the endorser must have been a bona fide user of it at the time of the endorsement. Enforcement of this provision is inconsistent at best and, in truth, testimonials are largely self-regulated. The Consumers Union (ConsumerReports.org, 2006) declared, "Most broadcasters, publishers, and Internet service providers don't make sure those 'real' people exist or verify their claims. (The big three networks clear ads before they run, but local ads are often unchecked.)"

There is a loophole in the use of testimonials. Advertisers can put atypical uses in the ad if it "clearly and conspicuously" discloses that their situation is unusual. Advertisers frequently use the disclaimer "Results vary" or "Results may not be typical," often in small print or in a rapidly delivered verbal disclaimer.

Testimonials may come from athletes, movie stars, physicians, or everyday users of the product. Some more absurd endorsements can be seen in old magazine advertisements for cigarettes in which a brand is endorsed by physicians for their health benefits compared with other brands.

Marketers are using celebrities in more stealthy forms of endorsements. As consumers become more cynical, the trend is to brand celebrities with merchandise by having them wear products in public appearances or during interviews. There is nothing to indicate to the audience that the celebrities are paid spokespeople.

Athletes are often virtual billboards. For example, NASCAR drivers and their cars are covered with ads. Professional tennis players wear patches bearing the name and logo of a product. Tiger Woods has worn a cap with a Nike swoosh. The Penn State University football jerseys also display the swoosh. These are a form of endorsement of the products by linking them directly with the wearer.

The consumer should be skeptical about endorsements. We should ask why an athlete, for example, is better qualified to judge a mattress than anyone else. We should also understand that even if the testimonial comes from a user of the product, the endorsement of that person does not guarantee that the experience is typical. Many advertisements carry disclaimers that state that the experience of the endorser may not be typical. Claims concerning the efficacy of any drug or device as defined in the Federal Trade Commission Act "shall not be made in lay endorsements unless (1) the advertiser has adequate scientific substantiation for such claims and (2) the claims are not inconsistent to the drug or device that is the subject of the claim" (15 U.S.C. 55, 45 FR 3872, January 18, 1980).

Testimonials are inherently selective. Few of us would be anxious to tell about a health product that did not work, especially after spending large sums for it. However, people are often very interested in sharing even the smallest improvement, often attributing it to a pill, lotion, or other treatment.

Weasel Words

Weasel words create the illusion of a promise but permit the advertiser to "weasel out" of the deal (Barrett, London, Baratz, & Kroger, 2007). Here are a few examples with replies from a healthy skeptic:

- Lose *up to* 30 pounds in a month. (Wouldn't a loss of zero pounds be in this range?)
- Product is *part of a healthy breakfast*. (Which part? Would the breakfast be just as healthy without the product? Would another product make the meal healthier?)
- Pain reliever *helps to* end headaches. (How much help is it? What other factors are in play?)
- Body wash is *new and improved*. (Was it so bad before? Improved in which qualities? If it is "improved," how can it also be "new"?)
- Product is *clinically tested* to be more effective. (What were the results of the tests? Does the product work as claimed? Tested maybe, but did the product pass or fail the test? More effective than what?)

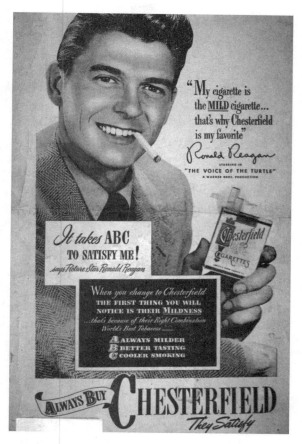

Famous actors have, for years, been used to market cigarettes. Here, an actor who was a future president acted as a shill for a tobacco company.

- *Four of every five doctors agree* that the product is effective. (Were only five doctors interviewed? How was the sample selected? Were the doctors compensated for their opinions? Do they own stock in the company?)

Weasel words heighten the expectations of the potential user without actually promising anything. They can be used to draw attention away from adverse evidence.

Attention Grabbers

On the other end of the spectrum are **attention grabbers**, words and phrases that offer power to the advertisement. Examples of common attention grabbers are:

- "All natural"
- "Amazing breakthrough"
- "Hospital tested"
- "Money-back guarantee"

Attention grabbers may appeal to a variety of senses. Pictures or video of attractive people or scenes or of people performing unusual or impossible feats can be attention grabbers. A catchy tune or just loud music can serve to grab our notice. Restaurants sometimes fry onions, allowing the aroma to waft out of vents, to attract customers.

Appeal to Basic Human Weaknesses and Fears

Many advertisements appeal to human weaknesses, fears, and frailties. Advertisements exploit individuals' fears of social or sexual inadequacy. A wide range of products, including deodorants, baldness "cures," alcoholic beverages, mouthwash, impotency cures, breast enlargers, and penis stretchers (or "natural male enhancers," as one commercial described its product), attempt to convince us that our social and sex lives will improve dramatically if we just buy the product. If your life is drab or you are afraid of loneliness, there are products and services that will purportedly change your future.

Fear can be a strong motivator to purchase. Exploitation of fear is a common advertising tool. Fear of aging is often exploited by marketers. Following the terrorist attacks of 2001 and subsequent periods of heightened threats, marketers seized on our fears to sell us anything from duct tape to weaponry.

Visual Imagery

Visual imagery is a time-tested method of promoting products. It is often accompanied by puffery. The marketer is at an advantage if an image favorable to the product can be placed in the mind of the consumer. Visual imagery can be enhanced if it is linked with an auditory cue, such as a jingle that you cannot seem to get out of your mind.

One product was billed as the "fluoride eraser," complete with images of an eraser wiping stains away from teeth. Pastoral settings often are used to present a safe, clean image of a product. The Marlboro Man sitting atop his horse surveying the open range provided the image of the independent "I'm my own man" cowboy. These visual images are very effective.

Statistics

Statistics are commonly used in advertisements with no context. They often are accompanied by graphs or other images. Sometimes they are reinforced with puffery. It is virtually impossible to present a valid argument using data in a short 30-second advertisement. In fact, it is very difficult to do so in a full-length infomercial. This is the reason that statistics are used only briefly and almost never with any unbiased interpretation. Graphs are easily formatted to present impressions that are inaccurate.

Marketers never use data that are neutral or unfavorable to their product. They also seldom make their data or the study from which they came available for consumer inspection. Consumers should never confuse association with causation. Just because two things are linked by some vague statistical reference does not mean that one caused the other.

Comedy

Comedy or humor is an old methodology in advertising. It makes the ad memorable. The antics and accent of the Geico gecko keep us chuckling as the

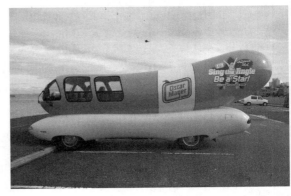

Humor is an effective tool in marketing products and services.

little green character sells insurance. Clips of inane behavior glue us to the television between scenes of real programming. Many people find advertising less obtrusive if it contains a good laugh.

Starting in 1925, motorists would eagerly await the next series of Burma-Shave signs containing a few words each and forming a rhyme delivering a chuckle and always ending with the name of the product displayed on the last sign. The Oscar Mayer Weinermobile always causes laughter as it motors down city streets. Billboards frequently attract our attention with color but hold it with humor.

Ads containing comedy are seldom informative. They are a form of puffery. They would be considered misleading only if the average person would not get the joke and would take the ad message literally. Yet, they are effective at keeping a product in our consciousness.

Sex

Sex has become almost a universal marketing tool. It is difficult to drive down a major street or highway without seeing billboards of scantily clad people, always very attractive, and sometimes not directly related to the product. Television ads make use of sex in myriad ways. Who can forget the Pepsi commercial of the 1990s in which a newborn flirts with model Cindy Crawford? Whether it be the women of Victoria's Secret or the hunk being admired as he

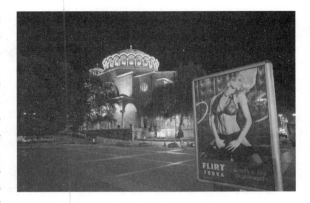

Is the consumer supposed to believe that this product will help her look like the model in the ad? Or is the male consumer to believe that this woman will be attracted to him if he drinks the right brand of vodka?

washes his car, sex sells and marketers know it. As the examples in these photo ads demonstrate, women are more frequently sexualized in advertisements than men.

Product Placement

Product placement is an old technique, dating to at least the 1950s. It is a rapidly growing method of slipping products into films and television programs. In this practice, also known as "embedding," advertising occurs when a product or brand gains exposure in a film, television program, photo, video game, book, or even in an advertisement for another product. It is becoming more attractive to television advertisers in an era when DVR users frequently skip commercials. In some cases, the logo or name of a product is placed in the background of a scene. News anchors may display a beverage from a sponsoring company on their desks. Advertisements for a product, rather than the product itself, may appear in scenes; this is called advertisement placement. In the majority of placements, the product is clearly visible; at other times it is referenced verbally; and sometimes it is only implied.

It is not necessary for a specific brand to be displayed. Smoking on film can be enhanced by its association with desirable characters, personalities, or characteristics. Drinking the same

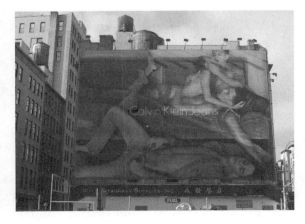

Does this billboard suggest that using Calvin Klein products will lead to group sex?

beverage, say beer, as a movie hero can be an attractive idea.

Overall, event marketing and paid product placement in various media accounted for about $3.61 billion in 2009, a reduction over the previous year, mainly because of the effects of the economic recession. Product placement is forecast to be the most rapidly growing segment of paid advertising through 2014 (PQ Media, 2010).

Television has become a fertile ground for embedding products. When the ladies of Wisteria Lane walked down the runway in a charity fashion show on ABC's *Desperate Housewives*, they wore Halston gowns; their kitchens are furnished by Thermador and Bosch. The Seinfeld show made reference to Snapple and Junior Mints. General Motors donated the $55,000 Hummers driven by the characters in CBS's *CSI: Miami*. The agents in Fox's *The X-Files* always drove Fords. Holly and Tina of the WB program *What I Like About You* competed to be the Herbal Essence girl, a plot point followed by a commercial for the shampoo. NBC's *The Office* displays Staples products, and Hooters has been identified as the office caterer.

Music videos are well designed for product placement. Lady Gaga's video for the song "Telephone" includes 10 product placements and generated more than four million views in its first 24 hours. Her video for "Bad Romance," which also includes several placements, had been viewed over 230 million times as of June 2010 (PQ Media, 2010).

The tobacco industry has been the undisputed villainous master of this technique for decades. For example, Dovemead Limited received financial incentives from the Philip Morris Company to place over 30 images of the Marlboro name or package, sometimes with primary characters using the product, in the 1979 movie *Superman II: The Movie* (Spengler, 1979). American actor Sylvester Stallone received $500,000 for his use of Brown & Williamson Company cigarette products in several of his movies (Ripslinger, 1983; Stallone, 1983). This practice has increased since the 1998 Master Settlement Agreement prohibited direct advertising to youth. It is not

a coincidence that tobacco product placement continues to appear in movies that are attractive to young people.

Product placement is apparently effective. In a longitudinal study of U.S. adolescents, Sargent et al. (2007) found that exposure to smoking in movies predicted risk of becoming an established smoker, behavior that is linked with adult dependent smoking and its associated morbidity and mortality.

The Federal Communications Commission (FCC) has established rules that require one sponsorship announcement be made at the time of broadcast. Such disclosures are usually tacked on to the end of a show so inconspicuously that viewers may rarely notice. The FCC is considering strengthening the notification requirements.

The Scope of Advertising

America's marketers spent $143.3 billion in advertising in 2005 (TNS Media Intelligence, 2006). This included over $25 billion in local newspapers, almost $22.5 billion in network television, over $21.6 billion in consumer magazines, and over $15.8 billion on cable television. Internet display advertising increased by 13.3 percent over the previous year to $8.3 billion. By 2009, according to *Advertising Age*, **measured marketing** of the 100 leading national advertisers was $125.3 billion, a considerable drop blamed largely on the recession. In 2009, about 19 percent of advertising each went to network television and magazines, followed by newspaper at 16.5 percent and cable television networks at 15.4 percent (Johnson, 2010). It is inevitable that much of this advertising was for health products and services, those products that purport to be healthful, and others that affect health.

The food, beverage, and restaurant industries spent $11.26 billion on advertising in 2004 (Endicott, 2005). By 2011, the food and beverage industry was forecast to spend over $1.1 billion on online advertising alone (eMarketer, 2010). By contrast, the federal and California "5 A Day" programs to encourage consumption of fresh fruits and vegetables spent only $9.55 million on communications (California Pan-Ethnic Health Network, 2005).

Advertising of Prescription Drugs

Advertisement of prescription drugs was once targeted only to health care professionals. Pharmaceutical salespeople would visit physicians' offices, make their pitch, and leave samples. Medical journals carried many advertisements, but those journals were read mostly by health care providers. Conferences and conventions were home to booths occupied by pharmaceutical representatives. Typical consumers or patients were usually left out of the marketing picture. They were expected to get information about prescription drugs from their doctors.

In 1983, all this changed. The U.S. Food and Drug Administration, feeling that its regulations provided sufficient safeguards to protect the public, approved direct advertising of prescription medications to consumers. These ads are known as direct-to-consumer (DTC) advertisements. At that point, the United States joined New Zealand as the only industrialized countries to allow DTC ads for prescription drugs (Marketing Week, 2006). During the 1990s, print ads proliferated. While DTC drug advertising formally started on television in 1996, it actually began in 1983 when Boots Pharmaceuticals, a British company, ran ads for its then prescription-only ibuprofen product, Rufen. Advertisements increasingly appeared in magazines, newspapers, and television. By 2005, total spending on network and cable television ads totaled $2.6 billion (Media Week, 2006).

Manufacturers of prescription drugs spent $11.4 billion on advertising in 2005, a decline of 3.5 percent from 2004. However, the share directed toward consumers increased by 5 percent in 2005 to $4.2 billion (Kaiser Family Foundation, 2007) and to $4.8 billion in 2007. Drug makers reduced their spending on DTC

advertising by 8 percent to $4.4 billion in 2008, the first reduction since the late 1990s (Winstein & Vranica, 2009).

Advertising works. Pharmaceutical manufacturers were the nation's most profitable industry from 1995 to 2002 and ranked second in 2006 with profits of 19.6 percent, compared with 6.3 percent for all Fortune 500 firms (Kaiser Family Foundation, 2007).

The FDA has regulated the advertising of prescription drugs since 1962, under the Federal Food, Drug, and Cosmetic Act and related regulations. The regulations establish detailed requirements for ad content. The FDA's Division of Drug Marketing, Advertising, and Communications (DDMAC) oversees two types of promotion for prescription drugs: promotional labeling and advertising. Advertising includes commercial messages broadcast on television or radio, communicated over the telephone, or printed in magazines and newspapers.

The FDA recognizes three types of DTC advertisements. They are:

- Product-claim ads, the most common type, that mention a drug's name and the condition it is intended to treat, and describe the risks and benefits associated with taking the drug
- Reminder ads, often used as an alternative to product-claim ads when manufacturers have decided not to present much information, that give only the name of the product, but not the conditions for which it is used, its effectiveness, or safety information
- Help-seeking ads, also used to avoid presenting much information and often called disease-awareness ads, that mention only the medical condition, such as high cholesterol or diabetes, and then direct you to ask your doctor about treatments

Prescription drug ads considered product-claim ads must contain information in a brief summary relating to both risks and benefits. Recognizing the time constraints of broadcast ads, FDA regulations provide that a broadcast advertisement may include, instead of a brief summary, information relating to the major risks. The ad must also make "adequate provision" for distributing the FDA-approved labeling in connection with the broadcast ad. This refers to the concept of providing ways for consumers to find more complete information about the drug. Most ads fulfill this requirement by including a toll-free telephone number, a Web site address, or a link to a concurrently running print ad. They also encourage consumers to talk to their health care providers (Rados, 2004). It is a matter of debate whether these methods are sufficient to be "adequate."

If it determines that a company is not following the rules, the FDA may issue two types of letters. Warning letters are sent to companies that have violated the law repeatedly or that have committed serious regulatory violations in their advertising. These letters typically request corrective advertisements to ensure that the audience receives truthful and accurate information. During the 12-month period ending in August 2005, the FDA sent 17 warning letters to advertisers, compared with about four to five letters in recent years (Heavey, 2005). The other type of letter, called "untitled," is usually sent to companies for first-time offenses or for less serious violations. Although spending on DTC advertising has increased dramatically in the past 10 years, in 2004, only four FDA staffers were reviewing such advertisements. The proportion of broadcast advertisements that underwent FDA review before airing declined from 64 percent in 1999 to 32 percent in 2004 (U.S. Food and Drug Administration, 2005). Recently, the FDA has picked up the intensity of its enforcement. In 2010, the FDA launched the "Bad Ad" program. The purpose is to train and situate physicians to detect and report misleading medical product promotions, including those sent to doctors.

Both print and broadcast prescription drug ads directed at consumers may only make claims that are supported by scientific evidence. This would imply that they are of the informative type of advertising. However, the FDA does not generally require prior approval of DTC ads, although companies are required to submit their ads to the FDA at the time they begin running. Unless the company specifically requests review, ads containing erroneous information could be disseminated before the FDA scrutinizes them.

Despite the oversight of the FDA, the primary reason for the reduction in advertising spending may be attributed to fewer new drugs and heightened scrutiny of drug-marketing practices by a few members of Congress.

While DTC ads are largely informative, they may also contain puffery. Television commercials touting the effectiveness of medications for erectile dysfunction set against a sunset with a middle-aged couple looking dreamily into each other's eyes or extolling the benefits of an arthritis remedy as a grandfather roughhouses with his grandchildren are puffery at its best.

Testimony before a Senate committee (Lurie, 2005) stated that DTC advertising has been concentrated on new, expensive drugs for conditions that are bothersome and incurable. Only one of the top 50 DTC-advertised drugs was an antibiotic. This is presumably because patients who take antibiotics are generally cured and have no need for long-term treatment. Most DTC ads are targeted at seniors. Generic drugs, which are frequently the most cost-effective method for treating medical conditions, are absent from DTC advertisements.

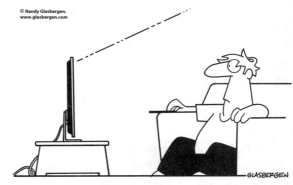

"Sick and tired of all the drug commercials on TV? Ask your doctor about new Drucomexx, to relieve that sick and tired feeling!"

Source: © Randy Glasbergen, used with permission from www.glasbergen.com.

DTC medication advertising generates revenue. According to a study by the Kaiser Family Foundation, "DTC advertising produces a significant return for the pharmaceutical industry: every additional $1 the industry spent on DTC advertising in 2000 yielded an additional $4.20 in sales" and was responsible for 12 percent of the increase in prescription drug sales, or an additional $2.6 billion (Rosenthal, Berndt, Donahue, Epstein, & Frank, 2003).

Advertising companies realized another source of dollars with the rise of **unbranded advertisement**, often called "educational" or "disease awareness" ads. For example, Pfizer made huge purchases of advertising time for its unbranded ads in erectile dysfunction and cholesterol categories. The move to unbranded range was motivated by the industry's adoption of new advertising guidelines that call for a greater level of patient education. This was undoubtedly motivated, at least in part, by the need to protect the pharmaceutical companies from liability suits.

Because advertising for prescription drugs is often informational, ads may increase awareness of possible treatments and play a role in generating questions by patients. Many doctors say patients' having seen a DTC ad had a positive impact on their interaction with patients. A study reported by the FDA (Aiken, 2005) supported some of the Pharmaceutical Research and Manufacturers of America (PhRMA) claims in finding that physicians believed that DTC ads increase patients' awareness of possible treatments and play a role in generating patient questions. A high percentage of doctors said the patient's having seen a DTC advertisement had a positive impact on interactions.

DTC ads do not convey information about risks and benefits equally well (Aiken, 2005). Since they are required to have a brief summary of the risks, they usually state side effects and **contraindications**, although frequently in such rapid cadence that it is difficult to understand, let alone contemplate and weigh the risks. One of the ways the FDA allows extra information to be shared with consumers is for all the ads to contain a toll-free phone number and/or a Web site.

Most ads state that you need to see a physician for a prescription and recommend talking with your doctor to determine if the product is right for you, undoubtedly an attempt to reduce legal liability.

The president of the National Consumers League expressed concern about these practices, stating, "People need to be careful with ads that it isn't just hype that they're going to feel better, with no objectivity of the downsides" (Rados, 2004). Certainly, a healthy dose of skepticism is advisable in considering information contained in any advertisement.

While it can be argued that DTC advertising is educational in nature, there is no doubt that such ads display imagery that is primarily emotive, therefore puffery. For example, a couple holding hands while lying in separate bathtubs overlooking a picturesque landscape during an ad for an erectile dysfunction drug certainly goes beyond the educational function.

Critics of DTC drug advertising make several claims. They often assert that the doctor-patient relationship is harmed. They claim that the advertising pressures health professionals to prescribe particular medications, and patients often insist that providers prescribe drugs that are heavily advertised. Some patients expect a prescription because of a DTC ad, and advertising may lead to overprescribing. Mintzes (2003) found that physicians often accede to patients' requests for prescriptions driven by DTC ads but are left feeling uneasy about it. In many cases, physicians must spend valuable time explaining to patients why they may have gotten incorrect impressions from advertisements.

Some DTC advertisements are misleading or dangerous. Advertisements by the manufacturers of Cox-2 inhibitors such as Vioxx claimed that these drugs relieved pain while protecting the stomach. For most patients, the purported stomach protection offered by these drugs was irrelevant because most patients tolerated conventional pain relievers without stomach pain. Nevertheless, an estimated two-thirds of the growth in Cox-2 use between 1999 and 2000 was among such patients (Hollon, 2005). With as many as 140,000 serious cardiovascular events due to Vioxx alone (Findlay, 2001), the dangers of these promotions are apparent. Vioxx was withdrawn from the market.

According to Lurie (2005), a November 2004 advertisement by AstraZeneca on its Web site and in print attempted to mislead the public by misrepresenting the FDA. In an advertisement for the cholesterol-lowering drug Crestor, a drug associated with muscle and kidney damage, AstraZeneca claimed, "We have been assured today at senior levels in the FDA that there is no concern in relation to CRESTOR's safety." The FDA was on record stating that "[the Agency] has been very concerned about Crestor since the day it was approved and we've been watching it very carefully" (Wolfe, 2004).

Many have called for strict regulation of DTC drug advertising, but lobbyists work hard to oppose governmental regulation. Frequently, voluntary guidelines are proposed as an alternative to governmental regulation, accompanied by claims that industries can police themselves. It should be obvious that where the profit motive is in play, voluntary self-regulation is suspect.

Pharmaceutical Research and Manufacturers of America is an advocacy or lobbying organization that represents pharmaceutical companies. PhRMA published guidelines for DTC for its members in 2005 (PhRMA, 2005). Among the guidelines are that DTC information should be accurate and not misleading, should make claims only when supported by substantial evidence, should reflect balance between risks and benefits, and should be consistent with FDA-approved labeling, standards for which are already in the FDA regulations. Other PhRMA guidelines indicate that ads should responsibly educate the consumer about the medicine and the condition for which it is prescribed, foster communication between patients and health care professionals, be altered or discontinued should new and reliable information indicate a serious previously unknown safety risk, be submitted to the FDA for release for television broadcast, provide balanced presentation of both the benefits and risks associated with the medicine, and be placed to avoid audiences that are not age appropriate for the messages involved.

Supporters of DTC advertising assert that patients with undertreated conditions might receive treatment they otherwise would not have received and that the doctor-patient communication improves because of patients' exposure to the ads. Others disagree. Gilbody, Wilson, and Watt (2005), in a comprehensive review of studies on DTC advertising, concluded, "No empirical research has demonstrated better communication [between patients and physicians] and improved health outcomes."

Critics claim that because the pharmaceutical companies exist to make a profit, to yield maximum return for their shareholders, and to sell as much of their products as possible, information is geared to these ends. Because of their financial conflicts of interest, pharmaceutical companies are perhaps the least trustworthy sources of information about their own drugs (Commercial Alert, 2010). Two drug advertising executives at FCB Healthworks wrote, "The ultimate goal of DTC advertising is to stimulate consumers to ask their doctors about the advertised drug and then, hopefully, get the prescription" (Loden & Schooler, 1998). Given this goal, it is not surprising that some physicians believe that DTC ads confuse patients about benefits and risks.

Others contend that DTC advertising creates a culture of disease and fear. Parry (2003), a marketing executive, said that pharmaceutical companies are "fostering the creation of a condition and aligning it with a product." A Reuters Business Insight article (Coe, 2003) explained that drug companies can "create new disease markets" through "medicalization of many natural processes." Parry criticizes this practice as "raising the level of awareness about something we don't even know we have until we began looking at it further." As an example, GlaxoSmithKline is accused (Moynihan & Cassels, 2005) of taking the notion of shyness and turning it into social anxiety disorder by hiring a public relations firm to establish social anxiety disorder as a way of "cultivating the marketplace" even before the launch of their drug Paxil. Later, GlaxoSmithKline issued a pamphlet claiming that "social anxiety disorder is a lot more common than you think . . . 1 out of every 8 Americans suffers from social anxiety disorder. The good news is that it is treatable."

Another example is the misuse of heavily marketed drugs to treat erectile dysfunction, such as Viagra, Cialis, and Levitra. St. John (2003) wrote that there is "an increasing number of sexually healthy men, many in their 20's, 30's, and 40's, who doctors and sex therapists say are using impotence drugs . . . as psychological palliatives against the mighty expectations of modern romance." Still, the vast majority of patients who ask about a brand have the condition that drug treats (Aiken, 2005; Rados, 2004).

Not all DTC ads target seniors with chronic conditions. The makers of prescription acne medication Differin broadcast ads for the acne medication both on the Internet and on MTV. The advertisements directed teen viewers to a portion of the Differin Web site to receive free music downloads. The viewer was exhorted to obtain a "Teen Survival Handbook" and to take a self-test on acne called "Zit 101." The ad played to teenage fears ("Remember: There are thousands of pores on your face, which means your skin has the potential to 'give birth to' thousands of microcomedones.") and notions of empowerment ("Fight Acne with Free Music. How Cool is That?"). The Web site carried an entire section on "Talking to Parents About Acne" (Lurie, 2005).

DTC advertising prompts millions of consumers to ask their doctors for prescriptions for specific brand-name drugs. As a result, it is important that the FDA acts effectively to minimize the public's exposure to misleading DTC advertisements (General Accounting Office, 2002). It remains to be seen if Congress or the FDA will try to reign in the DTC advertising carried on by drug companies. So far, the evidence is not impressive. There was an 85 percent decline in enforcement actions involving drug companies between 1998 and 2004 (Lurie, 2005). The number of letters sent by the FDA to pharmaceutical manufacturers regarding violations of drug-advertising regulations fell from 142 in 1997 to only 21 in 2007 despite an increase in spending on DTC ads of 330 percent (Donohue, Cevasco, & Rosenthal, 2007).

Lax enforcement and regulation may be tied to a common Washington phenomenon—lobbying and political donations. The pharmaceutical and health products industry has spent more than $800 million in federal lobbying and campaign donations at the federal and state levels in a recent seven-year period, a Center for Public Integrity investigation found. From 2000 to 2006, the top drug corporations and their employees and PhRMA gave more than $10 million to 527 organizations, tax-exempt political committees that operate in the gray area between federal and state campaign finance laws (Ismail, 2006). Such expenditure is obviously meant to make sure that the point of view of the donors is given high priority in government.

The cost of health care is being driven up as patients request newer, more expensive medications seen in DTC ads instead of older, generic alternatives that, in many cases, are just as effective. The General Accounting Office (2002) agreed that "DTC advertising appears to increase prescription drug spending and utilization," primarily because of increased utilization, not increased prices.

Consumers should remember that the primary reason for any advertisement is to sell the product. It is never safe to assume that you are receiving the full story from an ad. First, it is not usually possible to provide all relevant information in a 30-second television or radio commercial, on a billboard, or in a magazine advertisement. Second, marketers may not want consumers to know information that may reflect negatively on the product. Do not rely on advertisements for information. Seek information from your physician and pharmacist, read a reliable drug reference book, and seek additional information from the company.

Advertising of Nonprescription Drugs

Nonprescription drugs are also called over-the-counter (OTC) drugs. These are products that can be purchased without a prescription. Very few restrictions are placed on the sale of these products. They are advertised in many media, including television, radio, newspapers, magazines, and the Internet.

The ads for OTC drugs often use testimonials, puffery, and imagery. The wording of the OTC ads can be confusing and even misleading, but they tend to be mostly truthful. They may not contain all of the information necessary to make a good decision about the product. An example of wording that may mislead the consumer is the use of "new" or "extra-strength" when they are identical or similar to rival products.

In the 1970s, the Food and Drug Administration carried out a review of ingredients in nonprescription drugs. The review indicated that most OTC products contain at least one effective ingredient. However, ads often do not identify the active ingredients contained in the product.

Smart consumers are wary of the many drug ads that appear on television. It is easy to conclude that most of life's problems can be solved by drugs, and the marketers do nothing to dispel that conclusion.

Targeting Special Groups

Advertisers are adept at targeting groups. One favorite target group is women and girls. The Virginia Slims cigarette marketing campaign is one of the longest running and most effective. It plays on the anti-authority, rebellious attitude with which cigarette-smoking teenage girls identify. It also served as the primary sponsor for the women's professional tennis tour for decades.

Marketers have attempted to attract health-conscious customers to all types of products. Historically, consumers who fit the mold of those who will spend a little more or endure some degree of inconvenience in order to use healthier products are usually better educated with a fair amount of disposable income. The tobacco industry saw the economic benefits of this approach early with magazine ads that implied or even stated the health benefits of one brand over another. Some, as far back as the 1940s, made reference to the amount of nicotine, an addictive

drug, the product contained. Ironically, it was discovered years later that the tobacco companies had purposely manipulated the amount of nicotine in their products to make it easier for youth to become addicted consumers. Ads that were widely published in 1946 and 1947 proclaimed, "More Doctors Smoke Camels than Any Other Cigarette" to imply health benefits (see the example earlier in this chapter).

Commercial diet programs have concentrated on women with their before-and-after photos and their appeals to look sexy. Some have concentrated on adolescents, whose sense of body image is most vulnerable. Recently, some diet programs have used more male and minority testimonials.

Food manufacturers exploited health, happiness, and contented family early in advertising history. This continues with television ads for kids' meals, depictions of products with less sugar (less than what?), fewer calories (often than marketers' other brands, but not less than is recommended by health authorities), and families and friends who socialize around tables laden with deep-fried chicken or meat-lovers pizza.

Savvy food companies and marketers target people by race with ethnic-oriented media outlets and programs. In 2004, the food, beverage, and candy industries spent over $260 million to pitch their products to Hispanic-oriented broadcast television networks, cable stations, and Spanish-language magazines and newspapers (Endicott et al., 2005). Advertising to Spanish-speaking populations is made easier by the fact that there are magazines, newspapers, and television programs that use Spanish exclusively.

In 2005, Kraft announced the launch of its first marketing effort targeting Asian Americans. This included print ads placed in Chinese newspapers and bilingual "brand ambassadors" deployed to retailers to provide information to shoppers on products such as Oreos, Kraft Barbecue Sauce, and Philadelphia Cream Cheese (Reyes, 2005). Besides the food and beverage sector, automobile, telecom, and health care marketers have also targeted the Asian American demographic.

The African American population has been a steady target. Perhaps the most notorious example was the marketing of Uptown cigarettes by the R.J. Reynolds Tobacco Company directed toward urban African Americans, an effort quickly quashed by a diverse group of health, religious, and community organizations led by African Americans in Philadelphia. Advertising of malt liquor is more frequently targeted toward African Americans, while wine is more frequently advertised to Latinos.

Food companies work with ad agencies, market research firms, and consulting groups that specialize in developing digital strategies for targeting ethnic children and youth. These efforts have produced a variety of techniques tailored to specific ethnic groups, including African Americans and Hispanics, who are deemed less cynical about and more receptive to advertising (Anderson, 2006; Chester & Montgomery, 2007). For example, African American youth are considered particularly good candidates for "urban marketing" campaigns that employ peer-to-peer and viral strategies (Korzenny, Korzenny, McGavock, & Inglessis, 2007). Advertisers seek to take advantage of the fact that Hispanic and African American audiences are proficient at using mobile tools, such as text messaging. The Interactive Advertising Bureau (2007) explained, "Hispanics are best reached with an integrated multi-media message which entertains, engages, and provokes action."

Advertising to specific minority communities is not inherently negative. There are products that have higher preference in certain ethnic communities. Yet it is disturbing that a number of recent studies indicated that the types of food and beverages advertised to African Americans and Latinos are often less healthful than those marketed to general audiences (California Pan-Ethnic Health Network, 2005).

Marketing to Children

Numerous firms conduct marketing research focused on children as young as the preschool ages. These methods include photography, ethnography, and focus groups "in an Orwellian-sounding fashion to elucidate the psychological underpinnings of children's food choices, 'kid archetypes,' the 'psyche of mothers as the family gatekeeper,' and 'parent-child dyads of information'" (Nestle, 2006). This is obviously and unabashedly an effort to use research to exploit the suggestibility of young children. With the help of researchers and psychologists, advertisers now have access to in-depth knowledge about children's developmental, emotional, and social needs at different ages. Using research that analyzes children's behavior, fantasy lives, artwork, and even their dreams, companies are able to craft sophisticated marketing strategies to reach young people.

Producers recognized long ago the wealth that the children's market holds. Marketing to children is partly about creating "pester power"— that is, taking advantage of children's ability to nag their parents into purchasing items they may not otherwise buy. "Spokescharacters" such as the Keebler Elves; Tony the Tiger; Snap, Crackle, and Pop; the Burger King; and Ronald McDonald are examples of some of the strategies used to reach the youth market. Shameless marketers of high-calorie, high-sodium, and sugary foods to children justify it in such empty terms as "training" in consumer culture, as free speech, and as good for business.

Beginning in the early 1990s, food manufacturers launched the new product category "fun foods" to take advantage of children's increased spending power and independence. The category includes Heinz EZ Squirt and Kraft Easy Mac. Promoting directly to kids was cost effective because buying time in children's television programming was much less expensive than placing commercials in prime time (Parker, 2002). The number of new food and beverage products targeted to U.S. children and youth increased from 52 in 1994 to over 500 in 2003 (Williams, 2005).

A large number of television ads targeted to children are for food, most often candy, presweetened cereal, soft drinks, and fast food. A tiny minority of these commercials promote healthy foods. Given the amount spent advertising to kids, it is logical to conclude that television ads can influence children's purchases as well as those of their families. Following a study done through a congressional directive, the Institute of Medicine (IOM) of the National Academies concluded, "The dietary and health-related patterns of children and youth are influenced by the interplay of many factors, including genetics and biology, culture and values, economic status, physical and social environments, and commercial and media environments. Among these environments, the media, in its multiple forms and broad reach, plays a central socializing role for young people and is an important channel for promoting branded food and beverage products in the marketplace" (McGinnis, Gootman, & Kraak, 2006).

Children do not understand television commercials in the same way adults do. Most children younger than 6 years cannot distinguish between program content and commercials, and most children younger than 8 years do not understand the purpose of advertising to be selling products. Even children ages 8 to 10 who have the cognitive ability to understand the nature of advertising may not always discern the persuasive intent or understand the wording of a disclaimer (Kunkel, 2002). Advertisers are virtually free to take advantage of children's innocence.

Children are not born as consumers; they must be recruited and trained. Viewing children as sources of revenue and targets for marketing has important ethical implications. Very young children have little or no money, and parents of young children usually hold the power to purchase or not. Yet, these children are often the targets of advertisers. For example, restaurants offer playgrounds, clubs, toys, and games to attract young children and their parents. This means that the advertiser either can sell to the parent or can recruit the child into being the force that causes the parent to exchange money. As children grow up, they often have access to money to spend on their own. The purchase influence of children and youth is estimated at $500 billion for 2- to 14-year-olds (McGinnis, Gootman, & Kraak, 2006).

Brand awareness and loyalty drive the marketing to children. James U. McNeal, a well-known youth marketing consultant, stated that children become "brand conscious" at about 24 months of age, and by 3 years of age can make a connection that a brand can say something about their personalities—e.g., that they are strong, cool, or smart (Comiteau, 2003). This identification with brands is worth billions to companies. Four of the top six brands of which very young children show awareness are: Cheerios, McDonald's, Pop-Tarts, and Coke. By the time children reach first grade, they are typically loyal to one brand within each of the major categories of food they regularly consume such as soft drinks, candy, or cereal. Marketers count on us remaining emotionally attached to a brand as we grow into adulthood.

Much brand loyalty is encouraged by packaging that serves as a form of advertising. Marketers use front panel characteristics and cross-promotion activity features—e.g., movies to foods. Food packaging contains a wide variety of features such as characters likely to enhance the identification of children with the product. They are also used at the point of sale to capitalize on the impulsivity of children.

Licensing of products and linking them to popular characters through cross-promotions is an insidious way to market to children. Examples include SpongeBob Cheez-Its, Hulk pizzas, and Scooby-Doo marshmallow cereals. A *New York Times* business section article noted that "aiming at children through licensing is hardly new. What has changed is the scope and intensity of the blitz as today's youth become unwitting marketing targets at ever younger ages through more exposure to television, movies, videos and the Internet" (Kane, 2003).

This recruitment starts early. Many products that are sold for children originate in television or media. For example, many of the characters seen on commercial television or even educational programming such as Sesame Street are available as toys, making the program the commercial. There is a theme park known as Sesame Place in Pennsylvania that is built on the Sesame Street theme. To make matters worse, toys based on characters in mature entertainment are frequently marketed to children.

Movies are also often used to promote products. Toys associated with movies are stuffed into children's meals at fast-food restaurants. The movie is used to market the chain and its food, which is often not very nutritious. The movies themselves may contain songs, phrases, or images that stealthily promote products to children.

Product placement, the practice of placing the product in a movie, video game, "educational" material, or other medium, often targets youth. The product is not the primary focus of the medium, but it is subtly introduced to young viewers.

This is part of a larger picture in which, according to the Institute of Medicine (McGinnis, Gootman, & Kraak, 2006), food marketing intentionally targets children who are too young to distinguish advertising from truth and induces them to eat high-calorie, low-nutrient, but highly profitable "junk" foods. Marketing strongly influences children's food preferences, requests, and consumption. These choices are linked to increased body fat.

The majority of foods marketed to and for children are not nutritious and are high in calories. About one-third of American children and teens are overweight or obese, nearly triple the rate in 1963. Childhood obesity is now the top health concern among parents in the United States, topping drug abuse and smoking (American Heart Association, 2010).

Between 1994 and 2005, U.S. companies introduced hundreds of new children's food products. Half of them were candies or chewing gums, another one-fourth were other types of sweets or salty snacks. Only one-fourth are more healthful items, such as baby foods, bread products, or bottled waters. Companies support sales of "kids' foods," with marketing budgets totaling an estimated $10 billion annually (McGinnis, Gootman, & Kraak, 2006; California Pan-Ethnic Health Network, 2005).

Some examples of expenditures on advertising aimed at children are staggering. The Kellogg Company spent $22.2 million just on media advertising to support $139.8 million worth of Cheez-It crackers in 2004. McDonald's spent $528.8 million to support $24.4 billion in sales

(McGinnis, Gootman, & Kraak, 2006; California Pan-Ethnic Health Network, 2005). While these companies also market to adults, most of the advertisements for these products have kids in them.

According to the U.S. Department of Agriculture (Sebastian, Cleveland, Goldman, & Moshfegh, 2005), among 6- to 11-year-olds, the consumption of savory snacks increased 320 percent, consumption of pizza increased 413 percent, consumption of candy increased 180 percent, while consumption of vegetables decreased by 42 percent between 1977 and 2002. Among those ages 12 to 19 years, consumption of savory snacks increased by 320 percent, consumption of pizza increased by 208 percent, consumption of candy increased by 220 percent, and consumption of vegetables decreased by 32 percent in the same time period. Consumption of sodas (soft drinks) increased by 33.5 percent in the 6- to 11-year-olds and 58.5 percent in the 12- to 19-year-olds. This represented 50 percent of the total beverage intake for U.S. teens aged 12 to 19. Consumption of soft drinks has been linked to weight gain among children and adolescents (Berkey, Rockett, Field, Gillman, & Colditz, 2004).

In 2005, McDonald's spent over $742.3 million, Wendy's spent over $375.1 million, and Burger King spent over $268.8 million (down from $313.3 million in 2004) on advertising. The Coca-Cola Company spent $317 million advertising Coke and Diet Coke, while PepsiCo spent $262.7 million advertising Pepsi and Diet Pepsi (Advertising Age, 2006).

The statistics for food and beverage advertising bear out this comment from the National Cancer Institute (2000): "Commercial advertisers have learned that a consistent and prominent presence in the marketplace is key to achieving and holding market share." We can assume that advertisers of high-calorie, low-nutrition foods and drinks would not continue to spend large amounts of money if they did not think their ads were effective.

Robinson, Borzekowski, Matheson, and Kramer (2007) demonstrated the importance of brand loyalty in children. Using five pairs of identical foods and beverages in packaging from McDonald's and matched but unbranded packaging, children with a mean age of 4.6 years were asked to indicate if they tasted the same or if one tasted better. The children selected all five foods in the McDonald's packaging as tasting better than the unbranded products. The authors concluded that branding of foods and beverages influences young children's taste perceptions.

According to the Center for Science in the Public Interest (2003), marketers explicitly attempt to undermine family decisions about food choices by convincing children that they, not adults, should control these choices. These efforts can be seen in many television ads in which a parent, usually the father, is depicted as a buffoon who is out of touch with the world. Another tactic is to persuade children to eat foods made "just for them"—that is, not what adults are eating.

Advertising in schools has become commonplace. This advertisement takes several forms:

- Sponsorship of programs and activities, such as sports events or proms
- Exclusive agreements with product vendors such as soft-drink manufacturers
- Incentive programs, which link achievement of academic goals with the consumption of commercial products
- Appropriation of space for advertising in various forms on school property
- Sponsored educational materials, such as lesson plans and curricula furnished by commercial interests and frequently promoting products or ideas in the interests of their sponsors
- Electronic marketing, including dedicated school-based television channels with ads
- Fund-raising in conjunction with commercial product marketing
- Sales of name-brand products, including fast foods and soft drinks

School districts have become partners with the advertisers. Many school districts have signed contracts with soft drink companies. In exchange for making them the exclusive vendor, the companies paid large sums to schools or school districts. Some school districts have contracted with fast food companies to sell their products in school cafeterias. In response to these developments, 2005–2006 marked an expansion of local and state regulation to curtail the sale and marketing of low-quality foods in schools. This culminated in a voluntary agreement by the American Beverage Association and market leaders Coca-Cola and PepsiCo to ban sugared soft drink sales in schools. The agreement forestalled a threatened lawsuit by consumer groups against the industry. It did not, however, fundamentally challenge the overall legitimacy of marketing in schools (Molnar, 2006).

Commercialism in schools harms all students in various ways that include promoting poor health habits—e.g., consumption of sugar- and fat-laden snacks and soft drinks, distorting the curriculum, and eroding critical thinking skills (Molnar, 2003).

The advertising industry practices self-regulation through a set of guidelines enforced by the Children's Advertising Review Unit of the Council of Better Business Bureaus. These guidelines address approaches that are appropriate to use in marketing to children. Many consider them inadequate and poorly enforced. The Federal Trade Commission occasionally takes action against ads deemed unfair or deceptive.

The *Guidelines for Responsible Marketing to Children,* developed by the Center for Science in the Public Interest, marked a step forward. The guidelines are for food manufacturers, restaurants, supermarkets, television and radio stations, movie studios, magazines, public relations and advertising agencies, schools, toy and video game manufacturers, organizers of sporting or children's events, and others who manufacture, sell, market, advertise, or otherwise promote food to children. The guidelines provide criteria for marketing food to children in a manner that does not undermine children's diets or harm their health (Center for Science in the Public Interest, 2005). Still, it is worth asking how it can ever be responsible to market to children.

The CSPI guidelines say, for example, that products containing more than 35 percent of total calories, excluding nuts, seeds, and peanut or other nut butters, should not be advertised to kids. Low-nutrition drinks such as soft drinks, sports drinks, and fruit beverages containing less than 50 percent fruit juice should not be advertised to children under age 18. The guidelines also contain recommendations for marketing. Some examples are cited in the box.

EXAMPLES OF RECOMMENDATIONS FROM THE CSPI's *GUIDELINES FOR RESPONSIBLE MARKETING TO CHILDREN*

Marketing Techniques

When marketing foods to children, companies should follow these guidelines.

Product Characteristics and Overall Messages

- Companies should support parents' efforts to serve as the gatekeepers of sound nutrition for their children and not undermine parental authority. Marketers should not encourage children to nag their parents to buy low-nutrition foods.
- Companies should develop new products that help children eat healthfully, especially with regard to nutrient density, energy density, and portion size.

Specific Marketing Techniques and Incentives

- Companies should not advertise nutritionally poor choices during television shows: (1) with more than 15 percent of the audience younger than age 12; (2) for which children are identified as the target audience by the television station, entertainment company, or movie studio; or (3) that are kid-oriented cartoons.
- Companies should not use product or brand placements for low-nutrition foods in media aimed at children, such as movies, television shows, video games, Web sites, books, and textbooks.
- Companies should offer premiums and incentives (such as toys, trading cards, apparel, club memberships, products for points, contests, reduced-price specials, or coupons) only with foods, meals, and brands that meet the nutrition criteria described above.

Additional Guidance for Schools

- Schools are a unique setting. Parents entrust their children into schools' care for a large proportion of children's waking hours. Also, schools are dedicated to children's education and are supported by tax dollars. Companies should support healthy eating in schools and not market, sell, or give away low-nutrition foods or brands anywhere on school campuses, including through:
  - logos, brand names, spokescharacters, product names, or other product marketing on/in vending machines; books, curricula, and other educational materials; school supplies; posters; textbook covers; and school property such as scoreboards, signs, athletic fields, buses, and buildings
  - educational incentive programs that provide food as a reward (for example, earning a coupon for a free pizza after reading a certain number of books)

(continues)

- incentive programs that provide schools with money or school supplies when families buy a company's food products
- in-school television, such as Channel One
- direct sale of low-nutrition foods
- free samples or coupons
- school fundraising activities
- banner ads or wallpaper on school computers

Source: Center for Science in the Public Interest. (2005). *Guidelines for responsible marketing to children.* Washington, DC: Author.

Perhaps the most insidious advertising aimed at children is that done by cigarette companies. Before the 1998 Master Settlement Agreement (MSA) between the major tobacco companies in the United States and the attorneys general of 46 states, the companies denied advertising to children while doing so with impunity. Joe Camel and the Marlboro Man were advertising icons that were very effective at leading youth to smoking. Can the tobacco companies' motives be more obvious than an advertising campaign for one brand that used the slogan "The Perfect Recess" or another that used wall-mounted posters announcing "back-to-school specials"? These two examples came after the industry agreed in the MSA to stop advertising to children.

The MSA prohibits tobacco manufacturers from taking "any action, directly or indirectly, to target Youth within any of the Settling States in the advertising, promotion or marketing of Tobacco Products." As a blanket youth-targeting ban, this provision was intended to apply to all types of advertising, including transit ads, billboards, and magazines. Whereas transit ads and billboards were explicitly and completely banned in the MSA, application of the youth-targeting ban to magazines was not clearly specified (Chung et al., 2002). Youth magazines are those having either more than two million youth readers (under age 18) or more than 15 percent youth readership (U.S. Department of Health and Human Services, 1996). Several studies following the MSA ban demonstrated that neither advertising in youth magazines nor advertising expenditures in them

decreased (Chung et al., 2002; King & Siegel, 2001; Turner-Bowker & Hamilton, 2001). Thus, the companies ignored the intent of the MSA and continued to advertise cigarettes to youth and adolescents.

Product placement in movies and television programs that are popular with youth is a favorite strategy of the tobacco industry. Many youth advocates have spoken out against this practice. Bowing to the pressure, in summer of 2007, The Walt Disney Company announced that it would ban smoking in its family movies and discourage it in others.

A common theme in ads aimed at youth is that smoking is daring, gutsy, and a sign of independence and nonconformity, all characteristics valued by adolescents. For example, the phrase "Light My Lucky" highlighted a Lucky Strike cigarettes advertising campaign that featured photos of young, defiant-looking women staring directly into the camera.

In 2009, Congress passed and President Barack Obama signed the Family Smoking Prevention and Tobacco Control Act. The principal feature of the new law is the granting to the FDA the power to regulate tobacco products. It also requires tobacco manufacturers to release all marketing research documents to the FDA. The act prohibits using flavoring other than menthol, including fruit flavors, clove, cinnamon, and vanilla, flavors that had been used to attract youth to smoking. The law also outlaws promoting tobacco products as lower-risk alternatives to traditional products, thus eliminating claims of "low tar" and "light."

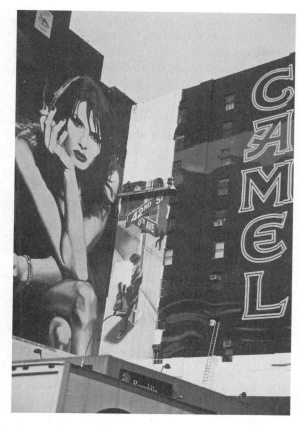

A large Camel cigarette advertisement featuring a defiant young female smoker is being painted over.

In June 2010, the Youth Access and Advertising Rule took effect. This rule severely restricts the way tobacco companies can advertise and sell cigarettes and smokeless tobacco products, especially marketing efforts designed to appeal to children and teens. We must always be mindful of the history of the tobacco industry of evading laws and breaking agreements that apply to marketing, especially to youth.

Tobacco is not the only drug product that is actively marketed to kids. Extrapolating from Federal Trade Commission data and other sources, the Center on Alcohol Marketing and Youth (2007) at Georgetown University concluded that the alcohol industry spent approximately $6 billion on advertising and promotion in 2005. Much of this is television advertising on sports programming and other entertainment enjoyed by youth. Apparel such as caps and tee shirts with alcohol logos are ubiquitous. There are also many ads in sports magazines and other types of publications that attract large youth readership. The Center (2006) found that, although alcohol advertising in magazines decreased from 2001 to 2005, alcohol advertising on television increased 41 percent for youth during the same period and much of the increase resulted from a steep rise in advertising distilled spirits. Unfortunately, the federal government has left it mostly to the alcohol advertisers to set their own standards and enforce them.

Those placing ads must believe they work if the record of their location is any indication. Garfield, Chung, and Rathouz (2003) concluded that magazine advertising by the beer and liquor industries is associated with adolescent readership and that the number of ads for beer and distilled spirits tended to increase with a magazine's youth readership. In a sample of radio advertising for the 25 leading alcohol brands in the summer of 2004, more than two-thirds of youth exposure to alcohol advertising came from ads placed in youth-oriented programming (Jernigan, Ostroff, Ross, Naimi, & Brewer, 2006).

Research clearly indicates that alcohol advertising and marketing have a significant effect on influencing both youth and adult expectations and attitudes, and help to create an environment that promotes drinking. A national study (Snyder, Milici, Slater, Sun, & Strizhakova, 2006) concluded that greater exposure to alcohol advertising contributes to an increase in drinking among underage youth. A study of New Hampshire middle school students found that ownership of alcohol-branded merchandise was significantly associated with increased likelihood of having initiated drinking one to two years later (McClure, Dal Cin, Givson, & Sargent, 2006). A study of product placement in movies found that youth with higher exposure to movie alcohol use were more likely to have started drinking 13 to 26 months later (Sargent, Wills, Stoolmiller, Gibson, & Gibbons, 2006). An increase in viewing television programs containing alcohol commercials in seventh grade is associated with an excess risk of beer use, wine/liquor use, and three-drink episodes in eighth grade (Stacy, Zogg, Unger, & Dent, 2004). Reduction in alcohol advertising will reduce alcohol use (Saffer & Dave, 2006).

What can parents and other consumers do about their kids' exposure to these ads? First, parents should take responsibility for what their children watch on television and read and see on the Internet. Marion Nestle (2006), Professor of Nutrition, Food Studies, and Public Health at New York University, has called for the following measures:

- Let the merchant know that you do not want it to market to your children.
- Shop with your feet. Don't patronize companies that sell products harmful to children. Let those companies know of your actions.
- Join an advocacy group. In January 2006, advocacy groups announced a Massachusetts lawsuit to enjoin Kellogg and Viacom, owner of Nickelodeon, a cable television network for children, from promoting foods to children (Center for Science in the Public Interest, 2006). Pressure from advocacy groups resulted in the voluntary removal of trans-fats from food on the menus of several chains and passage of legislation in some cities and states requiring removal.
- Enlist the help of elected officials. There is a thin line between freedom of speech protections and advertising harmful to children. Often the threat of legislation encourages marketers to make changes.
- Educate your children. Help them understand that you, not the advertiser, are their authority on nutrition and consumerism. Teach them skills necessary to make healthful decisions when you are not there. Speak with them about the subtle psychological ploys used in advertisements. Help them differentiate informative ads from puffery and misleading ads.
- Advocate that your school district adopt drug prevention programs that have evidence of effectiveness in reducing experimentation in youth, including experimentation with alcohol and tobacco.
- Go to your local board of education meetings and speak out on school nutrition and on the sale of unhealthy foods and drinks to children on campus. Encourage policies and best practices that promote availability and marketing of foods and beverages that support healthful diets.
- Encourage organizations such as parent-teacher organizations, local boards of education, private-sector businesses, and athletics associations to advocate for nutritional choices in schools and curtailing of marketing unhealthful products at schools and school events.
- Advocate for restrictions or bans on the use of cartoon characters, celebrity endorsements, health claims on food packaging, stealth marketing, and marketing in schools and for actions that promote media literacy, better school meals, and consumption of fruits and vegetables.

Such consumer action has already had some effect. In 2005, Kraft Foods, Kellogg, and The Walt Disney Company made commitments to limit advertising to children under the age of 12. In November 2006, 11 major food and drink makers—McDonald's, The Coca-Cola Company, PepsiCo, Kraft Foods, Cadbury Schweppes USA, Campbell's Soup, Kellogg, General Mills, Hershey, Unilever, and Masterfoods USA—agreed to adopt new voluntary rules for advertising. The companies said they would devote at least half their advertising to children to promote healthier diets and lifestyles. In July 2007, fearing federal government intervention, 11 of the nation's biggest food and drink companies that account for about two-thirds of television food advertisements directed to children agreed to adopt additional new rules to limit advertising to children under the age of 12. Seven of the companies pledged to no longer use licensed characters, such as those from popular movies and television programs, to advertise online or in print media unless they are promoting their healthier products. However, the "healthier products" mentioned in the agreement are not necessarily healthful products, only those that are relatively healthier than the companies' other products. The remaining four companies claimed to not advertise at all to children under 12. The companies can still use the licensed characters in their packaging. Some parent and health groups welcomed these measures, but many consider them only a good start.

The Boston-based Campaign for a Commercial-Free Childhood and the Center for Science in the Public Interest threatened to sue the Kellogg Company and Nickelodeon. Kellogg responded by announcing in June 2007 that it would restrict the use of its licensed characters such as Shrek in its advertising, and either reduce the amount of calories, fat, sugar, and sodium in its products or stop marketing them to children younger than 12. This action builds on a fall 2006 statement by The Walt Disney Company that it would limit the use of its characters in marketing junk food to children and a 2005 move by Kraft Foods to stop advertising products high in fat and sugar to children younger than age 11 (Tong, 2007).

Unmeasured Media

Advertising Age (Endicott, 2005) identified a category of advertising expenditures that it termed **unmeasured media**. This category includes strategies for which ad buy data may not be accessible, such as direct mail, sales promotion, couponing, catalogs, and special events. Unmeasured media also includes the use of product placement, advertising immersed in games, branded Internet environments, Web-based cross promotions, and cell phone and text messaging ads. Most accounting of advertising spending, including that detailed in previous sections of this chapter, do not take into account unmeasured media.

Still another method of unmeasured media is the enlistment of consumers to tout products. For example, the Tremor Group, an organization formed by Procter & Gamble, recruited 275,000 teens to create "buzz" about a variety of brands and products through online modes such as instant messaging and chat rooms. Reportedly, the Tremor Group has used this network to promote Coke and Pringles (Wells, 2004).

The estimated company-wide 2004 unmeasured media was $227.7 million for Burger King, $161.1 million for The Coca-Cola Company, $747.6 million for McDonald's, and $400.7 million for PepsiCo (Endicott, 2005). It is not clear how much was spent on individual products by these companies. It is clear that these strategies are a significant and growing part of food and beverage advertising. Since we are unable to track this type of advertising with much detail, we cannot say how much of it is directed toward children and adolescents.

Infomercials

An **infomercial** is a broadcast advertisement filling an entire program slot, often repeating the same body of content several times. It is usually listed in program guides as "paid programming." Infomercials are sometimes difficult to identify. They have the look and feel of "talk shows" and sometimes even resemble news programs with "moderators" or "reporters" who are usually paid actors. Products are praised by "experts" who are, of course, paid for their appearances. Testimonials are common. The Better Business Bureau (1996) provided some clues that a program might be an infomercial:

- The program's commercials are similar to its program content.
- Generally, any program that provides ordering information for a specific product is a paid advertisement.
- The program includes sponsor identification, although this may not be easily apparent. An identified sponsor who has a financial interest in the products is a tipoff.

Infomercials, although not named that until much later, originated in radio as early as 1950, before television displaced radio as the primary home entertainment medium. Two products advertised in 15-minute radio infomercials during the 1950s were:

- "Pro-Tam," guaranteed to melt off the pounds if you sprinkled it on your food. It was hawked in a question-and-answer format that mimicked a popular general-interest program of the time, *The Answer Man*. Pro-Tam was simply a protein powder.
- A product claimed to prevent hair loss. Listeners were urged to avoid alcohol-based hair products ("If alcohol could grow hair, a lot of people I know would have fur-lined stomachs.") and use a substance produced by "the animal that grows hair most like humans do: the sheep." The product was lanolin (Center for Media and Democracy, 2004).

Television infomercials began to flourish in 1984 when the Reagan administration lifted the Federal Communications Commission's restriction on how much time each hour could be devoted to commercials. Cable television, with its abundance of low-cost time, provided a fertile ground for infomercials.

Infomercials were soon targeted for criticism. They seem designed to lead viewers to believe that they are watching a program such as a talk show or investigative news report. They even carry "commercials" within the commercial that promote the product the infomercial is selling. The products themselves are often a waste of consumer money—weight-loss schemes, get-rich-quick promotions, "cures" for baldness and impotence. More recently, products promoted on infomercials may be fitness equipment, health and beauty products, work-at-home programs, and self-help and motivational products (Better Business Bureau, 1996). Dietary supplements are also often promoted in this medium, and weight loss remains a staple.

In 1991, the National Infomercial Marketing Association was founded with nine members. In 1997, it changed its name to the Electronic Retailing Association. The ERA is the trade asso-

ciation for companies that use direct response to sell products and services on television, online, and on radio. It claims to represent nearly 400 members in 45 countries. The ERA provides research to its members to help them get an advantage against their competition. The ERA established an Electronic Retailing Self-Regulation Program (ERSP), ostensibly to ensure ethical standards and best business practices. The ERSP allows direct response professionals a forum to review claims independently of federal regulation. This program allows advocacy and consumer groups, direct response marketers, and other interested parties the opportunity to refer suspect advertisements in an effort to remove offenders from the airwaves expeditiously (ERA, 2006).

The ability of the ERA to monitor and affect the quality and character of infomercials, online pop-up ads, e-mails, home-shopping channels, and other modes of advertising is questionable, especially given that the organization's rules state, "ERA will not refer or recommend the review of any specific matters to ERSP and will not encourage others to refer matters to ERSP" (ERA, 2006), although members may refer matters to the ERSP. Richard Cleland, an assistant director at the Federal Trade Commission's Division of Advertising Practices, said in 2005 that it is too early to say whether the ERSP is effective, but he commended the ERSP policy of requiring changes to questionable ads or referring cases to the Federal Trade Commission as "an impressive commitment." Conversely, Gary Ruskin of Commercial Alert, a watchdog organization, said, "The purpose of most advertising self-regulation is to provide a fig leaf to the advertising industry" (ConsumerReports.org, 2005).

However effective the industry's self-regulation may be, infomercials must adhere to the basic principles of advertising law or risk becoming the subject of action by authorities, principally the Federal Trade Commission. However, the FTC lacks the resources to effectively combat abuses that sometimes appear in infomercials.

Consumers should understand that the information in infomercials is not always accurate.

People appearing in them may not be what they seem—that is, doctors, scientists, or even real users of the products. The quality of products advertised in this medium may be poor. Offers that come with money-back guarantees are often hollow; you may not be able to find the company by the time you discover the poor quality of the product.

Often, you can buy them only by calling a toll-free number for "a limited time." Ask yourself: Does it make sense that the profit from a high-quality product would be maximized by marketing it only in 30-minute time slots and selling it in a limited sales environment—i.e., phone calls—for a limited amount of time? Of course not!

AN INFOMERCIAL STAR FALLS AND RISES

Kevin Trudeau is one of the most prolific users of infomercials, promoting a number of products in this medium. He is an attractive, articulate person who comes across as an earnest advocate for the health of the consumer. Playing the victim, Trudeau alleges that the medical establishment and the government want to silence him because the products he promotes will reduce the profits of conventional medicine if widely used.

Trudeau has a sordid past. In 1990, he pleaded guilty to larceny in a Cambridge, Massachusetts, state court after being charged with depositing $80,000 in worthless checks. The following year, he also pleaded guilty to credit card fraud in federal district court in Boston, resulting in a prison term of nearly two years. The federal charges involved the use of credit card numbers from customers of a memory improvement course Trudeau was promoting at the time.

The Federal Trade Commission filed a lawsuit against Trudeau in 1998, charging him with making false and misleading claims in infomercials for products he claimed could cause significant weight loss, cure serious addictions, and enable users to achieve a photographic memory. The case was resolved with a stipulated court order barring Trudeau from making false claims for products in the future. He was also ordered to pay $500,000 in consumer redress and establish a performance bond in the same amount to assure compliance.

The FTC filed another complaint against Trudeau in 2003, alleging that he and some of his companies made claims for Coral Calcium Supreme that were false and unsubstantiated. He had claimed that the product can cure cancer and other serious diseases and that a purported analgesic called Biotape can permanently cure or relieve severe pain. The court entered a preliminary injunction that prohibited him from continuing to make the challenged claims about Coral Calcium Supreme and Biotape. When Trudeau continued to make the claims, he was found in contempt of the injunction. In 2004, a court order directed Trudeau to pay $2 million to settle charges regarding false claims he made about the coral calcium product. The order banned him from infomercials except for those for informational publications such as books, provided that he "must not misrepresent the content" of the books.

Seizing on the initial exemption that allowed Trudeau to promote books, he was soon appearing in infomercials promoting his book *Natural Cures They Don't Want You to Know About*. According to the chairperson of the New York State Consumer Protection Board, "This book is exploiting and misleading people who are searching for cures to serious illness. What they discover is page after page of pure speculation." Trudeau used his infomercial about the book

(continues)

to tout a cancer cure that is not even mentioned in the book. The book jacket contains a list of endorsements that include a quote from a former commissioner of the U.S. Food and Drug Administration who died several years before the publication of the book. Despite the deception and speculation, the book soon became a best seller. In 2005, probably in response to widespread criticism that his book did not contain what it promised, Trudeau published a second edition that included alleged "natural cures" for more than 50 diseases and conditions. In 2006, he published a third book called *More Natural "Cures" Revealed*, in which he claims to have gotten his inside information from a "secret society" that gave him "health secrets, access to the inner circles of the rich and powerful, and the ability to live a life of luxury."

In 2007, the court found Trudeau in contempt of court—i.e., "in flagrant violation" of the court's order. The court found that Trudeau had misled thousands of consumers with false claims. The court banned Trudeau "or any person acting in concert with him, from participating in the production or publication of any infomercial for any product, including books, in which Mr. Trudeau or any related entity has an interest, for a period of three years." The court also imposed a judgment of more than $5 million against Trudeau.

Undaunted, Trudeau continues to appear in infomercials. Trudeau's recent infomercials promote his books on debt and "free money." They follow his typical formula of claiming to provide information that the government does not want you to know.

Sources: Barrett, S. (2004). Analysis of Kevin Trudeau's "Natural Cures" infomercial. http://www.infomercialwatch .org/tran/trudeau.shtml

ConsumerAffairs.com. (2004). Kevin Trudeau banned from infomercials. http://www.consumeraffairs.com /news04/2005/trudeau_infomercials.html

ConsumerAffairs.com. (2005). Consumer agency trashes Trudeau's "Natural Cures" book. http://consumeraffairs.com /news04/2005/trudeau_cpb.html

Federal Trade Commission. (2004). Kevin Trudeau banned from infomercials. http://www.ftc.gov/opa/2004/09 /trudeaucoral.shtm

Federal Trade Commission. (2008). Kevin Trudeau banned from infomercials for three years, ordered to pay more than $5 million for false claims about weight-loss books. http://www.ftc.gov/opa/2008/10/trudeau.shtm

Internet Advertising and Marketing

The Internet is now almost as far-reaching as television. Many entrepreneurs have made millions by advertising on the Web. Web sites and search engines make handsome profits advertising the products and services of others. Pop-up ads were the bane of Internet users in the 1990s until effective protection was developed.

Many consumers have become accustomed to purchasing everything from books to movie tickets to automobiles on the Web. Many people do their banking and pay their bills online.

There are predators in cyberspace. Complicated programs have been designed to hack into Web sites or steal individuals' private information from their own computers. Community Web sites and dating sites that promote personal interaction have been used to trap unsuspecting persons into dangerous activities. One scam involves the crook contacting the individual and striking up an online friendship. After sufficient trust is developed, the victim is convinced to accept merchandise ordered by the crook and charged to someone else's credit card. The person is then expected to ship the illegally gotten goods to another address, usually in another country, where it is sold for a profit by the criminal or his or her accomplices.

Other criminals set up bogus businesses and "sell" products to unsuspecting people who may think they are getting a bargain. Not only do they not receive the product or receive an inferior product, their credit card numbers are given to a stranger.

Drugs and products described as "natural" are marketed on the Web. Some of the sellers are located outside the United States and are not subject to federal regulation. Many sell inferior products. Immediately after a 2008 segment on the popular television news magazine *60 Minutes* about resveratrol, a component in red wine being studied for effects on longevity, Web sites sprung up to sell products supposedly containing the substance. It is impossible to know, before purchase and chemical analysis, exactly what is contained in such products. This example illustrates the speed with which entrepreneurs can exploit the World Wide Web.

There are a number of steps a consumer can take to reduce the chance of being defrauded or buying useless products on the Web. These protective steps are discussed at length in Chapter 1. However, it is worth summarizing them again here.

- Know the seller. Always look for a physical address and telephone number.
- Purchase with a credit card. If the product does not arrive or is defective, you can request a chargeback from your credit card company.
- Know exchange/return policies before you buy.
- Read policies on shipping/handling. Know when to expect the product, what will happen if it is out of stock, and your costs. If it is late, contact the company immediately.
- Attempt to determine if other charges apply and review your receipt when it arrives.
- Request an e-mail order form with all charges itemized.
- Contact the merchant immediately if there is a problem.
- Keep all your records, including the names and identification numbers of all the people with whom you speak, their titles, and the dates and times of the conversations.
- Do not be embarrassed to call authorities or tell acquaintances of your experience.

If you think you have been scammed through an online promotion or you have witnessed a fraudulent or misleading infomercial, there are places you can turn.

- Many cities and states have consumer protection agencies that investigate complaints.
- Your state attorney general may have a special office to investigate consumer complaints.
- The Federal Trade Commission at www.ftc.gov will take a report and decide to investigate. The toll-free telephone number is 1-800-FTC-HELP (382-4357).
- The Federal Bureau of Investigation at www.fbi.gov may investigate fraud complaints.
- Your local Better Business Bureau may offer to resolve your complaint.
- The U.S. Postal Service is responsible for investigating fraudulent use of the mail, including private delivery companies.
- The Federal Communications Commission operates a Consumer and Governmental Affairs Bureau that responds directly to consumers' inquiries and complaints. To file a complaint, go to http://www.fcc.gov/cgb/consumers.html.
- The Electronic Retailing and Self-Regulation Program accepts complaints at http://www.savvyshopper.org.

SUMMARY

Advertising is ubiquitous in Western society. It has become impossible to escape constant exposure to marketing. There are three main types of advertising—informative, misleading or deceptive, and puffery. Informative ads provide useful information. Misleading ads intentionally deceive. Puffery uses exaggeration and imagery, but an informed consumer should not be deceived.

Marketers use a variety of techniques to attract attention and to convince consumers of the need to purchase goods and services. Examples include testimonials, weasel words, appeals to human weaknesses, visual imagery, comedy, and sex.

Drugs are marketed in many ways. Both nonprescription and prescription drugs are marketed directly to consumers. Where prescription drugs are concerned, the practice is controversial. Some feel it leads to patients pressuring physicians for drugs they do not need, while others feel it strengthens doctor-patient communication. It is very lucrative for the drug makers and, although regulated by the FDA and scrutinized by Congress, it is probably here to stay.

Marketers apply the study of human behavior to their work. They use the information to target advertising, in both form and product, to groups of people and to individuals. They are especially adept at targeting children through a variety of techniques. Products such as fast food, cereal, soft drinks, and tobacco are marketed to children, although not always in obvious ways.

Infomercials are program-length commercials. They often market inferior products and services, using testimonials, flawed science, and outlandish claims. Regulation of infomercials is mostly voluntary.

The Internet is a far-reaching marketing engine. Consumers should exercise care in shopping on the Web because there are many unscrupulous merchants operating under the protective cover of the Internet. There are a number of agencies that attempt to police Web-based commerce, and consumers should not hesitate to report fraud to those agencies.

KEY TERMS

Attention grabber: words and phrases that offer power to the advertisement and attract interest

Bait-and-switch: when advertised goods or services are withdrawn from the market and other, more expensive and sometimes inferior, goods or services are substituted and offered for sale

Contraindication: a specific situation in which a drug, procedure, or surgery should not be used

Deceptive advertising: advertising that intentionally deceives or confuses the consumer

Endorsement: the use of opinions of experts, including individuals and organizations, or users of products to promote the products

Infomercial: a broadcast advertisement filling an entire program slot

Informative advertising: advertising that provides the shopper with useful information about the product

Measured marketing: marketing activity that has clearly defined and agreed-upon measurements that support the company's business objectives

Misleading advertising: advertising that intentionally deceives or confuses the consumer

Misrepresentation: false or misleading claims made by an advertiser about its products or services

Palming off: when an advertiser creates an impression that its products or services are those that are furnished by a competitor

Product disparagement: when an advertiser intentionally makes false or misleading negative remarks about a competitor's goods or services, causing the competitor to lose sales

Product placement: promotion by the use of real commercial products and services in media, where the presence of a particular brand is the result of an exchange of money

Puffery: the use of exaggeration, hyperbole, or imagery to market products

Testimonial: the use of statements of users of the product to market it

Unbranded advertisement: communications disseminated to consumers or health care practitioners that discuss a particular disease or health condition, but do not mention any specific drug or device or make any representation or suggestion concerning a particular drug or device; also called disease awareness advertisements

Unmeasured media: a category of advertising that includes strategies for which ad buy data may not be accessible, such as direct mail, sales promotion, couponing, product placement, catalogs, and special events

Visual imagery: using visual means to promote a vivid conscious experience of something not physically present

Weasel words: the use of vague words to create the illusion of a promise or commitment

Word-of-mouth marketing: the use of peer-to-peer communication to market a product

STUDY QUESTIONS

1. What are the objectives of advertising?
2. Define and explain the following types of advertising: informative, misleading/deceptive, puffery.
3. Why are testimonials and endorsements questionable ways to learn about a product?
4. What are "weasel words" and how are they used in ads?
5. How are statistics used and misused to make points in ads?
6. What is product placement? Is it effective?
7. What are the three recognized types of direct-to-consumer prescription drug ads?
8. How do advertisers target children? Is this ethical?
9. List forms of advertising that occur in schools.
10. Give examples of cigarette and alcohol advertising to youth.
11. What can parents do to protect children from inappropriate advertisements?
12. What is an infomercial? How do you recognize one?
13. What are some of the problems with infomercials?
14. List some steps you can take to reduce the risk of being defrauded when shopping on the Internet.

REFERENCES

Advertising Age. (2006). *Top 200 megabrands*. Retrieved from http://adage.com/datacenter/article/article_id-110575

Aiken, K. J. (2005). *Direct-to-consumer advertising of prescription drugs: Looking back, looking forward*. U.S. Food and Drug Administration. Retrieved from http://www.fda.gov/cder/ddmac/Presentations/Societyforwomenshealth

American Heart Association. (2010). *Overweight in children*. Retrieved from http://www.heart.org/HEARTORG/GettingHealthy/Overweight-in-Children_UCM_304054_Article.jsp

Anderson, J. (2006). *Multimedia clicks in*. Retrieved from https://www.imediaconnection.com/content/10534.imc

Barrett, S., London, W. M., Baratz, R. S., & Kroger, M. (2007). *Consumer health: A guide to intelligent decisions*, 8th ed. New York: McGraw-Hill.

Berkey, C., Rockett, H., Field, A., Gillman, M., & Colditz, G. (2004). Sugar-added beverages and adolescent weight change. *Obesity Research, 12*, 778–788. doi:10.1038/oby.2004.94

Better Business Bureau. (1996, November). *Infomercials*. Retrieved from http://www.bbbsilicon.org/topic021.html

California Pan-Ethnic Health Network, Consumers Union. (2005). *Out of balance: Marketing of soda, candy, snacks and fast food drowns out healthful messages*. Retrieved from http://consumersunion.org/pdf/OutofBalance.pdf

Center on Alcohol Marketing and Youth. (2006). *Still growing after all these years: Youth exposure to alcohol advertising on television, 2001–2005*. Washington, DC: Author.

Center on Alcohol Marketing and Youth. (2007). *Alcohol advertising and youth*. Retrieved from http://www.camy.org/factsheets/index.php?FactsheetID-1

Center for Media and Democracy. (2004). *Infomercials*. Retrieved from http://www.sourcewatch.org/index.php?title=Infomercial

Center for Science in the Public Interest. (2003). *Pestering parents: How food companies market obesity to children*. Washington, DC: Author.

Center for Science in the Public Interest. (2005). *Guidelines for responsible marketing to children*. Washington, DC: Author. Retrieved from http://www.cspinet.org/marketingguidelines.pdf

Center for Science in the Public Interest. (2006). *Parents and advocates sue Viacom & Kellogg* [press release]. Washington, DC.

Chester, J., & Montgomery, K. (2007). *Interactive food & beverage marketing: Targeting children and youth in the digital age*. Retrieved from http://www.ftc.gov/os/comments/behavioraladvertising/071018chesterandmontgomery.pdf

Chung, P. J., Garfield, C. F., Rathouz, P. J., Lauderdale, D. S., Best, D., & Lantos, J. (2002). Youth targeting by tobacco manufacturers since the Master Settlement Agreement. *Health Affairs, 21*(2), 254–263.

Coe, J. (2003). The lifestyle drugs outlook to 2008, unlocking new value in well-being. Datamonitor. *Reuters Business Insights*. Retrieved from http://www.globalbusinessinsights.com/content/rbhc0109m.pdf

Comiteau, J. (2003, March 24). When does brand loyalty start? *Adweek*. Retrieved from http://www.adweek.com/aw/magazine/article_display.jsp?vnu_content_id=1848001

Commercial Alert. (2010). *Stop drug ads: Learn more*. Retrieved from http://stopdrugads.org/learn_more.html

ConsumerReports.org. (2005, May). *Infomercial industry polices itself (Wait! there's more! call now!)*. Retrieved from http://www.consumerreports.org/co/personal-finance/infomercials-police-themselves-50

ConsumerReports.org. (2006, January). *Product testimonials*. Retrieved from http://www.consumerreports.org/cro/money/news/2006/01/product-testimonials-106

Donohue, J. M., Cevasco, M., & Rosenthal, M. B. (2007). A decade of direct-to-consumer advertising of prescription drugs. *New England Journal of Medicine, 357*(7), 673–381.

Electronic Retailing Association. (2006). *ERA*. Retrieved from http://www.retailing.org

eMarketer. (2010). *CPG online: Food and beverages party on*. Retrieved from http://www.emarketer.com/Reports/All/Emarketer_2000389.aspx

Endicott, R. C. (2005). 50th annual 100 leading national advertisers. *Advertising Age*. Retrieved from http://www.adage.com/images/random/Ina2005.pdf

Endicott, R. C., Brown, K., MacDonald, S., Schumann, M., Ryan, M., Sierra, J., & Wentz, L. (Eds.). (2005). *Hispanic fact pack: Annual guide to Hispanic advertising and marketing. Advertising Age* in association with the Association of Hispanic Advertising Agencies. Retrieved from http://www.adage.com/images/random/hispfactpack05.pdf

Findlay, S. (2001). *Prescription drugs and mass media advertising, 2000*. Washington, DC: National Institute for Health Care Management Research and Educational Foundation. Retrieved from http://www.nihcm.org/DTCbrief2001.pdf

Garfield, F., Chung, P. J., & Rathouz, P. J. (2003). Alcohol advertising in magazines and adolescent readership. *Journal of the American Medical Association, 289*(18), 2424–2429.

General Accounting Office. (2002, October). *Prescription drugs: FDA oversight of direct-to-consumer advertising has limitations*. GAO-03-177. Washington, DC: Author.

Gilbody, S., Wilson, P., & Watt, I. (2005). Benefits and harms of direct to consumer advertising: A systematic review. *Quality and Safety in Health Care, 14*, 246–250. doi:10.1136/qshc.2004.012781

Heavey, S. (2005, September 19). *US FDA steps up action on misleading drug ads*. Retrieved from http://news.healthhelp.org/us_fda_steps_up_action_on_misleading_drug_ads

Hoffman, I. (2004). *Advertising slogans: Fact vs. puffing*. Retrieved from http://www.ivanhoffman.com/slogansw.html

Hollon, M. F. (2005). Direct-to-consumer advertising: A haphazard approach to health promotion. *Journal of the American Medical Association, 293*(16), 2030–2033. doi:10.1001/jama293.16.2030

Interactive Advertising Bureau. (2007). *Reach U.S. Hispanics through online marketing*. Retrieved from http://www.iab.net/resources/docs/Hispanic_Presentation_Final.pdf

Ismail, A. (2006). *Drug lobby second to none: How the pharmaceutical industry gets its way in Washington*. Center for Public Integrity. Retrieved from http://www.publicintegrity.org/rx/report.aspx?aid-723

Jernigan, D. H., Ostroff, J., Ross, C. S., Naimi, T. S., & Brewer, R. D. (2006). Youth exposure to alcohol advertising on radio—United States, June–August 2004. *MMWR, 55*, 937–940.

Johnson, B. (2010). *Top outlays plunge 10% but defying spend trend can pay off*. Retrieved from http://adage.com/print?article_id=144555

Kaiser Family Foundation. (2007). *Prescription drug trends*. Retrieved from http://www.kff.org/rxdrugs/upload/3057_06.pdf

Kane, C. (2003, December 8). TV and movie characters sell children snacks. *New York Times*.

King, C., III & Siegel, M. (2001). The Master Settlement Agreement with the tobacco industry and cigarette advertising in magazines. *New England Journal of Medicine, 345*(7), 504–511.

Korzenny, F., Korzenny, B. A., McGavock, H., & Inglessis, M. G. (2007). *The multicultural marketing equations: Media, attitudes, brands, and spending*. Tallahassee, FL: Center for Hispanic Marketing Communication, Florida State University.

Kunkel, D. (2002). Eating and eating disorders. In V. Strasburger & B. Wilson (Eds.). *Children, Adolescents and the Media*. Thousand Oaks, CA: Sage, 237–270.

Loden, D. J., & Schooler, C. (1998, April). How to make DTC advertising work harder. *Medical Marketing and Media*.

Lurie, P. (2005). *Testimony before the Senate Special Committee on Aging on the impact of direct-to-consumer drug advertising on seniors' health and health care costs*. HRG Publication #1751. Retrieved from http://www.citizen.org/publications/pring_release.cfm?ID=7402

Marketing Week. (2006, November 23). *And now a word from our pharmaceutical manufacturer*. Retrieved from http://firstsearch.oclc.org/WebZ/

McClure, S., Dal Cin, S., Givson, J. M., & Sargent, J. D. (2006). Ownership of alcohol-branded merchandise and initiation of teen drinking. *American Journal of Preventive Medicine, 39*(4), 54–65.

McGinnis, J. M., Gootman, J. A., & Kraak, V. I. (Eds.). (2006). *Food marketing to children and youth: Threat or opportunity?* Washington, DC: National Academies Press.

Media Week. (2006, May 1). *Prescription drugs.* Retrieved from http://firstsearch.oclc.org/WebZ

Mintzes, B., Barer, M. L., Kravitz, R. L., Bassett, K., Lexchin, J., Kazanjian, A., . . . Marion, S. A. (2003). How does direct-to-consumer advertising (DTCA) affect prescribing? A survey in primary care environments with and without legal DTCA. *Canadian Medical Journal, 169*(5), 405–412.

Molnar, A. (2003, Fall). School commercialism hurts all children, ethnic minority group children most of all. *Journal of Negro Education.* Retrieved from http://findarticles.com/p/articles/mi_qa3626/is_200310/ai_n9248821

Molnar, A. (2006). The ninth annual report on schoolhouse commercialism trends: 2005–2006: Executive report. Tempe: Arizona State University.

Moynihan, R., & Cassels, A. (2005). *Selling sickness: How the world's pharmaceutical companies are turning us into patients.* New York: Nation Books.

National Cancer Institute. (2000). *5 a Day for Better Health program evaluation report.* Retrieved from http://www.cancercontrol.gov/5ad_exec.html

Nestle, M. (2006). Food marketing and childhood obesity—a matter of policy. *New England Journal of Medicine, 354*(24), 2527–2529.

Parker, P. (2002). *An eye on the multicultural future.* ClickZ Network. Retrieved from http://www.clickz.com/showPage.html?page=1033911

Parry, V. (2003, May 1). The art of branding a condition. *Medical Marketing and Media, 38*(5), 43. Retrieved from https://files.pbworks.com/download/twm/WdlUz3/sdsuwriting/8280746/Parry%20art%20of%20branding%20a%20condition.pdf

Pharmaceutical Research and Manufacturers of America. (2005). *PhRMA Guiding Principles to Consumer Advertisements About Prescription Medicines.* Washington, DC: PhRMA.

PQ Media. (2010). *New PQ Media report finds U.S. branded entertainment spending on consumer events & product placement dipped only 1.3% to $24.63 billion in 2009 & on pace to grow 5.3% in 2010, exceeding most advertising & marketing segments.* Retrieved from http://www.pqmedia.com/about-press-20100629-gbem2010.html

Rados, C. (2004, July–August). Truth in advertising: Rx drug ads come of age. *FDA Consumer Magazine.* Retrieved from http://www.fda.gov/fdac/features/2004/404_ads.html

Reyes, S. (2005, July 25). Targeting: Kraft initiative woos Asian American moms. *Admerasia.* Retrieved from http://www.admerasia.com/draftmom.html

Ripslinger, J. F. (1983, June 14). [Re: Stallone Tobacco Use Agreement]. Retrieved from http://tobaccodocuments.org/youth/AmBWC19830614.Lt.html

Robinson, T. N., Borzekowski, D. L. G., Matheson, D. M., & Kraemer, H. C. (2007). Effects of fast food branding on young children's taste preferences. *Archives of Pediatrics and Adolescent Medicine, 161*(8), 792–797.

Rosenthal, M. B., Berndt, E. R., Donahue, J. M., Epstein, A. M., & Frank, R. G. (2003). *Demand effects of recent changes in prescription drug promotion.* Menlo Park, CA: Henry J. Kaiser Family Foundation.

Saffer, H., & Dave, D. (2006). Alcohol advertising and alcohol consumption by adolescents. *Health Economics, 15*(6), 617–637.

St. John, W. (2003, December 14). In an oversexed age, more guys take a pill. *New York Times.*

Sargent, J. D., Stoolmiller, M., Worth, K. A., Dal Cin, S., Wills, T. A., Gibbons, F. X., . . . Tanski, S. (2007). Exposure to smoking depictions in movies. *Archives of Pediatric and Adolescent Medicine, 161*(9), 849–856.

Sargent, J. D., Wills, T. A., Stoolmiller, M., Gibson, J., & Gibbons, F. X. (2006). Alcohol use in motion pictures and its relation with early-onset teen drinking. *Journal of Studies on Alcohol, 67*(1), 617–637.

Sebastian, R., Cleveland, L., Goldman, J., & Moshfegh, A. (2005). Changes over 25 years in the dietary intakes of children 6-19 years [abstract]. *The Federation of American Societies for Experimental Biology Journal, 19*(14): A87.

Shin, A. (2006, December 12). *FTC moves to unmask word of mouth marketing.* Retrieved from http://www.washingtonpost.com/wp-dyn/content/article/2006/12/11/AR2006121101389.html

Snyder, L. B., Milici, F. F., Slater, M., Sun, H., & Strizhakova, Y. (2006). Effects of alcohol advertising exposure on drinking among youth. *Archives of Pediatrics and Adolescent Medicine, 160*(1), 18–24.

Spengler, P. (1979, October 18). [Re: Superman II- Movie]. Bates: 2024938787-2024938789. Retrieved from http://tobaccodocuments.org/youth/AmCgPMI19701018.Lt.htm

Stacy, A. W., Zogg, J. B., Unger, J. B., & Dent, C. W. (2004). Exposure to television alcohol ads and subsequent adolescent alcohol use. *American Journal of Health Behavior, 28*(6), 498–509.

Stallone, S. (1983, April 28). [Re: Agreement Between B&W and Sylvester Stallone to Promote B&W Products in Films]. Retrieved from http://tobaccodocuments.org/youth/AmBWC19830428.Lt.html

TNS Media Intelligence. (2006). *TNS Media Intelligence reports U.S. advertising expenditures increased 3.0 percent in 2005.* Retrieved from http://www.tns-mi.com/news/02282006.htm

Tong, V. (2007, June 21). Snack makers hope health push averts regulation. *Associated Press.*

Turner-Bowker, D., & Hamilton, W. L. (2001). *Cigarette advertising expenditures before and after the Master Settlement Agreement: Preliminary findings.* Retrieved from http://www.state.ma.us/dph/mtcp/report/mag.htm

The Lanham (Trademark) Act of 1947, 15 U.S.C. §301 *et seq.* (1947).

U.S. Department of Health and Human Services, Food and Drug Administration. (1996). Regulations restricting the sale and distribution of cigarettes and smokeless tobacco to protect children and adolescents. *Federal Register, 61*(168), 44395–44445.

U.S. Food and Drug Administration. (2005). *Prescription Drug User Fee Act (PDUFA): Adding resources and improving performance in FDA review of drug applications.* Washington, DC: Author.

University of Texas. (2000). *Advertising law and ethics.* Retrieved from http://advertising.about.com/gi/dynamic

Wells, M. (2004, February 2). Kid nabbing. *Forbes .com.* Retrieved from http://www.forbes.com/free_forbes/2004/0202.084.html

Williams, J. (2005). *Product proliferation analysis for new food and beverage products targeted at children 1994-2004.* Austin: University of Texas.

Winstein, K. J., & Vranica, S. (2009, April 16). Drug firms' spending on consumer ads fell 8% in '08, a rare marketing pullback. *Wall Street Journal.*

Wolfe, S. M. (2004). *Letter to FDA urging action on misleading CRESTOR advertising by AstraZeneca.* HRG Publication #17120. Retrieved from http://www.citizen.org/publication/release.cfm?ID=7347

Consumer Protection

Chapter Objectives

The student will:

- List the responsibilities and consumer protection authority of the Federal Trade Commission, the Consumer Product Safety Commission, the Environmental Protection Agency, the U.S. Department of Agriculture, and the U.S. Postal Inspection Service.
- Discuss the functions of patient safety organizations and the reasons for their establishment.
- Discuss consumer protection services provided by state and local governments.
- Explain the purposes and consumer protections services offered by the Better Business Bureau, Consumer Federation of America, Consumer Union, AARP, National Consumers League, National Consumer Protection Technical Resource Center, and Public Citizen.
- Explain accreditation and certification.
- Describe the functions of accreditation agencies and the benefits of accreditation.

Consumers are often vulnerable to marketplace deception and fraud. Company policies, warranties, and guarantees may seem to protect consumers, but they may often serve the interest of the company. Insurance companies and health care providers, motivated by profits, may not always act in the best interests of patients. It is important to have agencies and organizations that serve as a proactive force to minimize the chances that consumers will be victimized. Despite these safeguards, consumers sometimes believe they have been treated unfairly by a merchant or health care provider. The consumer or patient may need assistance in resolving problems. This can be a daunting task because some merchants and companies may seem too big for a single individual to challenge, and health care providers may be perceived as having too much authority and expertise to be confronted.

Federal and state laws give governments many legal mechanisms to protect consumers and punish those who violate those laws. In addition, the law gives consumers the right to seek a remedy when they have been treated unfairly by a merchant or advertiser. State regulatory agencies and professional associations may discipline health care providers who fail to render proper and respectful care to patients. There are also nongovernmental agencies that offer protective services and provide information for consumers so that they can guard their health and financial welfare. Some agencies provide accreditation and certification to facilities and organizations that perform health services. This chapter will describe consumer protection in the context of the agencies that are charged with these responsibilities.

Federal Consumer Protection

U.S. Federal Trade Commission

Laws have been written and the courts have ruled that advertisements cannot deceive the public. The Constitution gives the federal government the power to regulate interstate commerce, including advertising. That power to regulate advertising is vested in the Federal Trade Commission (FTC). The U.S. Congress enacted two major statutes, the Federal Trade Commission Act and the Lanham Act, that provide for the exercise of this regulatory power.

The FTC Act states that false advertising is a form of unfair and deceptive commerce. False advertising includes advertisements that make untrue statements or attempt to leave untrue impressions. It includes advertisements that make representations that the advertiser has no reasonable basis to believe, even if the representations turn out to be true. An example would be an advertisement for a computer printer that stated the machine used less ink than any comparable printer. The advertiser would have committed false advertising if it had no reasonable basis to believe the truth of this claim, even if it turned out to be true. This consumer protection does not extend to puffery because the consumer would not reasonably be expected to believe the depiction.

Under the FTC Act, the commission's authority to regulate advertising is broad. The authority allows the FTC to issue regulations barring advertisements that could be misleading even if true. A well-known example involves advertisements for the pain reliever Anacin. The maker of Anacin ran ads claiming that clinical tests showed that their product delivered the same headache relief as the leading pain relief medication. The ad failed to mention that at the time, aspirin was the leading pain relief medication, and that Anacin was aspirin with added caffeine. The FTC determined that the ad was misleading.

In another example, the FTC filed for permanent injunctions to prohibit the makers of Ab Energizer, AbTronic, and Fast Abs from making false or deceptive advertising claims, to stop them from engaging in other deceptive marketing practices, and to require them to pay compensation to consumers. The FTC alleged that the advertising statements they used ("Now you can get rock-hard abs with no sweat," "Lose 4 inches in 30 days guaranteed," "30% more effective than normal exercise," and "10 minutes = 600 sit-ups") were all misleading and deceptive. The makers of the products paid millions of dollars to settle the cases brought in a U.S. district court in Nevada.

The FTC also has power to order corrective advertisements that inform future customers about certain unfavorable facts about a product not revealed in previous ad campaigns. For example, Listerine was hyped as a cold and sore throat remedy for several years. The FTC forced the manufacturer to run corrective ads that stated that Listerine did not cure colds or relieve sore throats.

The Division of Advertising Practices (DAP) of the FTC coordinates the commission's actions with federal and international law enforcement agencies that share authority over health and safety products and services. The DAP also monitors advertising and marketing of alcohol, tobacco, violent entertainment media, and food targeted to children.

The FTC has sole authority to enforce the FTC Act. However, private consumers or even competitors can bring a legal action regarding false advertising under the Lanham Act. A violation under the Lanham Act requires that the plaintiff, the party bringing the suit, prove the following: (1) the advertiser made false statements of fact about its product; (2) the false advertisements actually deceived or had the capacity to deceive a substantial segment of the target population; (3) the deception was material in that it is likely to influence the purchasing decision; (4) the falsely advertised product was sold in interstate commerce; and (5) the plaintiff was injured or is likely to be injured as a result of the deception (as in *United Industries Corp. v. Clorox Co.,* 1998). The plaintiff is not required to show an actual loss in the form of injury. All that is needed is a reasonable basis for the belief that the plaintiff is likely to be damaged as a result of the advertising.

The DAP enforces the Children's Online Privacy Protection Act, which is meant to give parents control over information that online companies can collect about their children and how that information can be used. It also enforces the Federal Cigarette and Smokeless Tobacco Acts, which require the FTC to review and approve tobacco company plans for rotating and displaying the health warnings on tobacco labels and in ads.

Consumer Product Safety Commission

Deaths, injuries, and property damage from consumer product incidents cost the nation more than $800 billion annually. The U.S. Consumer Product Safety Commission (CPSC) is an independent federal regulatory agency that works to save lives and improve safety by reducing the risk of injuries and deaths associated with consumer products. It does this by:

- Developing voluntary industry standards
- Issuing and enforcing mandatory standards or banning consumer products if no feasible standard would adequately protect the public
- Obtaining the recall of products or arranging for their repair
- Conducting research on potential product hazards
- Informing and educating consumers through the media, state and local governments, and private organizations, and by responding to consumer inquiries (U.S. CPSC, 2010)

The CPSC is charged with protecting the public from unreasonable risks of serious injury or death from more than 15,000 types of consumer products under its jurisdiction. These are mostly products used in and around the home and in sports, recreation, and schools, including those that pose a fire, electrical, chemical, or mechanical hazard or that can injure children. Some examples include toys, cribs, power tools, cigarette lighters, and household chemicals. The CSPC does not

monitor automobiles and other on-road vehicles, tires, boats, alcohol, tobacco, firearms, food, drugs, cosmetics, pesticides, and medical devices. The CPSC contributed significantly to the 30 percent decline in the rate of deaths and injuries associated with consumer products over the past 30 years (U.S. CPSC, 2008). By way of example in 2010, after issuing several recalls on dropside infant cribs because of deaths caused by the cribs, the CPSC issued new mandatory standards for cribs that will: (1) stop the manufacture and sale of dangerous, traditional drop-side cribs; (2) make mattress supports stronger; (3) make crib hardware more durable; and (4) make safety testing more rigorous (U.S. Consumer Product Safety Commission, 2010).

Individuals are encouraged to file complaints and reports with the CPSC, either online or by mail, e-mail, fax, or phone. When a person reports a problem, he or she will receive a letter from the CPSC's National Injury Information Clearinghouse, describing how the CPSC will use the information. The person making the complaint may ask to remain anonymous. The complaint will be sent to the manufacturer of the product. The CPSC may or may not investigate the product complaint. The CPSC receives about 10,000 reports of product-related injuries and deaths a year from consumers and others. Due to the small staff size, relatively few complaints are investigated. If the CPSC investigates a product, an investigator will contact the complaining person by phone or mail. Based on the investigation, the CPSC has the power to recall the product.

The CPSC announces recalls of products that present a significant risk to consumers either because the product may be defective or because it violates a mandatory standard issued by the CPSC. At this point, the product may no longer be sold. Recalls are posted on the CPSC's Web site.

The CPSC publishes many documents about a variety of products. These publications are available on the commission's Web site (www.cpsc.gov). The National Injury Information Clearinghouse disseminates statistics and information relating to the prevention of death and injury associated with consumer products.

EXAMPLES OF RECALLS POSTED IN JULY 2010 BY THE CONSUMER PRODUCT SAFETY COMMISSION

Baja Motorsports Mini Bikes recalled about 308,000 minibikes and go-carts due to fire and burn hazards.

A recall was issued by the CPSC in cooperation with Health Canada and Tots in Mind, Inc., for about 20,000 Cozy Indoor Outdoor Portable Playard Tents Plus Cabana Kits because of strangulation hazards.

About 82,000 drop-side cribs were recalled by Pottery Barn Kids due to entrapment, suffocation, and fall hazards. The CPSC issued proposed rules for crib construction.

Star Asia USA recalled about 9,000 wire feed welders because of burn hazards.

U.S. Food and Drug Administration

The U.S. Food and Drug Administration (FDA) is responsible for protecting the public health by assuring the safety, efficacy, and security of human and veterinary drugs, biological products, medical devices, our nation's food supply, cosmetics, and products that emit radiation. The FDA is also responsible for advancing public health by helping to speed innovations that make medicines and foods more effective, safer, and more affordable. The FDA helps the public get the accurate, science-based information needed to use medicines and foods to improve health.

The authority granted the FDA under the Federal Food, Drug, and Cosmetic Act (FFDCA) covers products that represent nearly one-fourth of every dollar spent in the United States. The FFDCA governs the safety and accurate labeling of a trillion dollars' worth of products annually. These products include prescription and nonprescription drugs, cosmetics, medical devices, blood and tissue products, and most of the food supply. The agency regulates about 80 percent of the U.S. food supply, including all produce, seafood, and cheeses and excluding meat and poultry. The FFDCA does not empower the FDA to regulate advertising, alcohol, drugs without medical uses, health insurance, pesticides, restaurants and grocery stores, or drinking water other than bottled. Since its passage in 1938, the FFDCA has been amended dozens of times.

The FDA ensures that regulated products are honestly, accurately, and informatively represented to the public. This applies to truthfulness and completeness in product labeling and some marketing communications. The FDA has authority to require certain information on product labels, including standardized nutritional content boxes on food products and information on drug labels about side effects and drug interactions. The FFDCA forbids **misbranding**, and it provides for both civil and criminal actions against inaccurate product labeling.

The FDA approach is mostly reactive—i.e., the agency responds to reports of problems in the food supply. In 2010, responding to a congressional assignment, the Institute of Medicine recommended a risk-based approach that included

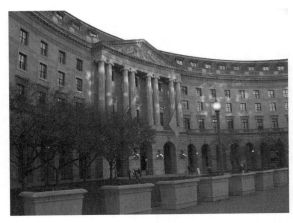

The U.S. Food and Drug Administration is located in Silver Spring, Maryland.

strategic planning, ranking hazards, targeted information gathering, and designing an intervention plan based on data. In essence, the IOM indicated that the FDA should be more proactive. The report also recommended that the FDA develop a set of universal standards and allow state and local authorities to implement them, especially inspections (IOM, 2010).

The work of the FDA can and should be improved. There are 76 million foodborne illnesses in the United States annually. Over 300,000 people are hospitalized and 5,000 die each year because of foodborne illnesses.

Some of the FDA's specific responsibilities include:

- Licensing biologic products and licensing manufacturing establishments
- Maintaining the safety of the nation's blood supply
- Supporting research to establish product standards and develop improved testing methods of biologics and other products
- Promoting safety of cosmetics and enforcing laws against misbranded cosmetics
- Approval of new drugs
- Assuring the accuracy of nonprescription and prescription drug labeling
- Setting and enforcing drug manufacturing standards

- Setting and enforcing standards for food labeling
- Ensuring the safety of all food products except meat and poultry
- Premarket approval of new medical devices
- Setting and enforcing manufacturing and performance standards for medical devices
- Tracking reports of medical device malfunctioning and serious adverse reactions
- Establishing and enforcing safety performance standards for radiation-emitting electronic products such as microwave ovens, television receivers, diagnostic technology, x-ray equipment, laser precuts, and cabinet x-ray systems, such as baggage x-rays at airports
- Assuring safety of ultrasonic therapy equipment, mercury vapor lamps, and sunlamps
- Accrediting and inspecting mammography facilities
- Setting and enforcing standards for veterinary products, including livestock feeds, pet foods, and veterinary drugs and devices

In order to pursue its mission, the FDA inspects processing plants and other facilities that produce or store products under its jurisdiction. The FDA often issues recalls of foods, drugs, and cosmetics that may pose a risk to the public.

EXAMPLES OF FDA RECALLS

Recalls of products regulated by the Food and Drug Administration may be voluntary, FDA requested, or FDA mandated. Examples of recalls are:

- In September 2010, Abbott Laboratories voluntarily recalled Similac powdered infant formula. The company identified a common warehouse beetle, both adult and larvae, in the finished product at a Michigan plant. The FDA determined that consumption of the beetle might cause gastrointestinal distress but posed no immediate health hazard.
- In August 2010, it was determined that eggs from Wright County Eggs and Hillandale Farms in Iowa were contaminated with *Salmonella enteritidis* bacteria. Wright County products are sold in 22 states and Mexico; Hillandale eggs are shipped to 14 states. Over 500 million eggs were recalled.
- In March 2010, Symbiq One- and Two-Channel Infusers were recalled. The infusers pump drugs, nutrients, blood, and other fluids into patients through numerous routes.

(continues)

The potential for unrestricted flow of fluids caused by faulty infusers could result in critical patient injury or death.

- In March 2007, more than 150 brands of pet foods were voluntarily recalled because of contamination with melamine and melamine-related compounds. Melamine is an industrial chemical with no approved use as an ingredient in animal or human food. After reports of several animal deaths and illnesses, the FDA traced the problem to products imported from China. Testing showed that a vegetable protein imported from China mislabeled "wheat gluten" and "rice protein concentrate" contained the melamine compounds. As a result of work by the FDA's Office of Criminal Investigation, two Chinese nationals and the businesses they operated and a U.S. company and two officers were indicted by a federal grand jury.

MedWatch, an FDA program, lists recalls and safety information.

The FDA has the responsibility to approve medications for public use. Pharmaceutical companies present findings of testing for safety and efficacy. Expert advisory committees make recommendations regarding the approval of these products, the accepted uses, and whether they are to be sold with or without a prescription. The FDA generally follows the recommendations of the advisory committees.

Consumers and medical and veterinary providers can submit reports about adverse events and products that may be below standards, including dietary supplements. Reports may be made online.

In June 2009, President Obama signed the Family Smoking Prevention and Tobacco Control Act. The act gave the FDA authority to regulate tobacco products but not to ban existing tobacco products. The agency must review new tobacco products before they go on the market. One of the first regulatory acts was to ban the use of the words "light," "mild," "medium," and "low" on cigarette packaging. The application of these words gave consumers the erroneous impression that the cigarettes labeled with these words pose less health risk than other cigarettes.

Patient Safety Organizations

The Patient Safety and Quality Improvement Act of 2005 was enacted in response to growing concern about patient safety in the United States.

The goal of the act is to improve patient safety by encouraging voluntary and confidential reporting of events that adversely affect patients (Agency for Healthcare Research and Quality, 2008).

The act created patient safety organizations (PSOs). PSOs collect and analyze confidential information reported by health care providers. Data are used to identify and address underlying causal factors of patient safety problems. There appears to be significant underreporting due to fear of discovery of peer deliberations and the fear that information contained in the reports could be used against providers in malpractice cases or in disciplinary proceedings. This results in an inability to compile sufficient patient safety event data for analysis. The act attempts to lessen these fears by providing federal legal privilege and confidentiality protections to information reported to or developed by PSOs. The act also significantly limits the use of this information in criminal, civil, and administrative proceedings. The Office for Civil Rights, under the Department of Health and Human Services, is responsible for enforcing confidentiality and privilege protections of the act. Once PSOs become accepted and information freely reported, they will be able to identify patterns of failures and propose measures to eliminate patient safety risks and hazards.

PSOs may be public or private entities, profit or not-for-profit entities, provider groups, such as hospital chains, and other organizations that establish special PSO components. Insurance companies or their affiliates are not eligible to be PSOs.

The act calls for the establishment of a Network of Patient Safety Databases to provide an interactive, evidence-based management resource for providers, PSOs, and others. The network is to be used to analyze national and regional statistics, including trends and patterns of patient safety events (Agency for Healthcare Research and Quality, 2008).

Environmental Protection Agency

The mission of the U.S. Environmental Protection Agency (U.S. EPA, 2009a) "is to protect human health and to safeguard the natural environment—air, water, and land—upon which life depends." The EPA's purpose is to ensure that:

- All Americans are protected from significant risks to human health and the environment where they live, learn, and work
- National efforts to reduce environmental risk are based on the best available scientific information
- Federal laws protecting human health and the environment are enforced fairly and effectively
- Environmental protection is an integral consideration in U.S. policies concerning natural resources, human health, economic growth, energy, transportation, agriculture, industry, and international trade, and these factors are similarly considered in establishing environmental policy
- All parts of society—communities, individuals, businesses, and state, local, and tribal governments—have access to accurate information sufficient to effectively participate in managing human health and environmental risks
- Environmental protection contributes to making our communities and ecosystems diverse, sustainable, and economically productive
- The United States plays a leadership role in working with other nations to protect the global environment

The EPA administers a wide range of laws and executive orders. Among these are the Atomic Energy Act, the Endangered Species Act, the Occupational Safety and Health Act, the Clean Air Act, the Clean Water Act, and the Resource Conservation and Recovery Act. Many of the agency's responsibilities and actions directly affect and protect consumers. We shall address a few of the laws that fall under the purview of the EPA, but only as illustrations of the agency's consumer protection responsibilities.

The Federal Food, Drug, and Cosmetic Act (U.S. EPA, 2009b) authorizes the EPA to set tolerances, or maximum limits, for pesticide residues on foods. Once a tolerance is established, exceeding the tolerance level is the trigger for enforcement actions, including seizure. In setting tolerances, the EPA must make a finding that the tolerance is "safe." Safe is defined as meaning that there is a "reasonable certainty that no harm will result from aggregate exposure to the pesticide residue." To make the safety finding, the EPA considers, among other things, the toxicity of the pesticide and its breakdown products, aggregate exposure to the pesticide in foods and other sources, and any special risks posed to infants and children. The EPA may grant exemptions in cases where the pesticide residues do not pose a dietary risk under reasonably foreseeable circumstances.

The Safe Drinking Water Act (SDWA) (U.S. EPA, 2009c) was established to protect the quality of drinking water in the United States. This law focuses on all waters actually or potentially designed for drinking use, whether above ground or underground. The act authorizes the EPA to establish minimum standards to protect tap water and requires all owners or operators of public water systems to comply. The 1996 amendments to SDWA require that the EPA consider a detailed risk and cost assessment, and the best available science, when developing these standards. State governments, which can be approved to implement these rules for the EPA, also encourage attainment of secondary standards, those that relate to monetary value, including damage to materials, recreation, natural resources, and community property. Under the act, the EPA also establishes minimum standards for state programs to protect underground sources of drinking water from endangerment by underground injection of fluids.

The EPA protects consumers by enforcing the Toxic Substances Control Act of 1976 (TSCA) (U.S. EPA, 2009d). This act grants the EPA authority to require reporting, record-keeping and testing, and restrictions relating to chemical substances. Certain substances are generally excluded from the TSCA, including food, drugs, cosmetics, and pesticides. The TSCA addresses the production, importation, use, and disposal of specific chemicals including polychlorinated biphenyls (PCBs), asbestos, radon, and lead-based paint. The TSCA compels the EPA to "compile, keep current, and publish a list of each chemical substance that is manufactured or processed in the United States." This inventory currently contains over 83,000 chemicals.

U.S. Department of Agriculture

The mission of the U.S. Department of Agriculture (USDA) is to "provide leadership on food, agriculture, natural resources, and related issues based on sound public policy, the best available science, and efficient management." The department's vision statement is: "We want to be recognized as a dynamic organization that is able to efficiently provide the integrated program delivery needed to lead a rapidly evolving food and agriculture system" (USDA, 2009). In carrying out its mission and vision, the USDA performs many consumer protection functions.

Perhaps nothing is more important than protecting children from hunger. The food assistance programs of the USDA's Food and Nutrition Service provide children and low-income people access to food, a healthful diet, and nutrition education. Nearly one-fifth of all Americans are assisted by these programs. The programs include the Women, Infants, and Children Program, known as WIC; the Supplementary Nutrition Assistance Program, formerly known as Food Stamps; the National School Lunch Program; the Fresh Fruit and Vegetable Program; and the Child and Adult Care Food Program.

The USDA furnishes a number of educational and outreach services for consumers and educators. These include a collection of educational materials for teachers, parents, and students featuring valuable learning tools on various aspects of agriculture, health, nutrition, and science as well as an extensive collection of resources for youth pertaining to all aspects of agriculture, including animals, nutrition, fire safety, and the outdoors. The Food and Nutrition Information Center, a leader in food and human nutrition information dissemination, provides credible and practical resources for nutrition and health professionals, educators, government personnel, and consumers.

The USDA's Food Safety Information Center provides online mechanisms for reporting problems with foods and for locating information about food-borne illnesses. The Center's Web site, www.foodsafety.gov, provides tips for preparation, cooking, and storage of food. It also contains information about recalls, inspection, and compliance.

The Food Safety and Inspection Service, a part of the USDA, is responsible for ensuring that the nation's commercial supply of meat, poultry, and egg products is safe, wholesome, and correctly labeled and packaged. The FSIS responds to complaints and reports of illness and contaminated foods. It frequently uses its authority to recall food products. When sanitary conditions or practices at slaughtering or processing facilities create health hazards, or for certain other violations, the FSIS will issue a Notice of Ineligibility requiring the business to stop operations. The business has the opportunity to correct the violations, contest the FSIS's actions at a hearing, or enter into a settlement or consent agreement with the FSIS. The Residue Violators Alert List is published monthly and contains names of individuals or firms responsible for repeat drug, pesticide, or other chemical residue violations in animals presented for slaughter. The FSIS Quarterly Enforcement Reports provide a summary of the enforcement actions FSIS has taken to ensure that products that reach consumers are safe, wholesome, and properly labeled (USDA, FSIS, 2009). The FSIS also certifies establishments that export food and food products to the United States and may, with justification, decertify those establishments.

United States Postal Inspection Service

The U.S. Postal Inspection Service is one of the country's oldest federal law enforcement agencies. Its history goes back to the eighteenth century when postmaster Benjamin Franklin was given the assignment of "regulating the several post offices and bringing the postmasters to account." The Service has a history of fighting criminals who attack our nation's postal system and misuse it to defraud, endanger, or otherwise threaten the public. The Postal Inspection Service is highly specialized, performing investigative and security functions. The Service provides assurance to American businesses for the safe exchange of funds and securities through the U.S. Mail; to postal customers of the "sanctity of the seal" in transmitting correspondence and messages; and to postal employees of a safe work environment (U.S. Postal Inspection Service, 2010).

Postal inspectors are federal law enforcement officers who carry firearms, make arrests, and serve federal search warrants and subpoenas. As they enforce more than 200 federal laws, inspectors work closely with U.S. attorneys, other law enforcement agencies, and local prosecutors to investigate postal cases and prepare them for trial. There are about 1,500 postal inspectors, supplemented by a security force of around 650 uniformed postal police officers who are assigned to critical postal facilities throughout the country. The officers provide perimeter security, escort high-value mail shipments, and perform other essential protective functions.

The Postal Inspection Service operates a forensic crime laboratory staffed with forensic scientists and technical specialists. They assist inspectors in analyzing evidence needed for identifying and tracing suspects and in providing expert testimony for cases brought to trial.

Postal inspectors cooperate with other law enforcement agencies in fighting crime. For example, postal inspectors work with Federal Bureau of Investigation agents and state and local police in confiscating shipments of illegal drugs and arresting persons suspected in these cases.

The Service investigates cases of mail fraud, mailbox vandalism, identity theft, false change of address, telemarketing fraud involving the mail, and other illegal activities. The actions and responsibilities of the Service were expanded several years ago to include private packaging and delivery services such as FedEx and UPS.

Mail fraud can take a number of forms. One infamous example was an advertisement for a "breast enlarger" that appeared in several magazines. Once the unsuspecting customer gave a credit card number on a toll-free number, she would be shipped only a hand-held magnifying glass. Another advertisement for the "universal coat hanger" turned out to be only a pair of tenpenny nails and a string. Though the culprits are often closed and moved on after shipping their fraudulent packages and collecting the money, postal inspectors have apprehended suspects in many of these cases.

Postal inspectors investigate allegations of charity fraud, a serious problem in the United States. Scam artists who use the mail to misrepresent charities may be prosecuted under the federal mail fraud statute. The penalty is a fine or up to five years' imprisonment, or both, unless a financial institution is affected. In that case the penalties may be a fine of up to $1 million or imprisonment for up to 30 years, or both. Before contributing to a charity, it would be wise to check it out at the Better Business Bureau's Wise Giving Alliance Web site.

A number of health insurance frauds have been revealed and pursued by postal inspectors. Elderly persons are most often the targets. Some policies offered to seniors through mailed advertisements and in other ways are offered by unscrupulous companies and salespeople. Recipients of these offers, especially elderly recipients, should discuss the offer with a knowledgeable friend or relative or with an accountant, attorney, or other trusted adviser. A wise consumer will also notify the local postmaster, the nearest postal inspector, the state insurance commissioner, or the office of the state attorney general about deceptive health insurance promotions received through the mail.

State and Local Governmental Protection

The constitution of each state gives its government the power to regulate commerce conducted solely within that state. Most also have laws banning false advertising. This is similar to the powers given to the federal government by the U.S. Constitution.

Although the structures of state and local governmental consumer protection differ, all states offer some form of protection services. Commonly, the office of the state attorney general bears responsibility for consumer protection. In the case of advertising and business practices, states usually only pursue complaints rather than seeking out violations. Many offices are poorly staffed, and consumer protection is sometimes not a high priority, since the attorney general is mandated to pursue a wide array of criminal and civil cases.

Some of the many consumer protection functions carried out by the state consumer protection offices are:

- Education, including pamphlets and tip and fact sheets
- Licensing and regulating various professions, including insurance agents and health care practitioners
- Offering consumer complaint phone lines and Web sites
- Investigating consumer scams, usually initiated by complaints
- Enforcing consumer protection laws through lawsuits or criminal prosecutions

Each of the 50 states and the District of Columbia have laws governing unfair and deceptive acts and practices (UDAP). These laws protect consumers from predatory, deceptive, and unscrupulous business practices. Health insurance, fitness centers, spas, cosmetology businesses, and businesses that market medications and dietary supplements are examples of health-related

businesses that fall under UDAP statutes. While state attorneys general can file charges against advertisers who violate state and local laws, they do so only in the most widespread and egregious cases. Relative to UDAP protections and their enforcement, Carter (2009) wrote, "The holes are glaring. Legislation or court decisions in dozens of states have narrowed the scope of UDAP laws or granted sweeping exemptions to entire industries. Other states have placed substantial legal obstacles in the path of officials charged with UDAP enforcement, or imposed ceilings as low as $1,000 on civil penalties. And several states have stacked the financial deck against consumers who go to court to enforce the law themselves." She cited the following specific findings:

- Court decisions in Michigan and Rhode Island have interpreted UDAP statutes as applicable to almost no consumer transactions.
- Insurance companies in 24 states enjoy immunity from UDAP laws.
- Five states—Colorado, Indiana, Nevada, North Dakota, and Wyoming—require the attorney general to provide proof that deceptive practices were done knowingly and intentionally before obtaining an injunction or other relief.
- Five states—Arizona, Delaware, Mississippi, South Dakota, and Wyoming—deny consumers the ability to recover their attorney fees even if they win a case under UDAP.
- Alaska's UDAP statute and court cases in other states require unsuccessful consumers to pay all or part of the attorney fees incurred by the business, even if the consumers filed suit in good faith.

Carter also noted that 43 states and the District of Columbia have UDAP statutes that include a broad prohibition against deception that is enforceable by both consumers and a state agency. Thirty-nine states and the District of Columbia have UDAP statutes that include at least a fairly broad prohibition against unfair and unconscionable acts. Only 27 states and the District of

Columbia give rulemaking authority to a state agency. Because of inadequate funding and staffing shortages, states often fail to enforce their UDAP laws.

Larger states attempt to localize consumer protection by providing consumer protection offices in the counties or cities. For example, California has 18 county and at least 3 city offices that provide consumer protection services.

Many large cities have provisions in their charters and statutes that address consumer interests, including false and deceptive advertising. Some have consumer protection agencies. For example, New York City has a Department of Consumer Affairs that mediates consumer complaints, licenses 55 industries, enforces the city's consumer protection law, litigates against businesses accused of violating the city's rules, and provides education about consumer rights and businesses' responsibilities.

State and local health departments also provide consumer protection by establishing and enforcing standards for food handling, the practice of cosmetology and barbering, and the operation of swimming pools and other recreational facilities. State or city codes often describe the standards of food storage, sanitation, and employee training. Inspectors visit businesses and evaluate their compliance with standards, but the visits provide only a "snapshot" of a business's practice rather than a long-term view of how it consistently performs. Citizens can report perceived infractions. Sometimes these reports result in unscheduled inspections. In extreme cases, businesses can lose their licenses to operate.

Establishments that produce food have the option to apply for federal or state inspection. States operate under a cooperative agreement with the Food Safety Inspection Service of the U.S. Department of Agriculture. States' programs must enforce requirements at least equal to those imposed under the Federal Meat Inspection Act and the Poultry Products Inspection Act. However, food produced under state inspection is limited to intrastate commerce. The FSIS provides up to 50 percent of the state's operating funds, as well as training and other assistance.

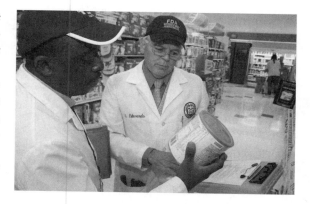

Food inspectors evaluate and enforce compliance with local and state ordinances relating to food preparation, food handling, equipment, and facilities. For many inspectors, education is a vital part of their work.

Nongovernmental Protection Agencies

Better Business Bureau

The Better Business Bureau (BBB) is a nonprofit, nongovernmental organization. It is dedicated to promoting good business practices and informing and protecting consumers. It has offices in more than 120 locations in the United States and Canada. The Council of Better Business Bureaus of the United States is located in Arlington, Virginia, and the Canadian Council of Better Business Bureaus is located in Toronto, Ontario.

The BBB has established the "Standards of Trust" to which member businesses are expected to adhere. They include transparency, so that the nature, ownership, policies, and procedures that affect the purchasing decision are identified; advertising honestly; responding quickly and professionally to marketplace disputes; safeguarding privacy; and conducting business commitments with integrity.

The BBB invites a business to be a member after determining that the business meets the Bureau's standards. The business is then accredited. Businesses pay a fee to be members of the BBB. Membership affords prestige and is an indication of integrity. There are hundreds of thousands of community businesses that voluntarily agree to abide by the BBB's ethical standards. BBB accreditation does not mean that the business's products or services have been evaluated or are endorsed by the BBB.

Consumer and Business Services

The BBB offers a wide array of services for consumers and businesses. For example, it publishes consumer alerts, available on its Web site. Examples of alerts describe scam artists targeting small businesses, phony Social Security scams, and **pyramid schemes** masquerading as gifting clubs. These alerts are updated regularly.

The Bureau also accepts complaints about businesses and their practices regardless of the membership status of the business. Complaints are presented to the business for information. If the business does not wish to resolve the complaint itself, the BBB offers conciliation, mediation, and arbitration services to try to reach a satisfactory conclusion. This is an alternative to going to court. Conciliation is an effort to encourage open communication and discussion leading to a resolution. In mediation, BBB provides a professionally trained mediator to talk with the parties and guide them in working out their own mutually agreeable solutions. Arbitration often follows when conciliation and mediation fail. An impartial arbitrator hears evidence from both parties and makes a decision that is binding on the parties. Local BBBs provide these services for local issues. Some BBB affiliates take advantage of contractual agreements with national companies to resolve disputes. In addition, unique programs have been developed to help customers with certain types of marketplace problems such as auto warranty/lemon law and moving and storage.

The BBB records the results of consumer complaints. Future consumers can request information about a business, and the BBB will provide the number of complaints and the number that were satisfactorily resolved, useful information to a consumer who is trying to select a company with which to do business.

The BBB provides free reports on businesses that include background, licensing, consumer experience, and government actions. These free reports are available even for businesses that have not been evaluated against BBB standards. Consumers should use this service before making large purchases.

The BBB is a partner in the U.S. Department of Defense Financial Readiness Campaign. A BBB Military Line offers a variety of free consumer services and materials to military personnel, retirees, Department of Defense civilian employees, and their families. Much of the news and information is specific to the branch of service—i.e., the Army, Navy, Air Force, Marine Corps, or Coast Guard. There is a BBB Military Line e-newsletter that contains information that promotes more prepared consumers and teaches how to avoid scams.

With the proliferation of Internet businesses, the Bureau established BBB*OnLine,* a program that offers two Web site honor programs, the Online Privacy Program and Reliability Seal Programs. The Privacy Program addresses how a Web site uses personally identifiable information it collects from Web site visitors. The Reliability Seal indicates that the company is a member of the local BBB, has met truth-in-advertising and other high business practice standards, has been in business for at least one year, and is committed to dispute resolution (BBB*OnLine,* 2010). Other BBB services, including accepting complaints and dispute resolution, are available through BBB*OnLine.*

Advertising Review

The BBB maintains a system of advertising review. An alliance of the Council of Better Business Bureaus, the Association of National Advertisers, the American Association of Advertising Agencies, and the American Advertising Federation forms the National Advertising Review Council (NARC). The NARC's mission is to foster truth and accuracy in national advertising through self-regulation. It attempts to provide a flexible alternative to government regulation while increasing public trust in the credibility of advertising. The system makes recommendations and reports on local and national advertising in the United States and Canada. In order to ensure the impartiality of the self-regulatory system, it is administered by the Council of BBBs. The NARC sets policy for the National Advertising Division (NAD) of the Council of BBBs, the Children's Advertising Review Unit (CARU), the National Advertising Review Board, and the Electronic Retailing Self-Regulation Program (ERSP).

One of the purposes of the NAD is to foster public confidence in advertising. The NAD reviews national advertising for truthfulness and accuracy. Policy and procedures for the NAD are established by the NARC. When a consumer complaint is filed, the NAD provides a written decision within 60 business days, usually while the ad campaign is still running. The NAD keeps confidential all data it receives in reviewing a case, unlike the procedure with judicial files. The speed and cost containment are beneficial to both advertisers and consumers.

The Children's Advertising Review Unit of the Council of BBBs, the children's branch of the advertising industry's self-regulation system, promotes responsible children's advertising as part of an alliance with the major advertising trade associations through the NARC. The CARU evaluates advertising that targets children and promotional material in all media to press for truthfulness, accuracy, and consistency with its Self-Regulatory Program for Children's Advertising and applicable laws. When child-directed ads are found to be misleading, inaccurate, or inconsistent with the Self-Regulatory Program for Children's Advertising, the CARU seeks change through the voluntary cooperation of advertisers (Better Business Bureau, 2010a). For example, in 2010, the CARU determined that a broadcast advertisement for Chuck E. Cheese did not adequately disclose which items were included in a birthday party package. Though it disagreed with the CARU's finding, the company changed its commercial.

When an advertiser disagrees with a decision made by the NAD or the CARU, the advertiser may appeal the ruling to the National Advertising Review Board (NARB), the appellant wing of the advertising industry's system of self-regulation. Policy and procedures for the NARB are established by the National Advertising Review Council (National Advertising Review Board, 2005).

The Electronic Retailing Self-Regulating Program is funded by the Electronic Retailing Association and managed as a separate self-regulatory program under the NARC and administered by the Council of BBBs. The mission of the ERSP is to enhance consumer confidence in electronic retailing. According to the BBB, "ERSP provides an effective mechanism for evaluating, investigating, analyzing, and resolving inquiries regarding the truthfulness and accuracy of performance claims in national **direct response advertising**." The ERSP maintains its own monitoring program from which cases can emerge. They may also originate from inquiries brought by competitors and consumers. The ERSP offers a swift system for review of advertising alleged to contain untrue or unsubstantiated claims (Better Business Bureau, 2010b).

Charity Reports and Standards

The BBB provides a list of charity reports completed by the BBB Wise Giving Alliance. The Bureau has developed Charity Accountability Standards that serve as a guide to ethical governance, fund-raising, and expenditure of resources. The BBB Web site contains reports on compliance with the standards by the agencies. Donors would be wise to visit the site and learn about a charity's compliance with the standards before deciding to give.

Consumer Federation of America

The Consumer Federation of America (CFA; 2010) is a membership organization of nearly 300 nonprofit organizations and over 50 million individuals. The sheer size of the CFA enables it to exert significant influence.

Advocacy is a major CFA role as it works to advance pro-consumer policy on a variety of issues before Congress, regulatory agencies, state legislatures, and the courts. The staff works with public officials to promote policies that benefit consumers and to oppose those that may be harmful. The CFA is also a research organization, investigating consumer issues, behavior, and attitudes to assist and inform policy makers, consumer advocates, and individual consumers. To support its education function, the CFA uses conferences, reports, books, brochures, news releases, a newsletter, and a Web site to disseminate information. The CFA also provides support to national, state, and local organizations committed to advocacy, research, and education about consumer issues.

Consumers Union

Consumers Union (CU) is an independent, nonprofit organization whose mission is to work for a fair, just, and safe marketplace for all consumers. CU publishes *Consumer Reports* and maintains ConsumerReports.org, a comprehensive source for unbiased information about products and services, health and nutrition, and other consumer concerns. CU also publishes two newsletters, *Consumer Reports on Health* and *Consumer Reports Money Adviser,* with combined subscriptions of more than eight million. In order to assist consumers in making health-related decisions, CU launched ConsumerReportsHealth.org and the Consumer Reports Health Rating Center in 2008. Consumers Union also has more than 600,000 online activists who help work to change legislation and the marketplace in favor of the consumer interest. Since its founding in 1936, Consumers Union has never taken any advertising or free merchandise (ConsumersUnion.org, 2010).

The organization maintains 50 state-of-the-art labs in Yonkers, New York, and a 327-acre auto test facility in East Haddam, Connecticut. Product testing and evaluation is a key CU function. Reports of this testing are presented in its publications and often in the news. Consumers should consult this valuable resource before making any major purchase.

CU also has three advocacy offices, in Washington, D.C.; Austin, Texas; and San Francisco, California. Advocating for product quality and safety is a major effort. Representatives of CU testify before federal and state legislative and regulatory bodies and petition government agencies.

AARP

AARP, formerly known as the American Association of Retired Persons, employs a variety of strategies to assist members in protecting themselves from fraud and deceptive practices. The organization publishes a magazine that contains informative articles about food, health, money, and family. The AARP Web site contains information about health in the retirement years. In addition, AARP maintains a powerful lobbying presence in Washington, influencing legislation that affects older persons.

National Consumers League

The National Consumers League (NCL) is a private, nonprofit advocacy group representing consumers on marketplace and workplace issues. The mission of the NCL is to protect and promote social and economic justice for consumers and workers in the United States and abroad. The NCL provides government, businesses, and other organizations with the consumer's perspective on concerns including child labor, privacy, food safety, and medication information (National Consumers League, 2010).

The NCL offers numerous publications designed to educate the public. Topics include what to do if your insurer denies your health claim, dietary supplements, generic drugs, food and drug interactions, mammograms, stress, irradiated food, and over-the-counter medications. The league also offers publications that help consumers avoid fraud.

The NCL operates a Fraud Center at www .fraud.org. The Center provides information about scams, telemarketing and Internet fraud, and counterfeiting. It also has news releases relating to fraud.

The NCL advocates on behalf of workers and consumers in both the United States and overseas. The League participates in nearly 50 coalitions, advisory committees, and boards. Representatives of NCL have given expert testimony, comments, and speeches representing consumers' perspectives on concerns including child labor, privacy on the Internet, food safety, and medication information.

The League commissions surveys and focus groups in order to expose consumers' attitudes and knowledge on issues, including those related to health. Results are used to help formulate the NCL's policies and advocacy work on behalf of consumers.

The NCL coordinates the Alliance Against Fraud in Telemarketing and Electronic Commerce. The Alliance is a coalition of interest groups, trade associations, labor unions, businesses, law enforcement agencies, educators, and consumer protection agencies. It promotes efforts to educate the public about various types of fraud, including telemarketing and Internet fraud. It publishes a quarterly electronic newsletter titled *Focus on Fraud*.

The National Coalition for Consumer Education is coordinated by the National Consumers League. It develops and provides educational materials and resources to consumer educators. The NCCE also sponsors LifeSmarts, a game-show competition for teens in grades 9 through 12 (General Services Administration, 2010).

The National Consumer Protection Technical Resource Center

The National Consumer Protection Technical Resource Center (NCPTRC) is funded by the U.S. Administration on Aging. It supports the Senior Medical Patrol Programs (SMP). SMPs help Medicare and Medicaid beneficiaries avoid, detect, and prevent health care fraud. They protect older persons and help preserve the integrity of the Medicare and Medicaid programs (NCPTRC, 2009). The SMPs use the skills and expertise of retired professionals to educate communities to take an active role in fighting health fraud and abuse, particularly in the Medicare and Medicaid programs. Thousands of volunteers and hundreds of partnerships help make SMPs work.

Health Research Group and Public Citizen

Health Research Group (HRG) is a division of the broader Public Citizen (PC) organization. HRG works for protection against unsafe food, drugs, medical devices, and workplaces. It also advocates for greater consumer control over personal health choices. HRG promotes openness and accountability in government and fights for the right of consumers to seek relief in the courts; for clean, safe, and sustainable energy sources; for social and economic justice in trade policies; for strong health, safety, and environmental protections; and for safe, effective, and affordable prescription drugs and health care (Public Citizen, 2009).

HRG publishes a monthly "Health Letter" on prescription drugs. It has published a well-respected critique of medications titled *Worst Pills, Best Pills* and maintains an informative Web site titled Worstpills.org.

Public Citizen, with a membership of 80,000, works in the judiciary, executive branch agencies, and the legislatures to protect consumers. For example, working with the Natural Resources Defense Council, PC won a lawsuit in 2009 against the Consumer Product Safety Commission, stopping the agency from allowing phthalate-laden children's products that were made before a ban of such items, to be sold after the ban took effect. In the same year, the U.S. Food and Drug Administration granted PC's 2008 petition requiring strong warnings to be issued to doctors and patients about the dangers associated with the use of botulinum toxin (Botox, Myobloc, Dysport). In 2008, bowing to pressure from PC, Congress passed the Consumer Product Safety Improvement Act that makes critical reforms to the Consumer Product Safety Commission.

Accrediting and Certification Agencies

Accreditation is a process that indicates that an institution meets certain predetermined criteria and that it achieves what it says it achieves. There are a number of agencies that provide accreditation and **certification** to health care organizations. These recognitions are a form of consumer protection because they indicate that an independent body has examined a health care organization and has been satisfied that the organization is performing according to strict criteria. They are valuable tools for consumers because they encourage facilities to find and fix systemic problems.

The Joint Commission

The Joint Commission (TJC) is a leader in developing the highest standards for quality and safety in the delivery of health care, and evaluating organizations' performance based on those standards. More than 18,000 health care organizations and programs are evaluated and accredited by TJC. Providers use the standards to guide their delivery of care and to improve performance. TJC accredits almost 12,000 psychiatric, children's, rehabilitation, and critical access hospitals as well as home care organizations, hospice care services, nursing homes, and other health care organizations that provide long-term care, behavioral health care, laboratory, and ambulatory care services. The Joint Commission has the capability and experience to evaluate health care organizations across the continuum of care (TJC, 2010). Consumers should attempt to learn if their health care facility is accredited prior to entering into an insurance contract that requires use of that facility.

TJC also provides certification. The Disease-Specific Care Certification Program was inaugurated in 2002. It is designed to evaluate clinical programs of every type and level of care. TJC-accredited organizations may seek certification for treatment of virtually any chronic disease or condition, including lung cancer, diabetes, brain injury rehabilitation, and chemical dependency. Certification is earned by programs or services that may be based within or associated with a health care organization. The Joint Commission has developed an advanced level of certification in several clinical areas—chronic kidney disease, chronic, obstructive pulmonary diseases, heart failure, inpatient diabetes, lung volume reduction surgery, primary stroke centers, and ventricular assist devices. These programs must meet the requirements for Disease-Specific Care Certification plus additional, clinically specific requirements and expectations.

The Health Care Staffing Services Certification Program evaluates a staffing firm's ability to provide qualified and competent staffing services for health care providers such as hospitals and nursing homes. Companies seeking this certification provide temporary clinical staff to health care facilities.

National Committee for Quality Assurance

The National Committee for Quality Assurance (NCQA) accredits health maintenance organizations and other managed care entities. NCQA Health Plan Accreditation helps employers and consumers distinguish among health plans based on quality and value. The NCQA process uses a unified set of standards for managed care organizations, including health maintenance organizations, preferred provider organizations, and point-of-service plans (see Chapter 4 for an explanation of insurance plans). The accreditation process evaluates the systems and processes employed by the health plan. More important, it also evaluates the results that the plan achieves on dimensions of care, service, and efficiency. A meticulous accreditation survey process includes onsite and offsite evaluations conducted by a team of physicians and managed care experts (NCQA, 2010).

URAC

The mission of URAC (formerly known as the Utilization Review Accreditation Commission), an independent nonprofit organization, is to promote continuous improvement in the quality and efficiency of health care management through accreditation and education. URAC offers a wide range of quality benchmarking programs and services designed to stay abreast of the rapid changes in the health care system. Its accreditation validates organizations' commitment to quality and accountability (URAC, 2010).

URAC accredits many types of health care organizations, including medical management organizations, health call centers, health plans (HMOs, PPOs, etc.), hospitals, and health Web sites. It offers accreditation and certification in over 16 areas, including drug therapy management, consumer education and support, health provider credentialing, and claims processing.

Community Health Accreditation Program

The Community Health Accreditation Program (CHAP) is an independent, nonprofit accrediting body that began as a joint endeavor of the American Public Health Association and the National League of Nursing. The program's purpose is to objectively validate the excellence of community health care practice through consistent measurement of the delivery of quality services. CHAP provides accreditation for community-based health care organizations, including organizations that provide health care supplies and equipment and hospice care.

CHAP has regulatory authorization to survey agencies providing home health and hospice services to determine if they meet the Medicare Conditions of Participation. This gives the program much power in determining if an agency is eligible for Medicare funding. This authority motivates providers to strive for continuous improvement. It also assists the public in determining which providers meet the standards of excellence (CHAP, 2010).

Other Accrediting or Certification Organizations

The American Heart Association recognizes institutions that treat heart attacks and/or strokes according to specific guidelines. These guidelines are backed by evidence of effectiveness.

The National Accreditation Program for Breast Centers is led by the American College of Surgeons and includes a consortium of 15 other organizations. The program recognizes breast cancer centers that adhere to 27 practice guidelines established by expert medical groups. For example, there are guidelines pertaining to physician credentials, diagnosing with standard-of-care needle biopsies rather than open surgery, ensuring that every patient is assigned a nurse to help her navigate the system, and medication timing. Reporting is followed by a site visit by the certifying groups' outside experts.

The Commission on Cancer is a program of the American College of Surgeons. There are 36 standards by which programs are evaluated. The key elements of success in achieving accreditation are state-of-the-art pretreatment evaluation, staging, treatment, and clinical follow-up for cancer patients; leadership of the hospital's cancer committee in setting goals, monitoring activity, evaluating patient outcomes, and improving care; cancer conferences for patient consultation and physician education; evaluating and improving patient outcomes through a quality improvement program; and the use of a cancer registry and database as the basis for monitoring the quality of care (American College of Surgeons, 2009). Between 70 and 80 percent of cancer patients receive treatment at a Commission-accredited hospital.

SUMMARY

There are a number of state and federal agencies that provide consumer protection. These agencies are established by law and enforce laws. Many of these agencies are charged with developing regulations and enforcing them. Examples of such federal agencies include the Federal Trade Commission, the Food and Drug Administration, and the Consumer Product Safety Commission.

Several private, nongovernmental agencies provide consumer protection services. These agencies are usually nonprofit organizations that depend on membership dues and fees for their financial support. They have no powers to enforce laws. Some of these agencies wield a lot of influence on consumer behavior. For example, many consumers use information from the Better Business Bureau or the Consumers Union before making a major purchase.

Some agencies provide credibility to service providers by bestowing accreditation and certification. These recognitions demonstrate that the providers adhere to previously agreed-upon standards of practice.

KEY TERMS

Accreditation: a process that indicates that an institution meets certain criteria and that it achieves what it says it achieves

Certification: a recognition that an individual, institution, or program meets certain criteria for excellence; usually more specific than accreditation

Direct response advertising: advertising in which the intermediary in the purchase process is eliminated and the only connection the consumer has to the product is the advertising and the only way a consumer can act on the advertisement or commercial is to return a coupon or make a phone call

Misbranding: advertising or labeling a product in a manner that is misleading

Pyramid schemes: fraudulent money-making schemes in which people are recruited to make payments to others above them in a hierarchy while expecting to receive payments from people recruited below them

STUDY QUESTIONS

1. What are the responsibilities of the Federal Trade Commission?
2. What are the responsibilities of the Consumer Product Safety Commission? How does it carry out its responsibilities?
3. What are the functions of the Food and Drug Administration?
4. What are patient safety organizations? Why were they established? What do they do?
5. What are the purposes of the Environmental Protection Agency? What are some of the laws it enforces?
6. What are the consumer protection responsibilities of the U.S. Department of Agriculture?
7. What consumer protection services are provided by the U.S. Postal Inspection Service?
8. How do state and local governments protect consumers?
9. What services are provided by the Better Business Bureau? How does the Council of Better Business Bureaus protect the rights of consumers and businesses?
10. What services are provided by the Consumer Federation of America?
11. How does the Consumers Union protect consumers? What services does it offer?
12. What is AARP and what does it do to protect its members?
13. How does the National Consumers League protect and promote social and economic justice?
14. What is the relationship between the National Consumer Protection Technical Resource Center and Senior Medical Patrol Programs? What do SMPs do?
15. What are Public Citizen and the Health Research Group? What do they do to educate and advocate for consumers?
16. What are accreditation and certification? What are some of the agencies that offer these services? Why are they important?

REFERENCES

Agency for Healthcare Research and Quality. (2008). *The Patient Safety and Quality Improvement Act of 2005.* Retrieved from http://www.ahrq.gov/qual/psoact.htm

American College of Surgeons. (2009). *Cancer program accreditation*. Retrieved from http://www.facs.org/cancer/coc/whatis.html

BBB*Online*. (2010). *Frequently asked questions*. Retrieved from http://www.bbbonline.org/Privacy/answer.asp

Better Business Bureau. (2010a). *Children's Advertising Review unit*. Retrieved from http://www.bbb.org/us/children-advertising-review-unit/

Better Business Bureau. (2010b). *Electronic Retailing Self-Regulation Program*. Retrieved from http://www.bbb.org/us/electronic-retailing-self-regulation-program/

Carter, C. L. (2009). *Consumer protection in the states: A 50-state report on unfair and deceptive acts and practices statutes.* Boston: National Consumer Law Center. Retrieved from http://www.consumerlaw.org/issues /udap/content/UDAP_Report_Feb09.pdf

Community Health Accreditation Program. (2010). *About CHAP.* Retrieved from http://www.chapinc.org /aboutus.htm

Consumer Federation of America. (2010). *About CFA.* Retrieved from http://www.consumerfed.org/about /default.asp

ConsumersUnion.org. (2010). *About Consumers Union.* Retrieved from http://www.consumersunion.org /about

General Services Administration. (2010). *Consumer Action Handbook.* Washington, DC: Author.

Institute of Medicine. (2010). *Enhancing food safety: The role of the Food and Drug Administration.* Washington, DC: National Academy of Sciences.

The Joint Commission. (2010). *Facts about joint commission accreditation and certification.* Retrieved from http:// www.jointcommission.org/AboutUs/Fact_Sheets/ facts_jc_acrr_cert.htm

National Advertising Review Board. (2005). *National Advertising Review Board.* Retrieved from http://www .narbreview.org

National Committee for Quality Assurance. (2010). *Health plan accreditation.* Retrieved from http://www.ncqa .org/tabid/689/Default.aspx

National Consumers League. (2010). *About NCL.* Retrieved from http://nclnet.org/mission

National Consumer Protection Technical Resource Center. (2009). *About us: Who are the SMPs?* Retrieved from http://smpresource.org

Public Citizen. (2009). *About Public Citizen.* Retrieved from http://www.citizen.org/about/

URAC. (2010). *About URAC.* Retrieved from http://www .urac.org/about/

U.S. Consumer Product Safety Commission. (2008). *CPSC overview.* Retrieved from http://www.cpsc.gov/about /about.html

U.S. Consumer Product Safety Commission. (2010). *Frequently asked questions.* Retrieved from http://www .cpsc.gov/about/faq.html

U.S. Consumer Product Safety Commission. (2010, January 17). *CPSC approves strong new crib safety standards to ensure a safe sleep for babies and toddlers* (press release). Retrieved from http://www.cpsc.gov /cpscpub/prerel/prhtml11/11074.html

U.S. Department of Agriculture. (2009). *About USDA: Mission statement.* Retrieved from http://www .usda.gov

U.S. Department of Agriculture, Food Safety and Inspection Service. (2009). *Regulatory enforcement.* Retrieved from http://origin-www.fsis.usda.gov/Regulations_& _Policies/Regulatory_Enforcement/index.asp

U.S. Environmental Protection Agency. (2009a). *Our mission and what we do.* Retrieved from http://www.epa.gov /epahome/whatwedo.htm

U.S. Environmental Protection Agency. (2009b). *Summary of the Federal Food, Drug, and Cosmetic Act.* Retrieved from http://www.epa.gov/lawsregs/laws /ffdca.html

U.S. Environmental Protection Agency. (2009c). *Summary of the Safe Drinking Water Act.* Retrieved from http:// www.epa.gov/lawsregs/laws/sdwa.html

U.S. Environmental Protection Agency. (2009d). *Summary of the Toxic Substances Control Act.* Retrieved from http:// www.epa.gov/lawsregs/laws/tsca.html

U.S. Postal Inspection Service. (2010). *Mission statement.* Retrieved from https://postalinspectors.uspis.gov /aboutus/mission.aspx

Glossary

Abuse (of drugs): the use of a drug in a manner, in amounts, or in situations such that the use of the drug causes problems or increases the chances that problems will occur; usually excessive or persistent usage without regard to accepted medical practice

Access to health care: the availability and timely use of health services to produce the optimum outcomes

Accreditation: a process that indicates that an institution meets certain criteria and that it achieves what it says it achieves

Acute care clinics: facilities, open to patients with less serious injuries, that accept patients without appointments

Adverse effects (of drugs): effects, other than those for which the drug is being taken, that may occur as a result of its use; also called side effects

Allopathy: methods of diagnosis, treatment, and prevention that have undergone extensive testing in multiple trials and have been shown to exceed agreed-upon standards of safety and effectiveness; also called conventional medicine

Alternative therapy: treatment methods that have not been verified by unbiased clinical trials; a remedy that has not been shown by scientific study to be safe and effective but is used in place of conventional medicine

Analgesics: drugs that relieve pain without loss of consciousness

Anecdotal evidence: evidence based on unscientific observation and accounts of individuals' personal experiences

Attention grabber: words and phrases that offer power to an advertisement and attract interest

Bait-and-switch: when advertised goods or services are withdrawn from the market and other, more expensive and sometimes inferior, goods or services are substituted and offered for sale

Bariatric surgery: surgery performed on obese people for the purpose of helping them lose weight

Basal metabolic rate: the rate at which we burn calories when at rest

Bioavailability (of drugs): amount of the active ingredients of a drug that get into the bloodstream in a specific amount of time

Bioequivalent: describing two or more drugs that perform in the same manner; often used to describe a generic drug in comparison to its brand-name counterpart

Botanical: a plant or plant part valued for its medicinal or therapeutic properties

Brand name: a simple name for a drug applied by the manufacturer and approved by the Food and Drug Administration; the name used in marketing

Catastrophic insurance: a type of fee-for-service health insurance policy that is designed to give protection against momentous tragic health occurrences

Certification: a recognition that an individual, institution, or program meets certain criteria for excellence; usually more specific than accreditation

Chelate: chelator plus metal atom bound together

Chelator: a substance consisting of molecules that bind tightly to metal atoms, thus forcing the metal atoms to go wherever the chelator goes

Chemical equivalent: drugs that contain essentially identical amounts of identical ingredients in identical doses; the term is often used to compare generic drugs to their brand-name counterparts

Chemical name: the complete chemical description of the molecule making up a drug

Coinsurance: the amount the subscriber is required to pay for medical care after the deductible has been met

Community hospitals: nonfederal, short-term general and special hospitals whose facilities and services are available to the public

Complementary therapy: a therapy that has not been accepted as conventional medicine but is used together with conventional medicine

Contraindication: a specific situation in which a drug, procedure, or surgery should not be used

Conventional medicine: methods of diagnosis, treatment, and prevention that have undergone extensive testing in multiple trials and have been shown to exceed agreed-upon standards of safety and effectiveness; also called allopathy or allopathic medicine

Coordination of benefits: a clause in an insurance policy that restricts the total amount paid out by each insurer when there are multiple policies

Copayment: a flat fee that an insured person pays for each use of the health care system

Deceptive advertising: advertising that intentionally deceives or confuses the consumer

Deductible: a fixed amount of medical expenses the subscriber must pay each year before health insurance starts to pay

Dietary supplement: a product (other than tobacco) that is intended to supplement, or be an addition to, the diet and is not represented for use as a conventional food or as a sole item of a meal or the diet and that contains one or more of the following: vitamins, minerals, herbs or other botanicals, amino acids, or any combination of the above ingredients

Direct response advertising: advertising in which the intermediary in the purchase process is eliminated; the only connection the consumer has to the product is the advertising, and the only way a consumer can act on the advertisement or commercial is to return a coupon or make a phone call

Drug interaction: when the effect of a particular drug is altered when it is taken with another drug, a supplement, or with food

Effectiveness (of drugs): a reasonable expectation that, in a significant proportion of the target population, the pharmacological effect, when used under adequate directions for use and warnings against unsafe use, will serve a clinically significant function in the diagnosis, cure, mitigation, treatment, or prevention of disease

Elimination period: the period of time between the beginning of a disability and the time one is eligible for benefits

Endorsement: the use of opinions of experts, including individuals and organizations, or users of products to promote the products

Essential amino acids: those that cannot be manufactured by the body and must be consumed

Exchange: a marketplace of health insurance plans from which consumers may choose

Fad diet: a diet that has little or no nutritional value or scientific credibility and that usually has short-term popularity

Faith healing: a concept that religious belief can bring about healing, through prayers, touch, or rituals that evoke a divine power that cures disease or disability

Fee-for-service: charges are made for each single service that is provided; a type of insurance in which the subscriber pays for a service, submits a claim to the insurance company, and, if the service is covered in the policy, receives reimbursement

Fraud: an intentional act perpetrated to be deceptive in order to gain something of value

Generic name: a short, simple version of the chemical name of a drug

Glycemic index: a system that ranks carbohydrates in individual foods on a gram-for-gram basis in regard to their effect on blood glucose levels in the first two hours after a meal

Group plans: insurance plans, usually offered by employers or large organizations such as professional associations or unions, that allow employees or members to purchase insurance and that keep premiums down because of the large pool of persons covered

Half-truths: deceptive statements that contain some element of truth but are partly false

Health care fraud: an intentional deception or misrepresentation that an individual or entity makes knowing that the misrepresentation could result in some unauthorized benefit to the individual, to the entity, or to some third party

Health fraud: services or articles of unproven effectiveness that are promoted to improve health, well-being, or appearance

Health maintenance organization: type of prepaid medical service in which subscribers pay a monthly or yearly fee for all health care and the organization controls costs and access to specific services

High-deductible plan: a catastrophic insurance plan

Holistic approach: an approach to treatment that includes the entire person—mind, body, and spirit

Hospice care: medical services, emotional support, and spiritual resources for family members and people who are in the last stages of a terminal illness

Hospitalist: a physician who coordinates or assumes much of the care of a hospitalized patient

Impulse buying: a spur-of-the-moment, unplanned purchase

Indemnity insurance: a type of health insurance that requires the subscriber to pay certain charges, such as copayments and deductibles, and which allows the insured to choose his or her health care provider

Infomercial: a broadcast advertisement filling an entire program slot

Informative advertising: advertising that provides the shopper with useful information about the product

Integrative therapy: combining mainstream medical therapies for which there is some high-quality scientific evidence of safety and effectiveness with alternative or even ancient therapies

Ketogenic diet: a high-fat, high-protein diet that includes very few carbohydrates

Lifetime limits: the maximum amount an insurance policy will pay for health services for the life of an individual

Low-calorie diet: a diet providing between 800 and 1,500 calories per day

Major medical plan: insurance plan that covers major hospital and medical expenses

Managed care: a system of delivering and financing health care that is designed to reduce cost and control the use of health care

Measured marketing: marketing activity that has clearly defined and agreed-upon measurements that support the company's business objectives

Misbranding: advertising or labeling a product in a manner that is misleading

Misleading advertising: advertising that intentionally deceives or confuses the consumer

Misrepresentation: false or misleading claims made by an advertiser about its products or services

Misuse (of drugs): use of a drug for purposes for which it is not intended, for appropriate purposes but in improper doses, or in inappropriate combinations

Nonprescription drugs: medications that can be purchased without a prescription; also called over-the-counter drugs

Opportunity cost: something you give up when you decide to do something else

Palming off: when an advertiser creates an impression that its products or services are those that are furnished by a competitor

Phytomedicines: products made from botanicals that are touted to maintain or improve health; also called herbal products or botanical products

Placebo: substance used in medical treatment that has no pharmaceutical effect on the problem it is being used to treat

Placebo effect: a positive response to a product, device, or procedure that cannot be accounted for by pharmacologic or other direct physical action

Point-of-sale displays: displays of products set up at places where payment is made

Preexisting condition: a health problem that existed before one's health insurance goes into effect

Preferred provider organization: a type of managed care organization of health care providers and hospitals that have contracted with an insurer or a third-party administrator to provide health care at reduced rates to the insurer's or administrator's clients

Premium: the amount a person and/or employer pays for insurance coverage

Prescription drugs: medications that require a written order, called a prescription, that gives the user the legal right to purchase and use the drug

Primary care: the entry point for patients into the health care system; it includes diagnosis and treatment of acute and chronic illnesses; it is performed and managed by a personal physician in collaboration with other health professionals

Primary care physician: the physician who handles most of your care and who makes referrals to specialists

Product disparagement: when an advertiser intentionally makes false or misleading negative remarks about a competitor's goods or services, causing the competitor to lose sales

Product placement: promotion by the use of real commercial products and services in media, where the presence of a particular brand is the result of an exchange of money

Puffery: the use of exaggeration, hyperbole, or imagery to market products

Pyramid scheme: a fraudulent scheme in which people are recruited to make payments to others above them in a hierarchy while expecting to receive payments from people recruited below them

Quackery: promotion of health practices or remedies that have no compelling scientific basis

Reasonable, usual, and customary charge: a calculation by an insurer of what it believes is the appropriate fee to pay for a specific health care product or service in a specified geographic area

Regression fallacy: failure to recognize that health conditions change without treatment and ascribing changes in conditions to some therapy

Rescission: a practice used by insurance companies to drop people from coverage once they get sick

Safety: the relative freedom from harmful effect to persons affected, directly or indirectly, by a product when prudently administered, taking into consideration the character of the product in relation to the condition of the recipient at the time

Side effects (of drugs): effects, other than those for which the drug is being taken, that may occur as a result of its use; also called adverse effects

Single-payer health care: a system in which there is one insurer of health care, the government

Testimonial: a written or spoken statement by a person purported to have used a product or service extolling the virtues of the product or service

Unbranded advertisement: communications disseminated to consumers or health care practitioners that discuss a particular disease or health condition, but do not mention any specific drug or device or make any representation or suggestion concerning a particular drug or device; also called disease awareness advertisements

Unmeasured media: a category of advertising that includes strategies for which ad buy data may not be accessible, such as direct mail, sales promotion, couponing, product placement, catalogs, and special events

Very-low-calorie diet: a diet providing fewer than 800 calories per day

Visual imagery: using visual means to promote a vivid conscious experience of something not physically present

Vitalism: a doctrine that the processes of life are not explainable by the laws of physics and chemistry alone and that a force courses through the body that affects physical, mental, and spiritual health

Weasel words: the use of vague words to create the illusion of a promise or commitment

Word-of-mouth marketing: the use of peer-to-peer communication to market a product

Index

A

AARP, 139, 228
accreditation
    agencies, 230–231
    Better Business Bureau, 225
    and chiropractic, 121
    as consumer protection, 215
    and Food and Drug Administration, 219
    of hospitals and health plans, 36, 41
    and managed care, 79
    and National Practitioner Data Bank, 37
    and naturopathy, 116
    and point-of-service plans, 79
    and selecting a health care facility, 41
    and senior living facilities, 42
acute care clinics, 20
acupuncture, 122–125
    and chiropractic, 121
    and homeopathy, 122
    and naturopathy, 115, 124
    regulation, 124
    and traditional Chinese medicine, 128
    adverse effects of drugs, 89–90, 99
advertising, advertisements
    alcohol, 203–204
    attention grabbers, 188
    comedy, 188–189
    informative, 184
    Internet, 208–209
    misleading or deceptive, 184–185
    and nonprescription drugs, 196
    and prescription drugs, 191–196
    product placement, 189–190
    puffery, 184, 185–186
    in schools, 200–202, 204
    sex as advertising technique, 185, 188, 189
    and statistics, 188
    testimonials, 185, 186–187
    tobacco advertisement, 184, 190, 196–197, 202–203
    visual imagery, 188
Agatson, Dr. Arthur, 173
Agency for Healthcare Research and Quality, 12, 28
aging scams, 47, 60
Alli, 175
allopathy, allopathic medicine, 105, 112
alternative treatment, therapy, medicine
    and conventional medicine, 105–106, 112
    and placebo effect, 53
    popularity of, 129
    and reflexology, 125
American Academy of Orthopaedic Surgeons, 14
American Association for Ayurvedic Medicine, 117
American Association of Naturopathic Physicians, 114, 116
American Board of Medical Specialties, 11
American College of Physicians, 28
American College of Rheumatology, 124
American College of Surgeons, 231
American Dietetic Association, 139, 143, 170
American Heart Association, 28, 49, 174, 178, 231
American Medical Association, 69, 101, 122, 162
American Naturopathic Medical Association, 116
amino acids, 135–136, 147–148, 155
aristolochic acid, 131, 141, 153
aromatherapy, 128
Arthritis Foundation, 49
arthritis fraud, 58
assisted living, 41

Association of National Advertisers, 226
Atkins Diet, 171–174
Atkins, Dr. Robert, 171
attention grabbers, 47, 188
Ayurveda, 108, 116–117, 130, 139

B

bait-and-switch, 185
bariatric surgery, 178–179
Bayer, 135
behind-the-counter drugs, 100–101
Better Business Bureau, 225–227
    Children's Advertising Review Unit, 200–201
    and complaints, 49, 209
    and fitness products and services, 57
    and infomercials, 205–206
    Wise Giving Alliance, 223
bioavailability, 90, 92
bioelectromagnetic-based therapies, 108
bioequivalence, 108
biofeedback, 108, 115, 128
biofield therapies, 108
Blue Cross/Blue Shield, 28, 67
Body Mass Index (BMI), 159
botanicals
    as complementary and alternative therapy, 128
    as dietary supplement, 135, 136
    and herbs, 148
    and ingredient list, 152
brand name drugs, 90–92
Brinkley, Dr. John, 51, 52
Burzynski, Stanislaw R., 59
Bush, George W., 70, 100

C

caffeine, 150, 175–176
Campaign for Commercial-Free Childhood, 205
cancer fraud, 58–59
carbohydrate-restricted diets, 170–174
Carter, Jimmy, 70
catastrophic insurance, 77
celebrity advice about health, 57
Center for Alcohol Marketing and Youth, 203
Center for Food Safety and Applied Nutrition, 138

Center for Science in the Public Interest, 201, 205
Centers for Disease Control and Prevention, U.S., 60–61, 110
certification, 11, 37, 37, 230, 231
chemical equivalence, 92
chemical name of drugs, 90, 91
Child and Adult Care Food Program, 222
Children's Advertising Review Unit, 200, 227
Children's Online Privacy Protection Act, 217
chiropractic, 120–122
    as body-based method, 108
    and children, 110
    common therapies, 109
    and homeopathy, 121, 122
    and naturopathy, 116
    regulation, 121
Chopra, Deepak, 117
Christian Science, 126
Church of Scientology, 126–127
Clinton, Bill, 70
Cochran Database of Systematic Reviews, 138–139
coinsurance, 76
Combat Methamphetamine Epidemic Act, 100
comedy in advertising, 188–189
comfrey, 139, 149, 153
commercial weight loss programs, 162, 165–170, 178
Commission on Accreditation of Rehabilitation Facilities, 42
Commission on Cancer, 231
Commission on a High Performance Health System, 29–33
Commonwealth Fund, 29–32
Community Health Accreditation Program, 231
community hospitals, 19
complementary medicine, 105, 108, 112, 124, 129
Congressional Budget Office, 39, 70–71, 72
Consolidated Omnibus Budget Reconciliation Act (COBRA), 38, 70, 79–80
Consumer Federation of America, 227
Consumer Product Safety Commission, 217–218, 229
Consumer Product Safety Improvement Act, 229
Consumer Reports
    and chiropractic, 121–122
    Consumers Union, 228
    and dietary supplements, 137, 139
    and fitness products, 57

and Internet shopping, 15, 57, 121–122
Consumers' Checkbook, 41
Consumers Union, 178, 186, 228
conventional medicine, 105, 131
coordination of benefits, 76
copayments, 54, 73, 78
Council on Chiropractic Education, 121
Council on Naturopathic Medicine, 116
counterfeit drugs, 93, 95–97

D

deductible, 54, 73, 76, 77
dental insurance, 82
Department of Agriculture, U.S., 167, 222–223
Department of Education, U.S., 116, 121
Department of Health and Human Services, U.S., 37, 43, 56, 89, 220
diabetes fraud, 58
Dianetics, 126–127
Dietary Reference Intake, 143, 148
Dietary Supplement and Health Education Act, 49, 153–154
Dietary Supplement and Nonprescription Drug Consumer Protection Act, 155
Dietary Supplement Current Good Manufacturing Practices, 154
dietary supplements
    and allopathic physicians, 107
    athletes, 136, 140, 141, 143
    as biologically-based therapy, 108
    characteristics, 135
    as complementary and alternative therapy, 136
    and conventional medicine, 136
    definition, 128
    and drug interaction, 137, 140
    and herbal products, 127, 129, 148–149
    regulation, 149, 153–156
    research, 140–141
    safety, 137
direct-to-consumer advertising, 60, 93, 191–196
Directory of Medical Specialists, 11
disability insurance, 83
disease coverage insurance, 82
disparities, health, 33
Doctrine of Signatures, 49

Drug Enforcement Administration, 37, 84
drug interaction
    with dietary supplements, 137, 140
    and electronic health records, 31, 35
    guidelines, 91
    and nonprescription (over-the-counter) medications, 98, 99

E

echinacea, 110, 140, 150, 152
Eddy, Mary Baker, 126
ediets.com, 165, 170
effectiveness (of drugs), 87
Eldercare Locator, 41
electromagnetic fields, 128
electronic health (or medical) records, 31, 35
Electronic Orange Book, 92
Electronic Retailing Association, 206, 227
Electronic Retailing Self-Regulatory Program, 206, 209, 227
elimination period, 83
Employee Retirement Income Security Act (ERISA), 37, 70
Encyclopedia of Natural Medicine, 115
endorsements. *See* testimonials
Environmental Protection Agency, 221–222
ephedra, 139, 153, 155, 175
ephedrine, 175–176
Epilepsy Foundation of America, 49
esogenic colorpuncture, 128
exchanges, health insurance, 39–40, 72, 75

F

fad diets, 177–178
Family Smoking Prevention and Tobacco Control Act, 203, 220
faith healing, 126, 129
Federal Communications Commission, 190, 206, 209
Federal Food, Drug, and Cosmetic Act, 113
    advertising prescription drugs, 191
    and authority of the Food and Drug Administration, 218
    and dietary supplements, 148
    definition of drug, 152

and Environmental Protection Agency, 218

and homeopathic remedies, 113

Federal Trade Commission, U.S., 216–217

and commercial weight loss programs, 166

and deceptive advertising, 186

and dietary supplements, 138, 149

and endorsements, 201

and fitness fraud, 57

fraudulent advertising, 62

and genetic tests, 60

and infomercials, 206–207

and Internet complaints, 209

puffery, 185

and quackery, 52

and Trudeau, Kevin

Federal Trade Commission Act, 216

fee-for-service, 67, 76–77, 81

fitness fraud, 47, 56–57

flexible spending account, 84

Food and Drug Administration, U.S., 218–220

and acupuncture needles, 122, 124

advisories, 139

and counterfeit drugs, 96

and diabetes fraud, 58

and dietary supplements, 137, 138, 142, 152–156

and direct-to-consumer advertising, 191–196

and disposal of prescription drugs, 102

Family Smoking Prevention and Tobacco Control Act, 203

and genetic tests, 61

and health fraud, 47, 49

and homeopathy, 113

and influenza scams, 60

and Internet pharmacies, 93–95

and kava kava, 151

and l-tryptophan, 147–148

MedWatch, 97

and nonprescription drugs, 98, 100, 196

and prescription drugs, 88–89, 90, 92

and Public Citizen, 230

regulating bogus products, 62

reporting health fraud, 63

and Trudeau, Kevin, 162

and weight loss, 175–177

and weight loss fraud, 56

Food and Nutrition Information Center, 222

Food Safety Inspection Service, 222, 225

Fresh Fruit and Vegetable Program, 222

G

generic drugs, 91–92, 96, 192

genetic tests, 47, 60–61

germander, 149, 153

ginger, 140, 141, 151

gingko biloba, 140–141, 148, 151

ginseng, 49, 150, 152

glycemic index, 169

group health insurance, 67–68, 71

guided imagery, 105, 109, 128

Guidelines for Responsible Marketing to Children, 201–202

H

Health Care and Education Reconciliation Act (HCERA), 27, 32–36

and costs, 28, 73, 75

coverage and universality, 72–73, 75

and fraud, 73–75

immediate measures, 33

and insurance exchanges, 39–40, 72

and Medicaid, 81–82

and Medicare, 80–81

and models of universal health care, 38–40

and preexisting conditions, 75

as revision of Patient Protection and Affordable Care Act, 24, 68

Health Care Fraud Hotline, 55

Healthcare Integrity and Protection Data Bank, 36–37, 38

health care reform,

and cost of health care, 24

and insurance, 33

legislation of 2010, 68–75

and uninsured, 27–28, 30, 34

universal health care, 38

health education, 34

health fraud

identifying, 47–50

insurance, 54–56

and National Consumers League, 228

and the Patient Protection and Affordable Care Act, 28, 73–75
  reporting, 62–63
  and single payer model, 39
  testimonials, 131
Health Insurance Portability and Accountability Act (HIPAA), 37, 38, 70
Health Maintenance Organization Act of 1973, 39, 67, 69, 77
health maintenance organizations (HMOs)
  accreditation, 231
  comparison with other types of managed care, 79
  and managed care, 77–78
  and Medicare Advantage Plans, 81
  and Medicare Part C, 81
  and national health care system, 70
  and point-of-service plans, 78
  and preferred provider organizations, 78
  and technology, 28
Health Management Resources, 165
health reimbursement arrangements, 83–84
Health Research Group, 229
health savings accounts, 77, 83
health systems agencies, 70
HealthGrades, 12, 41
Healthy People 2010, 23
Healthy People 2020, 23
herbs and herbal supplements, 127, 129, 148–149
  and acupuncture, 122, 123
  and aromatherapy, 128
  and athletic performance, 136, 141
  and Ayurveda, 117
  as biologically based therapy, 108
  and chiropractors, 121
  and dietary supplements, 127–129, 135–136, 148, 155
  and drug interactions, 148
  and homeopathy, 112
  and naturopathy, 115
  research, 149
  and sexual enhancement, 59
  weight loss, 174, 176
high deductible health plan, 77, 83
Hill-Burton Act, 69
HIV/AIDS fraud, 57–58
holistic approach, 106, 112, 114

homeopathy, homeopathic therapy, 112–114
  and acupuncture, 112
  as alternative "medical" system, 108
  and chiropractic, 121, 122
  as common CAM therapy, 109
  and naturopathy, 115
  and popularity, 129
  and regulation, 113–114
hospice care, 20, 75, 80
hospitalist, 34–35
Hubbard, L. Ron, 126–127
human growth hormone, 60
hypnosis, 108

I

indemnity insurance, 33, 67, 76–77
Indian Health Service, 32, 74
influenza scams, 60
infomercials, 205–208
  and CAM remedies, 130
  and dietary supplements, 153
  and quackery, 50
  statistics, 188
  and weight loss, 161
informative advertising, 184
Institute of Medicine
  and advertising toward children, 198, 199
  Committee on the Consequences of Uninsurance, 34
  Committee on Identifying and Preventing Medication Errors, 12
  and Food and Drug Administration, 218–219
  and health insurance, 34
  and medical errors, 22
integrative therapy, 106, 112
International Food Information Council Foundation, 139
Internet pharmacies and prescriptions, 89, 93–95

J

Jenny Craig, 165, 167–168, 178
The Joint Commission, 7, 36, 230

K

kava, 139, 151

L

laetrile, 59, 143
Lane, I. William, 59
Lanham Act, 185, 216–217
licensure, licensing
  and acupuncture, 124
  and ayurveda, 117
  and chiropractic, 120–121
  and Food and Drug Administration, 96
  and Healthcare Integrity and Protection Data Bank, 37
  and homeopathy, 114
  and National Practitioner Data Bank, 36–37
  and naturopaths, 116
  and nurses, 27
  and Patient Protection and Affordable Care Act, 74
  and pharmacies, 93, 96
  and physicians, 11, 36, 106
  and senior living facilities, 42
  state licensing boards, 36
life expectancy at birth, 22
lifetime limits on insurance, 73
long-term care insurance, 83
low-calorie diets, 142, 148
l-tryptophan, 139, 147–148

M

major medical health insurance plans, 76–77
managed care
  accreditation, 231
  and cost management, 33
  and quality assurance, 38
  and regulation, 79
  types, 77–80
massage
  and acupuncture, 122
  and allopathic hospitals, 107
  as alternative "medical" system and manipulative and body-based method, 108
  as common complementary and alternative therapy, 109
  definition, 128
  and naturopathy, 115
  and popularity of alternative treatments, 129

  and reflexology, 126
Master Settlement Agreement, 190, 202
Medicaid, 81–82
  and choosing a physician, 11
  establishment of, 69
  fraud, 6, 28, 54–56, 73
  and Health Care and Education Reconciliation Act, 33, 71, 73–75, 80–81
  and health care reform, 68, 71
  and insurance exchanges, 72
  and medical errors, 23
  and national health care system, 70
  and National Practitioner Data Bank, 36–37
  and Patient Protection and Affordable Care Act, 71, 73–75
  percentage of health care expenditures, 16, 28
  reporting fraud, 12–13, 56, 62
  and senior living facilities, 43
  Senior Medical Patrol Programs, 229
  and State Children's Health Insurance Program, 82
  termination of participation, 36, 37, 38
  underpayment and costs, 28
  waste, 28
medical (and medication) errors, 11, 22, 23
medical specialties, 20–21
Medicare, 80–81
  and acupuncture, 124
  and choosing a physician, 11
  and Community Health Accreditation Program, 231
  and Consolidated Omnibus Reconciliation Act, 70
  establishment of, 69
  fraud, 6, 28, 54–56, 73
  and Health Care and Education Reconciliation Act, 33, 38, 73, 81
  and health reform, 71
  and medical education, 32
  and medical errors, 12
  and national health care system, 70
  and National Practitioner Data Bank, 36–37
  and naturopathic services, 116
  Part A, 80
  Part B, 80
  Part C, 80–81
  Part D, 35, 70, 81

and Patient Protection and Affordable Care Act, 38, 71, 73–75, 81

percentage of health care expenditures, 16, 28

reporting fraud, 12–13, 56, 62

and senior living facilities, 43

Senior Medical Patrol Programs, 229

and single payer model, 39

termination of participation (exclusion), 36, 37, 38

waste, 28

Medicare Advantage, 74, 80–81

Medicare Catastrophic Coverage Act, 70

Medicare Modernization Act, 70

Medifast, 168–169

Medigap, 81

meditation, 105, 108, 117, 128

Mediterranean Diet, 164, 170, 178

MEDLINE, 109

MedWatch, 63, 97, 137, 138, 219

mental healing, 108

Mexico, United States, and Canada Health Fraud Working Group, 56, 58

minerals, 135, 141–147, 155

Minimum Daily Allowances, 142

misleading or deceptive advertisement, 184–185

misrepresentation, 185

N

National Academy of Sciences, 143

National Accreditation Program for Breast Centers, 231

National Advertising Division of the Better Business Bureau, 227

National Advertising Review Board, 227

National Advertising Review Council, 226

National Association of Boards of Pharmacy, 93, 94, 96–97

National Association of Naturopathic Physicians, 115

National Ayurvedic Medical Association, 117

National Center for Complementary and Alternative Medicine

  and acupuncture, 123

  categories of CAM, 108

  and herbs, 149

  and homeopathy, 113

  and kava kava, 151

  and naturopathy, 114

  and Reiki, 188

  and research, 107

  and yoga, 108, 118

National Coalition on Substance Abuse and Addiction, 94

National Committee for Quality Assurance, 230

National Consumer Protection Technical Resource Center, 229

National Consumers League, 96, 193, 228

National Council Against Health Fraud, 114, 121

National Health Planning and Resources Development Act, 70

national health service (or system), 38–39, 70

National Health Service Corps, 32

National Infomercial Marketing Association, 206

National Injury Information Clearinghouse, 217

National Institutes of Health, 107, 138

National Practitioner Data Bank, 36–37

National Research Council, 143

National Task Force on the Prevention and Treatment of Obesity, 168

Natural Medicine Comprehensive Database, 136

naturopathy, 108, 114–116

nonprescription drugs, 97–100, 137. *See also* over-the-counter drugs

nursing home care

  accreditation, 230

  certification, 230

  as indication of quality, 30

  and long-term care insurance policies, 83

  and Medicaid, 81–82

  and Patient Protection and Affordable Care Act, 74

  selecting, 40, 41–43

  and selecting a health insurance plan, 75

Nursing Home Compare, 43

Nutrisystem, 165, 169, 170

O

Obama, Barack

  Family Smoking Prevention and Tobacco Control Act, 203, 220

  Health Care and Education Reconciliation Act, 27, 68, 70

  health care fraud, 74

Patient Protection and Affordable Care Act, 27, 68, 70

OPTIFAST, 165, 168

Orphan Drug Act, 97

orphan drugs, 97

osteopathic manipulation, 108

over-the-counter drugs. *See* nonprescription drugs

Overeaters Anonymous, 170

P

pain relievers, 100

palming off, 185

Patient Protection and Affordable Care Act (PPACA)
    and electronic health (or medical) records, 35
    and fraud, 73–75
    and health care costs, 28, 34, 73, 75
    health care reform, 27–28, 32–36, 68–75
    and health disparities, 24
    and health education, 34
    immediate effects, 71
    and insurance exchanges, 39–40, 72
    and mandated coverage, 73
    and Medicaid, 81–82
    and medical education and training, 32
    and Medicare, 80
    and preexisting conditions, 75
    and tort reform, 36
    and universal coverage of health care, 38, 38–40, 72–73

patient safety organizations, 220–221

Pauling, Linus, 59

Percent Daily Value, 143

Pharmaceutical Research and Manufacturers of America (PhRMA), 193, 194, 195

phenylpropanolamine (PPA), 176

Physicians Desk Reference, 88

placebo effect
    and acupuncture, 123, 124
    anecdotal evidence, 131
    and complementary and alternative medicine (CAM), 129
    and Doctrine of Signatures, 49
    and faith healing, 126
    and testimonials, 47, 53

point of service plans (POS), 78–79, 81, 230

Postal Inspection Service (U.S.), 149, 152, 223–224

Postal Service (U.S.), 62, 209

prayer, 107, 108, 126, 129

preexisting conditions,
    and Health Insurance Portability and Accountability Act, 70
    and Patient Protection and Affordable Care Act, 28, 71, 72, 73
    and selecting a health insurance plan, 75
    and traditional health insurance, 76, 77

preferred provider organization (PPO), 33, 78, 79, 231

premiums, insurance
    and flexible spending accounts, 84
    and fraud, 54, 55
    and group plans, 68
    and Health Care and Education Reconciliation Act, 28, 33, 72
    and health savings accounts, 83
    and insurance exchanges, 40
    and malpractice insurance, 32, 36, 39
    and managed care, 78–80
    and Medicare, 80–81
    and Patient Protection and Affordable Care Act, 28, 71, 72, 73
    and selecting a health insurance plan, 75
    and State Children's Health Insurance Program, 82
    and supplemental insurance, 82–83
    and traditional health insurance, 76–77
    and the uninsured, 27

Prescription Drug Marketing Act, 96

prescription drugs, 88–91. *See also* generic drugs
    abuse by teens, 92–93
    and advertising, 191–196
    and Canada, 95, 96
    cost, 27, 35, 87, 89
    counterfeit drugs, 95–97
    and dietary supplements, 59, 137
    erectile dysfunction, 59
    Food and Drug Administration approval, 89, 90
    guidelines for safe use, 91
    and high deductible health plans, 77
    and homeopathic remedies, 113
    and Internet, 93–94
    labels, 90
    and Medicaid, 82
    and medical errors, 12

Medicare Part D, 35, 70, 81
orphan drugs, 97
with over-the-counter drugs, 98
and Patient Protection and Affordable Care Act, 71
point-of-service plan, 79
and selecting a health insurance plan, 77
and *United States Pharmacopeia*, 91
PriceGrabber.com, 15
PriceSCAN.com, 15
primary care physician (PCP)
    choosing, 11–12
    and family medicine, 21
    getting the most from health insurance, 84
    and Health Care and Education Reconciliation Act, 73
    health maintenance organizations, 78
    and managed care, 79
    and Patient Protection and Affordable Care Act, 73
    and point-of-service plans, 78
    and preventive medicine, 32
    and selecting a hospital, 40
    and selecting a senior living facility, 41
product disparagement, 185
product placement, 189–190, 199, 202, 204, 205
professional standards review organizations, 69–70
progressive relaxation, 109
pseudoephedrine, 100–101
Public Citizen, 88, 229
PubMed, 138
puffery
    and advertising targeting children, 204
    and advertising techniques, 186
    characteristics, 185–186
    and comedy, 189
    and consumer protection, 216
    and direct-to-consumer drug advertising, 192–193
    and over-the-counter drug advertising, 196
    types of advertising, 184
    and visual imagery, 188
    and statistics, 188
pyramid scheme, 62, 226

Q

qi gong, 108, 128
quackery, 47, 50–57, 106

R

Reagan, Ronald, 70
reasonable, usual, and customary charges, 76
recission, 73
Recommended Daily Allowances, 142–143
reflexology, 108, 121, 125–126, 129
regression fallacy, 58, 124
Reiki, 108, 118
religious-based therapy, 126–127
retirement communities, 41
Rolls, Dr. Barbara, 169–170
Roux-en-Y Gastric Bypass, 179

S

Safe Drinking Water Act, 221–222
safety (of drugs), 87, 90, 94, 96
scientific method, 9
Senior Medical Patrol Programs, 229
sex in advertising, 185, 188, 189
Shiatsu, 128
side effects. *See* adverse effects
single payer model, 38, 39
Slim Fast, 12
South Beach Diet, 173, 174
St. John's wort, 130, 139, 150
State Children's Health Insurance Program, 28, 70, 71, 82
supplemental insurance, 82–83
Supplemental Nutrition Assistance Program, 222
supplements. *See* dietary supplements
support groups, 108

T

Take Off Pounds Sensibly (TOPS), 165, 170
testimonials (and endorsements), 186–187
    and complementary and alternative medicine, 131
    and dietary supplements, 136, 137
    and fitness fraud, 57
    and health fraud, 47, 62
    in infomercials, 205
    and misleading advertising, 185
    and nonprescription drugs, 196
    and weight loss, 56, 165, 178, 196

A Textbook of Natural Medicine, 115
therapeutic touch, 108, 128
tort reform, 35–36
traditional Chinese medicine, 128
travel health insurance, 83
Trudeau, Kevin, 161–162, 207–208

U

unbranded advertisement, 193
universal health care, 38–40, 70
unmeasured media, 205
URAC, 230
United States Pharmacopeia, 91

V

Verified Internet Pharmacy Practice Sites, 94, 97
very-low-calorie diets, 168
Veterans Administration, 28, 29, 74
vision insurance, 82
visual imagery, 188
vitalism, vital force, vital energy
    and acupuncture, 122
    and Ayurveda, 117
    and naturopathy, 114, 115
    and qi gong, 128
    and traditional Chinese medicine, 128
vitamins, 141–145, 147
    Dietary Supplement Health and Education Act, 153, 155
    dietary supplements, 135–136

fat soluble vitamins, 144
Food and Drug Administration advisories, 139
and herbs, 148
safe use, 137
water soluble vitamins, 144–145
Volumetrics, 169–170
Voluntary Guidelines for Providers of Weight Loss Products or Services, 166

W

walk-in clinics, 20
weasel words, 187–188
weight loss
    and dietary supplements, 137, 140, 142
    fraud, 47, 56
    guidelines, 163–164
    and nonprescription drugs, 175–177
    and online pharmacies, 94
    and prescription drugs, 91, 177
Weight Watchers, 165, 166–167, 170, 178
White House Office of National Drug Policy, 102
Women, Infants, and Children Program (WIC), 222
Worst Pills, Best Pills, 88, 229

Y

Yoga, 108, 109, 118–120

Z

zone therapy. *See* reflexology

Photo Credits

Chapter 1

Page 2 © Blend Images/ShutterStock, Inc.; **page 5** © Kenneth V. Pilon/ShutterStock, Inc.; **page 11** © Monkey Business Images/Dreamstime.com

Chapter 2

Page 20 © Digital Vision/age fotostock; **page 30** © Alexander Raths/ShutterStock, Inc.

Chapter 3

Page 52 Courtesy of the Kansas State Historical Society

Chapter 4

Page 68 © Xinhua/Landov

Chapter 5

Page 88 © Muellek Josef/ShutterStock, Inc.

Chapter 6

Page 107 © Niday Picture Library/Alamy Images; **page 119** © Andrejs Pidjass/ShutterStock, Inc.; **page 121** © Lisa F. Young/ShutterStock, Inc.; **page 122** © frotos /ShutterStock, Inc.; **page 125** Courtesy of Pamela McMahon, Journey to Wellness, Tucson, AZ.

Chapter 7

Page 140 Courtesy Karen Bergeron; **page 148** © Pradi /Dreamstime.com

Chapter 8

Page 166 © Lon C. Diehl/PhotoEdit, Inc.

Chapter 9

Page 183 Courtesy of European Pressphoto Agency; **page 184 (top)** © blickwinkel/Alamy Images; **(bottom)** Courtesy of Thomas J. Butler; **page 187** © HO Old /Thomson Reuters; **page 188** © ABN IMAGES/Alamy Images; **page 189 (top)** © Konrad Wothe/age fotostock; **(bottom)** © Stacy Walsh Rosenstock/Alamy; **page 203** © Joseph Reid/Alamy Images

Chapter 10

Page 218 © Jason Maehl/ShutterStock, Inc.; **page 225** Courtesy of the U.S. Food and Drug Administration

Unless otherwise indicated, all photographs and illustrations are under copyright of Jones & Bartlett Learning.